M000106690

The Future of Children

PRINCETON - BROOKINGS

VOLUME 16   NUMBER 1   SPRING 2006

Childhood Obesity

Introducing the Issue

Christina Paxson, Elisabeth Donahue, C. Tracy Orleans, and Jeanne Ann Grisso

Pediatricians, parents, and policy-makers alike are concerned about high and rising rates of overweight and obesity among U.S. children. Over the past three decades, the share of children who are considered overweight or obese has doubled, from 15 percent in the 1970s to nearly 30 percent today, while the share of children who are considered obese has tripled. The problem of childhood obesity has captured public attention and is regularly featured on the evening news, in school newsletters, and in articles in parenting magazines. Increasingly policymakers are recognizing the need for action. In 2004, the Institute of Medicine released a report calling the prevention of childhood obesity a national priority.[1]

Despite all the public attention, no one is sure which policies and programs will most effectively combat childhood obesity. The uncertainty reflects in part a lack of agreement about what caused obesity to increase in the first place. Theories abound. The "epidemic" in childhood obesity has been attrib-uted to various factors: increases in television and computer game use that have led to a new generation of "couch potatoes"; the explosive proliferation of fast-food restaurants, many of which market their products to children through media campaigns that tout tie-ins to children's movies and TV shows; increases in sugary and fat-laden foods displayed at children's eye level in supermar-kets and advertised on TV; schools that offer children junk food and soda while scaling back physical education classes and recess; working parents who are unable to find the time or energy to cook nutritious meals or su-pervise outdoor playtime; the exodus of gro-cery stores from urban centers, sharply re-ducing access to affordable fresh fruits and vegetables; and suburban sprawl and urban crime, both of which keep children away from outdoor activities. The problem is not the lack of explanations for the increase in childhood obesity, but the abundance of them. In such circumstances, deciding which of the possible causes to address first and which policies and programs will be most ef-fective is not easy.

www.futureofchildren.org

Christina Paxson is a senior editor of *The Future of Children*, the director of the Center for Health and Wellbeing, and a professor of econom-ics and public affairs at Princeton University. Elisabeth Donahue is associate editor of *The Future of Children* and a lecturer at Princeton Uni-versity's Woodrow Wilson School. C. Tracy Orleans is a senior scientist at the Robert Wood Johnson Foundation. Jeanne Ann Grisso is a senior program officer at the Robert Wood Johnson Foundation.

This issue of *The Future of Children* lays out the evidence on the multiple causes, consequences, and methods of dealing with childhood obesity. Now is an opportune time to assess what is and is not known. Many policymakers, having become convinced that childhood obesity is indeed a problem, are searching for effective ways to combat it. The Child Nutrition and WIC (Women, Infants, and Children) Reauthorization Act of 2004, for example, responding in large measure to the rise in childhood obesity, requires school districts that participate in the National School Lunch Program or School Breakfast Program to develop a local wellness policy by the beginning of the 2006–07 school year. Many states are developing broader programs aimed at curbing obesity and improving health among their citizens. The "Healthy Arkansas" initiative, launched in 2004, aims—ambitiously—to reduce the state's rate of childhood obesity from 11 percent to 5 percent. Other states are taking similar steps, many with the support of the Centers for Disease Control and Prevention (CDC), which in 2005–06 gave funds to twenty-one states to build capacity in the area of obesity and to seven more to implement programs. But while the policymakers' desire to reduce obesity is clear, state and federal budgets are stretched thin. It is crucial to develop programs and policies that are effective and can be implemented at reasonable cost.

Why Should We Care about Childhood Obesity?

Although there may not be universal agreement on what caused the increase in childhood obesity, there is fairly widespread consensus on several important points. The first is that obesity in general, and childhood obesity in particular, has serious adverse health consequences. Obesity causes many health problems, as Stephen Daniels documents in his article in this volume. Heart disease, high blood pressure, hardening of the arteries, type 2 diabetes, metabolic syndrome, high cholesterol, asthma, sleep disorders, liver disease, orthopedic complications, and mental health problems are just some of the health complications of carrying excess weight. The difficulty for children is twofold. First, many obese children today are developing health problems that once afflicted only adults. These children thus have to cope with chronic illnesses for an unusually extended period of time. Living with type 2 diabetes beginning around age fifty is one thing; living with it from age sixteen is quite another. Second, in obese children, such health problems as heart disease begin, almost invisibly, earlier in life than they do in normal-weight children. Even if the disease is not diagnosed until adulthood, it begins taking its physical toll sooner, perhaps resulting in more complications and a less healthy life. The possibility has even been raised that given the increasing prevalence of severe childhood obesity, children today may live less healthy and shorter lives than their parents.[2] Although this claim is controversial, it is dramatic enough to give us pause and reinforce the idea that childhood obesity is far more than a cosmetic concern.

The increase in obesity is an economic issue as well. Estimates of the costs of treating obese children are relatively small but rising rapidly. For example, Guijing Wang and William Dietz estimate that hospital costs of treating children for obesity-associated conditions rose from $35 million to $127 million (in 2001 constant dollar values) from 1979–81 to 1997–99.[3] Costs of treating adult obesity and its attendant health problems are far more substantial. Roland Sturm estimates that health care costs (including inpatient costs and costs of ambulatory care) of nonelderly obese adults are 36 percent greater than those of the non-obese, while costs for medicines are 77 percent greater.[4] The cost differences between obese and non-obese adults are even greater than those between smokers and nonsmokers. Eric Finkelstein and several colleagues conclude that in 1998 the nation spent between $51.5 and $78.5 billion on health care related to overweight and obesity among adults. The upper bound on these estimates, based on what the authors judge the better of their two data sources, corresponds to 9.1 percent of total annual medical spending in the United States.[5] Roughly half of this spending was publicly funded—paid for by all Americans through Medicaid and Medicare, the government's health programs for the poor and elderly. And ever higher rates of obesity will burden society with other costs. Obese adults may be more likely than their normal-weight counterparts to become disabled before retirement, lowering their earnings and raising the costs of the federal disability insurance system, and may require more nursing home care as they move into retirement.[6]

If the heaviest health and economic burdens of obesity are borne by adults instead of children, why should the focus be on childhood obesity rather than adult obesity? There are two key reasons to focus on children. First, those who are overweight and obese as adolescents are much more likely than others to become obese as adults.[7] Second, it is quite difficult for obese adults and children to shed excess weight. Although the health professions have developed new drugs and medical procedures for treating obesity-related health problems, these procedures are expensive and do not counter all such problems. Preventing obesity in childhood must be the centerpiece of plans to reduce both the health-related and economic costs of obesity.

A final point of broad consensus is that childhood obesity is best viewed as a societal problem reflecting the interactive influences of environment, biology, and behavior, rather than as an individual medical illness. Most agree that the nation has seen dramatic changes in the past thirty years in the ways Americans work, live, and eat. Broad societal and environmental trends have engineered routine physical activity out of everyday life for most Americans and made low-nutrition,

---

A final point of broad consensus is that childhood obesity is best viewed as a societal problem reflecting the interactive influences of environment, biology, and behavior, rather than as an individual medical illness.

---

energy-dense foods and beverages more accessible, affordable, and appealing than more healthful foods. Although reducing obesity requires changes in behaviors surrounding eating and physical activity, strategies that rely only on individual "self-control" are unlikely to be effective in environments that are conducive to poor eating habits and sedentary activity. This is especially true for children, who don't control the environments in which they live, learn, and play. In addition, children have a more limited capacity to make informed choices about what is healthful and what is not. For this reason, there is a clear rationale for modifying children's environments to make it easier for them to be physically active and to make healthful food choices, thus reducing their chances of becoming obese.

Defining obesity as a societal issue does not imply that all children are at equal risk of gaining too much weight. The articles in this volume indicate that some groups of children—in particular, children from low-income families and from ethnic minority groups—are at a higher risk of becoming obese. Evidence presented in this volume indicates that the obesity crisis is also a result of the interplay between people's genes and environments. While humans may be hardwired to overeat in times of plenty, those with a greater genetic propensity for weight gain may be more likely to gain weight in an environment that promotes or encourages unhealthful eating and minimal physical activity. The idea that susceptibility to obesity is genetic has led some to speculate that it will one day be possible to tailor interventions toward those with predispositions to obesity. For now, however, broader policies that alter children's environments are the only realistic options.

What Does This Volume Do?

This volume is a collection of articles that present up-to-date literature reviews and analyses written by leading researchers and experts from many disciplines. The goal of the issue is to promote effective policies and programs targeting childhood obesity by providing timely, objective information based on the best available research on this topic.

The development of effective strategies to prevent childhood obesity must be informed by an understanding of why obesity has risen so fast and so much in the past thirty years. Thus, we asked one pair of researchers to document the trends in childhood obesity, paying careful attention to the timing of the increase in obesity trends compared with the timing of changes in the environment that may have aided the increase in weight. We

asked another researcher to document the effects that these trends have had on the health of those who become obese as children.

To identify effective strategies for reducing rates of overweight and obesity among children, we focused on several broad domains of children's environments—the marketplace, the built environment, schools, child care providers, and homes—that might be modified to reduce obesity. We, therefore, asked researchers to present the best evidence on the role of each of these domains in the development of overweight and obesity and to assess strategies for keeping children at healthy weights. Finally, we asked a pair of researchers to consider issues that are unique to ethnic minority and low-income children, and another researcher to document how those in the medical community—particularly pediatricians—are handling the health problems that come with childhood obesity when prevention efforts fail.

Common Issues: Definitions and Standards of Evidence

Because childhood overweight and obesity are not always defined uniformly across studies, a note about definitions is warranted. Unless otherwise noted, all articles in this volume follow the common convention of defining overweight and obesity in terms of "body mass index," a measure of how much a person weighs relative to how tall that person is. Specifically, the body mass index (BMI) is equal to weight (in kilograms) divided by height (in meters) squared.[8] For adults, the CDC identifies those with BMI values at or above 25 but less than 30 as overweight but not obese and those with BMIs at or above 30 as obese. For example, an adult who is 5 feet and 9 inches tall would be considered overweight at between 169 and 202 pounds and obese at 203 pounds or more.

As Patricia Anderson and Kristin Butcher note in their article, however, the conventional definitions for children and adolescents are somewhat different, because normal BMI values change throughout childhood. Instead, children's levels of adiposity, or fatness, are assessed by comparing their BMI values with those of a fixed reference group of U.S. children of the same age and sex. Children at or above the 85th percentile of the BMI distribution—meaning that at least 85 percent of children of the same age and sex in the reference group had lower values of BMI—are often defined as being overweight, and those at or above the 95th percentile of the distribution for the reference group are often defined to be obese. Although researchers commonly agree that the 85th and 95th percentiles are appropriate cutoffs, not all use the same sets of labels to define children who exceed these cutoffs. The CDC and some researchers refer to children at or above the 85th percentile as being "at risk for overweight" and those at or above the 95th percentile as being "overweight."[9] Most of the articles in this volume, however, use the labels "overweight" and "obese" for parsimony and to be consistent with the adult definitions. Finally, in speaking generally, our authors often use the term "childhood obesity" to refer to both overweight and obesity as seen in both children and adolescents. The distinctions between overweight and obesity are made clear when it is important to do so.

Many of the articles in this volume review evidence on how various features of the environment are related to overweight and obesity. Assessing the quality of that evidence is important in developing effective programs and policies. For example, we may want to know whether children who are breast-fed are less likely to become obese. If so, "preventing obesity" can be added to the long list of benefits of breast-feeding. Similarly, we may want to establish whether children who live in neighborhoods with more fast-food restaurants or who attend schools with vending machines stocked with low-nutrient, high-calorie foods and beverages are more likely to become obese. For most of the topics discussed in this volume, we do not yet have evidence that firmly establishes cause-and-effect relationships. For example, in their article on the built environment, James Sallis and Karen Glanz note that evidence

The idea that susceptibility to obesity is genetic has led some to speculate that it will one day be possible to tailor interventions toward those with predispositions to obesity.

that people who live near parks are more physically active could suggest that easy access to parks is a cause of that physical activity. But it could also be that more physically active people choose to live near parks. So far, research has not conclusively established that proximity to parks reduces obesity.

Evidence on other topics is less equivocal, although often not definitive. Some studies carefully account for the factors that could be linked with obesity but that do not reflect causal relationships. Others rely on comparisons of individuals' behaviors and body weights before and after policy changes or programs are put into place. Finally, in a small but growing body of evidence based on experimental studies, children are randomly assigned to interventions, such as programs designed to reduce TV viewing or to improve nutrition, which may or may not be effective. Comparing the weights of children assigned to the intervention with the weights of those in a control group provides conclusive evidence of the specific intervention's effectiveness among the children being studied. Of course, as Sallis and Glanz point out, randomized interventions are rarely feasible for large-scale programs such as park construction or changes in a city's zoning laws. The quality of available evidence necessarily varies from topic to topic. For the articles in this volume, we have asked the authors to review the best evidence available on their topics and to make it clear how firmly the evidence establishes causal relationships.

What We Have Learned

Each article in the volume contains a detailed discussion of recent evidence on childhood obesity. We briefly summarize each article's chief findings below.

Documenting the Trends

Patricia Anderson and Kristin Butcher document trends in childhood obesity and examine the possible underlying causes of the obesity epidemic. They note that the increase in childhood obesity rates began between 1980 and 1988, and then they assess whether the timing of various changes in the children's environment coincides with the observed increase in obesity. Among the changes that have affected children's energy intake during the critical time period are increases in the availability of energy-dense, high-calorie foods at school; in the consumption of soda and other sugar-sweetened beverages; in the advertising of these products to children; and in dual-career or single-parent working families that may have also increased demand for food away from home or for preprepared

foods. Changes that have reduced energy expenditure over the critical time period include less walking to school and more travel in cars; changes in the built environment and in parents' work lives that make it more difficult for children to engage in safe, unsupervised (or lightly supervised) physical activity; and possibly more time spent in sedentary activities, such as viewing television, using computers, and playing video games. Anderson and Butcher find no single critical factor that has led to increases in children's obesity. Rather, many complementary changes have simultaneously increased children's energy intake and decreased their energy expenditure.

How Obesity Harms Children's Health

Stephen Daniels documents the heavy toll that the obesity epidemic is taking on the health of the nation's children. He notes that many obesity-related health conditions, such as type 2 diabetes and high blood pressure, that were once seen almost exclusively in adults are now being seen in children and with increasing frequency. Obesity affects many systems of the body—cardiovascular, pulmonary, gastrointestinal, orthopedic—and although adult obesity damages each, childhood obesity often exacerbates the damage. For example, the processes that lead to a heart attack or stroke often take decades to develop into overt disease. Obese children may thus suffer the adverse effects of cardiovascular disease at a younger age than their parents would despite the advent of new drugs to treat some of these problems. They also suffer from higher rates of depression, greater difficulty in peer relationships, and poorer quality of life than their normal-weight counterparts.

The Role of Markets

In the first of five articles that survey in detail the environments that may have contributed to increasing childhood obesity, John Cawley focuses on the role of markets. He first documents important market changes, such as increases in the costs of preparing foods at home relative to eating out, that may have contributed to the increase in obesity. He then lays out three economic rationales to justify government intervention in markets to reduce obesity. First, because free markets generally underprovide information, the government may intervene to provide consumers with information they need to make healthy choices. Second, because society bears the soaring costs of obesity, the government may intervene to lower the costs to taxpayers. Third, because children are not what economists call "rational consumers"—that is, they cannot evaluate information critically and weigh the future consequences of their actions—the government may intervene to educate them and help them make better choices. Cawley assesses an array of market-based policy interventions and concludes that the most promising policies are those that reduce advertising targeted to children, increase the incentives for food manufacturers and restaurants to provide more nutritious choices, and improve the quality of foods that schools provide to children, although further evidence on their cost-effectiveness is required.

Changes in the Built Environment
Over the past forty years, the built environment in the United States has changed in ways that have promoted sedentary lifestyles and less healthful diets. James Sallis and Karen Glanz conclude that although researchers have found many links between the built environment and children's physical activity, they have yet to find definitive evidence that aspects of the built environment promote obesity. For example, children and adolescents with easy access to recreational facilities are more active than those without such access, and few of these facilities exist in low-income neighborhoods. Likewise, safe and short routes to school make it easier for children to walk and cycle to school. But, given the paucity of research, researchers cannot yet establish conclusively that more access to recreation or more active commuting would reduce rates of obesity or even identify which kinds of environmental changes are most likely to promote greater physical activity. Recent changes in the nutrition environment, including greater reliance on convenience foods and fast foods, a lack of access to fresh fruits and vegetables, and expanding portion sizes, are also believed to contribute to the epidemic of childhood obesity. But, again, conclusive evidence that changes in the nutrition environment will reduce rates of obesity does not yet exist.

Changes in Schools
Mary Story, Karen Kaphingst, and Simone French demonstrate that U.S. schools offer many opportunities for developing obesity-prevention strategies. They explain that meals at school are available both through the U.S. Department of Agriculture's school breakfast and lunch programs and through "competitive foods" sold à la carte in cafeterias, vending machines, and snack bars. School breakfasts and school lunches must meet federal nutrition standards, but competitive foods are exempt from such requirements. While schools argue that budget pressures force them to sell popular but nutritionally poor foods à la carte, limited evidence shows that schools can offer students more healthful à la carte choices and not lose money. In fact, some states are limiting sales of nonnutritious foods, and many of the nation's largest school districts restrict competitive foods. Other pressures can compromise schools' efforts to provide comprehensive

physical activity programs. As states use standardized tests to hold schools and students academically accountable, schools view physical education and recess as lower priorities. Yet some states are promoting more physical activity in schools. In addition, randomized evaluations of a small number of school-based interventions have shown success at reducing weight gain among children. These interventions typically involve components that teach children about nutrition, promote reductions in television viewing, and engage children in physical activity. Many also involve parents to promote more healthful eating and greater physical activity when children are not in school. These studies indicate that school-based programs, policies, and environments can make a difference in childhood obesity.

Changes in Child Care

Mary Story, Simone French, and Karen Kaphingst also acknowledge that researchers know relatively little about either the nutrition or the physical activity environments in the nation's child care facilities, though existing research suggests that the nutritional quality of meals and snacks may be poor and activity levels may be inadequate. Part of the problem is that no uniform standards apply to nutritional or physical activity offerings in child care centers. With the exception of the federal Head Start program, which has federal performance standards for nutrition and physical activity, child care facilities are regulated by states, and state rules vary widely. One federal program—the Department of Agriculture's Child and Adult Care Food Program—provides funding for meals and snacks for almost 3 million children in child care each day. Providers who receive these funds must serve meals and snacks that meet certain minimal standards but not specific nutrient-based standards. With a large share of

young children attending child care and preschool programs, policymakers should place a high priority on understanding what policies and practices in these settings can prevent childhood obesity.

Changes in Parenting

Ana Lindsay, Katarina Sussner, Juhee Kim, and Steven Gortmaker review evidence on how parents can help their children develop and maintain healthful eating and physical activity habits—and thereby ultimately help prevent childhood obesity. They show how important it is for parents to understand how their roles in preventing obesity change as their children move through critical developmental periods, from before birth through adolescence. They point out that researchers, policymakers, and practitioners should also make use of such information to develop more effective interventions and educational programs that address childhood obesity right where it starts—at home. Although a great deal of research has been done on how parents shape their children's eating and physical activity habits, surprisingly few high-quality data exist on the effectiveness of obesity-prevention programs that center on parental involvement. The authors also review research evaluating school-based interventions that include components targeted at parents. The authors acknowledge that achieving the ultimate goal of preventing and controlling the growing childhood obesity epidemic will require programs and policies that are multifaceted and community-wide, but they emphasize that parents are central to these wider efforts. Research shows that successful intervention must involve and work directly with parents from the very early stages of child development and growth to make healthful changes in the home and to reinforce and support healthful eating and regular physical activity.

Targeting Interventions for Minority and Low-Income Children

Although rates of childhood obesity among the general population are alarmingly high, they are higher still in ethnic minority and low-income communities. Shiriki Kumanyika and Sonya Grier summarize differences in childhood obesity prevalence by race and ethnicity and by socioeconomic status. They then discuss how various environmental factors may have contributed to the higher obesity rates among disadvantaged and minority children. The authors show that low-income and minority children watch more television than white, non-poor children and thus are exposed to many more commercials for high-fat and high-sugar foods. They note that neighborhoods where low-income and minority children live typically have more fast-food restaurants and fewer vendors of healthful foods than do wealthier neighborhoods. Children in these neighborhoods often face many obstacles to physical activity, such as unsafe streets, dilapidated parks, and a lack of facilities. The authors see some promise in the schools that low-income and minority children attend. The national school lunch and breakfast programs, for example, provide important nutritional safety nets for many of the nation's poorer children. Also, state efforts to limit sales of sugar- and fat-laden foods at school could lead the way to effective obesity prevention—although the authors caution that these policies may impose a financial burden on poorer school districts.

When Prevention Fails: The Medical Community's Response

Sonia Caprio notes that although pediatricians are concerned about the problem of obesity, most are not equipped to treat obese children. The most effective treatment programs have been carried out in academic centers through an approach that combines a dietary component, behavioral modification, physical activity, and parental involvement. Such programs, however, have yet to be translated to primary care settings. Successfully treating obesity will require a major shift in pediatric care that makes use of the findings of these academic centers regarding structured intervention programs. To ensure that pediatricians are well trained in treating obesity, the American Medical Association is working with federal agencies, medical specialty societies, and public health organizations to educate physicians about how to prevent and manage obesity in both children and adults, incorporating evidence from new research as it is developed. The goal is to include such training as part of undergraduate, graduate, and continuing medical education programs. Effective treatment will also require changes in how obesity treatment and prevention services are financed. Currently, because insurance often does not cover obesity treatment, long-term weight-management programs are beyond the reach of most patients.

Implications

The research in this volume firmly establishes that increases in childhood overweight and obesity pose a real health threat for the nation's children. As the articles demonstrate, researchers have proposed many environmental and policy solutions—from building more sidewalks, to limiting soda sales in schools, to building more grocery stores in poor neighborhoods—to fix the problem. But evidence on the effectiveness of many of these proposed solutions will take time to develop. In the short run, it makes sense to focus attention on programs and policies that have a good chance of being effective and for which there are policy "levers" to produce change. A review of the evidence in this volume suggests four promising strategies. The first is to implement obesity-prevention initiatives that involve and benefit both children and their parents. The second is to improve nutrition and physical activity environments within schools. The third is to limit children's exposure to advertising. And the fourth is to improve the way pediatricians deliver preventive care and treatment for obesity and related conditions.

Implementing obesity-prevention strategies in after-school programs presents an attractive option for many schools, because it may present fewer conflicts with the schools' academic mandates.

Several articles in this volume discuss obesity-prevention programs that have been shown to work. These interventions, discussed in the two articles by Mary Story, Karen Kaphingst, and Simone French and in the article by Ana Lindsay, Katarina Sussner, Juhee Kim, and Stephen Gortmaker, have been implemented with children of varying ages, from preschoolers to adolescents. They are typically conducted within schools and child care centers and involve components that teach children and their parents about diet and television viewing and that engage children in physical activity. In some programs, such as "Planet Health"—which Mary Story and her colleagues discuss in their article on schools—parents and children are asked to work collaboratively to make such changes in the home environment as reducing TV time. Others combine in-school activ-

ities with informational materials sent home to parents. Although more work is required to tailor these interventions to children of various ages and demographic groups, the evidence indicates that obesity-prevention interventions can be effective at changing the behaviors of both children and their parents.

It makes sense to locate obesity-prevention programs in schools and child care centers, where instructors can reach both children and their parents, but many schools and child care centers lack the resources or skills to implement new programs. In addition, schools are under increasing pressure to devote time to academics rather than to health-oriented programs. These problems can be countered in part by providing schools and child care centers with the funds and training required to implement obesity-prevention programs. Another possible venue for obesity prevention is after-school programs. These programs serve a growing number of children, especially low-income and minority children who are at the highest risk of becoming obese. Implementing obesity-prevention strategies in after-school programs presents an attractive option for many schools, because it may present fewer conflicts with the schools' academic mandates.

Another promising strategy is to improve the foods that children eat at school. Because it is easier for policymakers to regulate what is served in the school cafeteria than to affect what is offered on the kitchen table, schools are a logical place to focus efforts to improve children's diets. Local, state, and federal policies affect what foods are now served in schools. The Department of Agriculture (USDA) enforces standards for the nutritional content of food sold in the national school lunch program, and schools that participate in this program are prohibited from selling foods of "minimal nutritional value" in school cafeterias during lunchtime. But, as Mary Story and her coauthors point out, the definition of "minimal nutritional value" includes only a small class of foods (such as soda and chewing gum) and excludes such foods as candy bars, cookies, and potato chips. Barring additional state or local regulations, schools that follow the USDA's regulations are free to sell these foods in their cafeterias and can sell food of minimal nutritional value outside of cafeterias, often in vending machines or student stores.

Many states and local school districts have chosen to impose requirements that are stronger than those the USDA enforces. By April 2005, twenty-eight states had taken steps to limit competitive foods sold in school cafeterias.[10] The National Conference of State Legislatures reported in May 2005 that a few states had enacted laws regulating vending machine sales in schools, and others had introduced legislation that would, if enacted, restrict vending machine sales.[11] The popularity of these initiatives is heightened by evidence, discussed by Mary Story and her coauthors, that schools that have shifted to more healthful foods in cafeterias and vending machines have been able to do so without losing revenue. An important question is whether these state efforts are sufficient, or whether it is time for the USDA to play a larger role in regulating sales of competitive foods. A strong case could be made for changes in federal policy if the states that are experimenting with new school nutrition policies show success in promoting more healthful eating and in preventing childhood obesity. Although less is known about the relationship between the nutritional quality of foods provided in child care centers and the development of obesity, the Child and Adult Care Food Program, which serves these set-tings, provides similar opportunities for federal policy to influence children's diets.

Schools may also take steps to increase children's physical activity. However, the evidence on the best way to do so is mixed. A recent study by John Cawley, Chad Meyerhoefer, and David Newhouse indicates that states that increased the time that students were required to spend in physical education classes did not show reductions in the share of children who were overweight.[12] Yet some interventions aimed at increasing physical activity in schools have been proven effective. The key to this puzzle may be that many physical education classes do not provide students with enough vigorous exercise to be effective. The study by Cawley, Meyerhoefer, and Newhouse found that increases in the required hours of physical education translated into much smaller increases in students' reports of time spent exercising. Researchers should place a high priority on identifying and implementing programs that effectively increase physical activity at school.

Another area that deserves immediate attention is commercial advertising aimed at children. Regulated at the federal level by Congress and the Federal Communications Commission, advertising aimed at children, particularly advertising that promotes unhealthful behavior, has traditionally been subject to limits that courts have found constitutionally permissible.[13] As John Cawley notes in his article in this volume, children view an average of 40,000 television ads a year. A child watching Saturday morning television may see one food commercial every five minutes, with most featuring such energy-dense, minimally nutritious foods as candy, sugared cereal, and fast food.[14] Although studies have not found a conclusive link between the content of advertising and obesity, they have shown that children find advertisements very persuasive and that, in turn, children successfully influence their parents' food purchases.[15] The evidence that Shiriki Kumanyika and Sonya Grier present in this volume indicates that low-income and minority children, who have a higher chance than other children of becoming obese, are exposed to more advertising than other children.

Obviously, one strategy for limiting children's exposure to advertising is to educate parents about television and encourage them simply to turn off the TV. The reality is, however, that even with limited television viewing, children are exposed to a great deal of advertising. Thus another strategy is to reduce advertising time for energy-dense foods aimed at children or to mandate that ads for junk food be balanced with advertising for healthy foods such as fresh fruits and vegetables. The most aggressive strategy would be to institute an outright ban on advertising for foods that are high in sugar, fat, and calories during children's programming, just as Congress has banned all tobacco advertising on television and radio.[16] Although the evidence of a link between obesity and advertising may not yet be strong enough to justify a ban on food advertisements geared toward children, the evidence that children are easily swayed by food commercials suggests that some limits are advisable.

A final area that clearly needs reform is the way pediatric medical care is delivered to prevent and treat childhood obesity. As Sonia Caprio documents, pediatricians are not being adequately trained to screen for, prevent, and treat childhood obesity. To remedy this deficiency, medical schools and pediatric residency programs need to train physicians how to prevent obesity as well as how to man-

age its associated health problems. In addition, doctors must be compensated for delivering obesity-related care. Although federal law does not prevent states from reimbursing providers for obesity prevention and treatment services through Medicaid and the State Child Health Insurance Programs (S-CHIP), neither does it mandate that they do so. Many states now offer little coverage for these services.[17] Moreover, some private insurance companies do not recognize obesity as a disease or reimburse treatment at low rates.[18] Thus some providers find themselves in the position of being able to claim reimbursement for treating specific health problems that stem from obesity, but not being reimbursed fully for treating obesity itself. States could mandate that Medicaid and private insurance cover obesity as a disease, with appropriate reimbursement for evidence-based counseling and biomedical interventions. Several states have already done so; according to Sonia Caprio's article in this volume, of the four bills introduced in states this year to require Medicaid treatment options, two became law. At the federal level, views about whether obesity is or is not a disease are also starting to shift. In July 2004, the Department of Health and Human Services removed language from the Medicare Coverage Issues Manual stating that obesity was not an illness. Removing this language paved the way for Medicare recipients—primarily elderly Americans—to be covered for obesity treatments that are shown to be effective. Policymakers should take similar steps for the public and private health insurance programs that cover children.

These policy recommendations are cautious, based on strategies that promise to yield the most results in the short term. But they are simply first steps in what is likely to be a long battle to reverse obesity trends. Numerous innovative policies and programs, not now supported by strong evidence, nevertheless hold promise. Among them are improving access to healthful foods in low-income neighborhoods by bringing in farmers' markets and grocery stores; constructing sidewalks so that children can walk or bike to school; building or enhancing hiking trails and parks so that children and their families can be more physically active; and requiring restaurants to provide more helpful nutrition information to consumers.

The only way to learn whether these strategies work is to experiment with them. Many states and communities are undertaking new programs that incorporate a wide array of obesity-prevention strategies. These initiatives can teach us about the most effective ways to reduce child obesity. But to realize their full promise, researchers must carefully and extensively evaluate these initiatives and then disseminate their findings widely. A prerequisite for any effective public health campaign is a solid base of knowledge about what can be done to improve health. Building this knowledge base will take time, attention, and funding, but it is essential to halting the rise in childhood obesity.

Notes

1. Jeffrey P. Koplan, Catharyn T. Liverman, and Vivica I. Kraak, eds., *Preventing Childhood Obesity: Health in the Balance* (Washington: National Academies Press, 2005).

2. S. Jay Olshansky and others, "A Potential Decline in Life Expectancy in the United States in the 21st Century," *New England Journal of Medicine* 352 (2005): 1138–45. An editorial in the same volume, however, cautioned that this claim may be overstated. See Samuel H. Preston, "Deadweight? The Influence of Obesity on Longevity," *New England Journal of Medicine* 352 (2005): 1135–37.

3. Guijing Wang and William H. Dietz, "Economic Burden of Obesity in Youths Aged 7 to 17 Years: 1979–1999," *Pediatrics* 109, 5 (2002): E81.

4. Roland Sturm, "The Effects of Obesity, Smoking, and Drinking on Medical Problems and Costs," *Health Affairs* 21, no. 2 (2002): 245–53.

5. Eric A. Finkelstein, Ian C. Fiebelkom, and Guijing Wang, "National Medical Spending Attributable to Overweight and Obesity: How Much, and Who's Paying?" *Health Affairs,* Supplemental Web Exclusives: W3-219-26.

6. Darius N. Lakdawalla, Jay Bhattacharya, and Dana P. Goldman, "Are the Young Becoming More Disabled? Rates of Disability Appear to Be on the Rise among People Ages Eighteen to Fifty-Nine, Fueled by a Growing Obesity Epidemic," *Health Affairs* 23, no. 1 (2004): 168–76; Darius Lakdawalla and others, "Forecasting the Nursing Home Population," *Medical Care* 41, no. 1 (2003) (Point/Counterpoint): 8–20.

7. Robert C. Whitaker and others, "Predicting Obesity in Young Adulthood from Childhood and Parental Obesity," *New England Journal of Medicine* 337 (1997): 869–73.

8. In imperial measurements, the calculation is (weight in pounds/height in inches [squared]) x 703.

9. Department of Health and Human Services, "2000 CDC Growth Charts for the United States: Methods and Development," *Vital and Health Statistics,* series 11, no. 246 (Hyattsville, Md.: National Center for Health Statistics, 2002).

10. U.S. Government Accountability Office, "School Meal Programs: Competitive Foods Are Widely Available and Generate Substantial Revenues for Schools" (Government Accountability Office, August 2005) (www.gao.gov/new.items/d05563.pdf [accessed December 5, 2005]).

11. www.ncsl.org/programs/health/vending.htm (accessed December 6, 2005).

12. John Cawley, Chad D. Meyerhoefer, and David Newhouse, "The Impact of State Physical Education Requirements on Youth Physical Activity and Overweight," Working Paper 11411 (Cambridge, Mass.: National Bureau of Economic Research, June 2005).

13. See Children's Television Act of 1990, P.L. 101-437; Children's Internet Protection Act, P.L. 106-554; *Code of Federal Regulations* 47, sec. 73.670 (1991 FCC rule limiting commercials aimed at children); 15 U.S.C. 1335 (congressional prohibition of advertisements for tobacco on radio and television). See also *People of State of California v. R. J. Reynolds Tobacco Co.* (2004), which let stand a lower court decision that sanctioned R. J. Reynolds for targeting youth with tobacco advertising in magazines with a teen audience of 15 percent or more—a violation of the tobacco litigation Master Settlement Agreement.

14. Krista Kotz and Mary Story, "Food Advertisements during Children's Saturday Morning Television Programming: Are They Consistent with Dietary Recommendations?" *Journal of the American Dietetic Association* 94, no. 11 (1994): 1296–1300.

15. J. Galst and M. White, "The Unhealthy Persuader: The Reinforcing Value of Television and Children's Purchase Influence Attempts at the Supermarket," *Child Development* 47 (1976): 1089–96; Howard L. Taras and others, "Television's Influence on Children's Diet and Physical Activity," *Journal of Developmental and Behavioral Pediatrics* 10 (1989): 176–80.

16. 15 U.S.C. 1335.

17. Adam Gilden Tsai and others, "Availability of Nutrition Services for Medicaid Recipients in the Northeastern United States: Lack of Uniformity and the Positive Effect of Managed Care," *American Journal of Managed Care* 9, no. 12 (2003): 817–21.

18. Andrew M. Tershakovec and others, "Insurance Reimbursement for the Treatment of Obesity in Children," *Journal of Pediatrics* 134 (1999): 573–78.

Childhood Obesity:
Trends and Potential Causes

Patricia M. Anderson and Kristin F. Butcher

Summary

The increase in childhood obesity over the past several decades, together with the associated health problems and costs, is raising grave concern among health care professionals, policy experts, children's advocates, and parents. Patricia Anderson and Kristin Butcher document trends in children's obesity and examine the possible underlying causes of the obesity epidemic.

They begin by reviewing research on energy intake, energy expenditure, and "energy balance," noting that children who eat more "empty calories" and expend fewer calories through physical activity are more likely to be obese than other children. Next they ask what has changed in children's environment over the past three decades to upset this energy balance equation. In particular, they examine changes in the food market, in the built environment, in schools and child care settings, and in the role of parents—paying attention to the timing of these changes.

Among the changes that affect children's energy intake are the increasing availability of energy-dense, high-calorie foods and drinks through schools. Changes in the family, particularly an increase in dual-career or single-parent working families, may also have increased demand for food away from home or pre-prepared foods. A host of factors have also contributed to reductions in energy expenditure. In particular, children today seem less likely to walk to school and to be traveling more in cars than they were during the early 1970s, perhaps because of changes in the built environment. Finally, children spend more time viewing television and using computers.

Anderson and Butcher find no one factor that has led to increases in children's obesity. Rather, many complementary changes have simultaneously increased children's energy intake and decreased their energy expenditure. The challenge in formulating policies to address children's obesity is to learn how best to change the environment that affects children's energy balance.

www.futureofchildren.org

Patricia M. Anderson is a professor of economics at Dartmouth College. Kristin F. Butcher is a senior economist at the Federal Reserve Bank of Chicago. This article reflects the views of the authors and not necessarily those of the Federal Reserve Bank of Chicago or the Federal Reserve System. The authors thank Blair Burgeen, Kyung Park, Alex Reed, and Diana Zhang for excellent research assistance and William Dietz, Diane Whitmore Schanzenbach, participants at the Future of Children conference, Christina Paxson, Elisabeth Donahue, Tracy Orleans, and J. A. Grisso for helpful comments.

The increase in childhood obesity has gained the full attention of health care professionals, health policy experts, children's advocates, and parents. All are concerned that today's overweight and obese children will turn into tomorrow's overweight and obese adults, destined to suffer from all the health problems and health care costs associated with obesity. In this essay, we document trends in children's obesity and examine the underlying causes of the obesity epidemic.

We begin by discussing definitions of overweight and obesity, noting some potential problems. We document trends in adult and childhood obesity, both worldwide and in the United States, over the past three decades, paying particular attention to the timing of the increase in obesity. We preface our analysis of obesity's causes with a brief review of research on children's energy intake and energy expenditure and on what affects children's "energy balance." Research findings support the idea that children who eat more "empty calories" and expend fewer calories through physical activity are more likely to be obese than other children. Finally we examine how the environment in which children are raised might have changed over the past three decades and how these changes might have upset the energy balance equation. Have changes in the food market, in the built environment, in schools and child care settings, and in the role of parents contributed to increased obesity? In particular, we examine whether the timing of the changes in children's environments coincides with the timing of the increase in obesity, making it likely that those changes are driving the increase in children's obesity rates.

Defining Obesity

Typically, obesity and overweight in adults are defined in terms of body mass index (BMI), which in turn is defined as weight in kilograms divided by height in meters squared (kg/m^2).[1] Guidelines issued by the National Institutes of Health consider an adult underweight if his or her BMI is less than 18.5, overweight if BMI is 25 or more, and obese if BMI is 30 or more.[2]

Use of BMI to assess overweight and obesity in children is more controversial. Because children are growing, the link between adiposity, or "true fatness," and the ratio of their weight to their height may be looser than that of adults. However, William Dietz and Mary Bellizzi, reporting on a conference convened by the International Obesity Task Force, note that BMI offers "a reasonable measure with which to assess fatness in children and adolescents."[3] They also conclude that a BMI above the 85th percentile for a child's age and sex group is likely to accord with the adult definition of overweight, and a BMI above the 95th percentile is consistent with the adult definition of obese.[4] Children are thus defined as being overweight or obese if they have a BMI above given age- and sex-specific percentile cutoffs. These cutoffs, which were set for a base population surveyed in the early 1970s before obesity began to increase, yield a specific, fixed BMI cutoff used to define overweight and obesity for boys and girls of each age.[5] Later in the article we will use these cutoffs to define obesity using the National Health and Nutrition Examination Surveys (NHANES), a nationally representative sample of U.S. children who were consistently weighed and measured between 1971 and 2002.[6] The data will show an increase in measured obesity over time if more children in each of the NHANES surveys have a BMI above this fixed cutoff number.

International Trends in Obesity

Obesity is a problem not just in the United States but worldwide. Comparing international obesity rates and trends using BMI, however, is complicated, as the relationship between "true fatness" and height and weight may differ for people in different environments. Some groups, for example, may simply have denser body composition than others. Definitions are particularly complicated in international comparisons of obesity in children. If age- and sex-specific growth patterns in Botswana differ from those in the United States, then obesity definitions based on the same BMI cutoffs are unlikely to yield useful comparisons. Nonetheless, a growing body of literature examining specific populations has concluded that obesity is increasing worldwide.

Table 1 lists adult obesity rates collected by the World Health Organization for selected countries and time periods.[1] Although different countries have different obesity rates, a common pattern across all countries listed, with the exception of Japan, is that adult obesity rates are rising. U.S. adult obesity rates are among the world's highest (compare the rates in table 1 with those in figure 1 on page 23). In 1995, for example, 15 percent of men and 16.5 percent of women in England were obese. In the United States (in the nearest time period for which data are available), the share was more than 20 percent for men and women combined. Only the former German Democratic Republic has obesity rates that are similar to those in the United States for similar years. The rates are still quite low in Japan, Finland, Sweden, and the Netherlands.

Many studies of individual countries have also noted increases in childhood obesity in recent years. Helen Kalies and two colleagues found that obesity rates rose from 1.8 to 2.8 percent among preschool children in Germany between 1982 and 1997.[2] Among children aged seven to eleven in England, the prevalence of overweight and obesity increased from less than 10 percent for both boys and girls in the mid-1970s to more than 20 percent for girls and more than 15 percent for boys by 1998.[3] In urban areas in China, the prevalence of obesity increased among children aged two to six from 1.5 percent in 1989 to 12.6 percent in 1997. In rural China over the same period, obesity rates fell.[4] Though childhood obesity is on the rise worldwide, the patterns differ, in expected ways, between developing and developed countries. In the former, obesity may coexist with undernutrition, with children in the relatively affluent urban areas more likely to be obese than their rural counterparts.

1. World Health Organization, "Obesity: Preventing and Managing the Global Epidemic" (Geneva: WHO, 1998).

2. Helen Kalies, J. Lenz, and Rüdiger von Kries, "Prevalence of Overweight and Obesity and Trends in Body Mass Index in German Pre-School Children, 1982–1997," *International Journal of Obesity* 26 (2002): 1211–17.

3. Tim J. Lobstein and others, "Increasing Levels of Excess Weight among Children in England," *International Journal of Obesity* 27 (2003): 1136–38.

4. Juhua Luo and Frank B. Hu, "Time Trends of Obesity in Pre-School Children in China from 1989 to 1997," *International Journal of Obesity* 26 (2002): 553–58.

Obesity in the United States

In the United States obesity rates have increased for all age groups over the past thirty years. Figure 1 shows the share of the U.S. population, by age group, that is obese based on the BMI cutoffs described above.[7] During 1971–74 about 5 percent of children aged two to nineteen years were obese. By 1976–80 the share obese was slightly higher, but between 1980 and 1988–94 the share obese nearly doubled. By 1999–2002 nearly 15 percent of U.S. children were considered obese. Al-

Table 1. Obesity Rates, by Country and Year

Country	Year	Prevalence of obesity (percent)	
		Men	Women
Australia (aged 25–64)	1980	9.3	8.0
	1989	11.5	13.2
Brazil (aged 25—64)	1975	3.1	8.2
	1989	5.9	13.3
Canada (aged 20–70 in 1978 and 18–74 in 1986–90)	1978	6.8	9.6
	1986–90	15	15
England (aged 16–64)	1980	6.0	8.0
	1995	15.0	16.5
Finland (aged 20–75)	1978–79	10	10
	1991–93	14	11
Former German Democratic Republic (aged 25–65)	1985	13.7	22.2
	1992	20.5	26.8
Japan (aged 20 and older)	1976	0.7	2.8
	1993	1.8	2.6
Netherlands (aged 20–29)	1987	6.0	8.5
	1995	8.4	8.3
Sweden (aged 16–64)	1980–81	4.9	8.7
	1988–89	5.3	9.1

Source: World Health Organization, "Obesity: Preventing and Managing the Global Epidemic" (Geneva: WHO, 1998). European countries: table 3.4, page 25; Western Pacific countries: table 3.7, page 28; the Americas: table 3.2, page 22. An individual is categorized as obese if he or she has a body mass index of 30 or above.

though the rates of obesity were higher for older children in every survey, all age groups showed an increase in obesity. Rates for boys and girls were nearly identical. Adult obesity also steadily increased, with the share of adults defined as obese larger than that of children in any given time period. Obesity rates increased for both men and women, though women had higher rates than men.[8]

Logically enough, increasing childhood obesity is related to increasing adult obesity. Obese children are much more likely than normal weight children to become obese adults. Obesity even in very young children is correlated with higher rates of obesity in adulthood. A study from the late 1990s shows that 52 percent of children who are obese between the ages of three and six are obese at age twenty-five as against only 12 percent of normal and underweight three- to six-year-old children.[9]

Although the obese share of the population is expected to increase with age, obesity today is increasing with age more quickly than it did thirty years ago. Researchers in 1971 trying to project what share of ten-year-olds that year would be obese by the time they turned forty in 2001 would have predicted the share to be between 10 and 15 percent. But in 1999–2002 the share was close to 30 percent. This change in the relationship between age and obesity has important implications for predicting what share of the population will have obesity-related health problems as the population ages.

The precise timing of the increase in obesity in the United States is also important for researchers attempting to identify its causes. As shown in figure 1, the obese share of the U.S. population for both children and adults was fairly stable between 1971–74 and 1976–80 and only began to increase thereafter. Thus, in

Figure 1. Percentage of U.S. Population That Is Obese

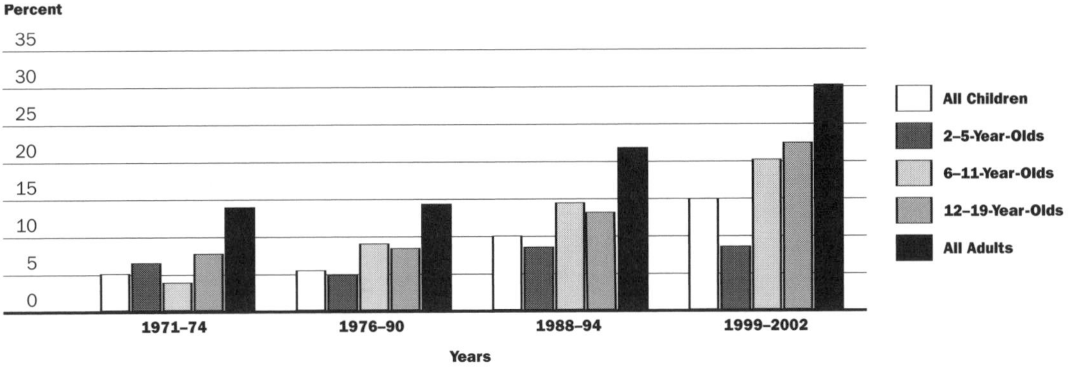

Source: Authors' calculations from National Health and Nutrition Examination Surveys (NHANES).

the search for causes of the obesity epidemic, researchers focus particularly on any environmental changes that began between 1980 and 1988 and continued during the 1990s.

Before beginning our analysis of these causes, we want to document a few more important features of the trend in obesity. As figure 2 shows, obesity rates are higher among minority and low-income children than among children as a whole.[10] Although obesity increased for all children, it increased more for children in low-income families and increased the most for African American children.

In addition to examining changes in obesity rates it is important to examine how the distribution of BMI has also changed. Obesity rates alone may be misleading because small changes in BMI may result in large changes in obesity rates. Suppose, for example, that in one year a large group of children with BMIs just below the obesity cutoff gained a few pounds, thus tipping over into the obese category. Obesity rates would increase, even though the underlying health of the population did not change much. Distribution of BMI is also important in comparing obesity rates between groups. For example, if obesity rates were higher among low-income children simply because a slightly higher fraction of children had

BMIs above the obesity cutoff, differences in obesity rates would not be expected to translate into differences in health outcomes.

An examination of the data indicates that movements of people from just below to just above the BMI cutoffs cannot explain changes in obesity in the 1990s. By 1999–2002 not only was a larger share of children obese, those who were obese were also heavier than in the past. Figure 2 charts changes in the percentage of children who are obese for all children, for low-income children, and for African American children; it also reports average BMI among the obese for these groups. Average BMI among all obese children increased little between 1971–74 and 1988–94, implying that the increase in obesity rates was mostly due to a higher fraction of children "tipping" over the obesity cutoff. But by 1999–2002 average BMI had increased among obese children. The increase in average BMI among obese children between 1971–74 and 1999–2002 corresponds to an increase in body weight for a 4'6" tall child from about 113.6 pounds to 116.1 pounds.

Figures 3 and 4 cast more light on the changing BMI distribution. They show the share of adults and children, respectively, that is overweight (but not obese) and the share obese.

Figure 2. Percentage of Children Who Are Obese and Average BMI among Obese Children, by Group

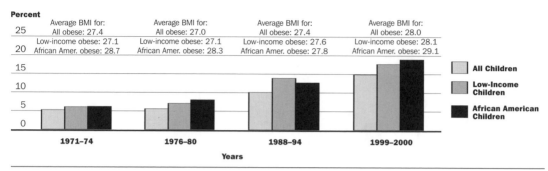

Source: Authors' calculations from National Health and Nutrition Examination Surveys (NHANES).

They also show BMI at the median of the distribution (half of the people are heavier) and at the 95th percentile of the distribution (5 percent of the people are heavier). After 1976–80 the share overweight and the share obese increase for both adults and children, but the share obese increases more rapidly. Similarly, although the median BMI increases after 1980, BMI at the 95th percentile increases more quickly.

Two examples illustrate the consequences of these changes in the distribution of BMI. An adult woman who is 5'4" tall, with a BMI at the median, would weigh 143.3 pounds in 1971–74. By 1999–2002 she would weigh 157.3 pounds, a gain of 14 pounds, or 9.8 percent. But a 5'4" tall woman with a BMI at the 95th percentile would go from 197.5 to 231.9 pounds over the same period—a gain of 34.4 pounds, or 17.4 percent. For children, the difference in the median and upper-tail weight gain is even more striking. A 4'6" child with the median BMI would gain 4.6 pounds over this period for a 6.3 percent increase (73.4 to 78.0 pounds). But a child at the 95th percentile would gain about 19 pounds for a 17.5 percent weight gain (108.3 to 127.3 pounds).

In short, BMI is becoming more unequally distributed: the heavy have gotten much heavier. Furthermore, obesity is not evenly distributed across socio-demographic groups. Indeed, given the pattern of changes in the BMI distribution, obesity appears to have much in common with other diseases: everyone may be exposed to a given change in the environment, but only those with a susceptibility to the given disease will come down with it. For those with a susceptibility to obesity, the conditions appear to be right for their disease to flourish.

A Question of Energy Balance

Clearly, overweight and obesity are increasing in children and adults. Less clear are the causes of this increase, although the basic physiology of weight change is well understood: weight is gained when energy intake exceeds energy expenditure. Although certain endocrinological or neurological syndromes, including Praeder Willi, Klinefelter's, Frohlich's, Lawrence Mood Biedl, Klein-Levin, and Mauriac syndromes, can lead to overweight—and although these syndromes are often tested for, especially in cases of childhood obesity—less than 5 percent of obesity cases result from these "endogenous" factors.[11]

Genetics also plays a big role in obesity. Recent studies have concluded that about 25 to 40 percent of BMI is heritable.[12] Identical

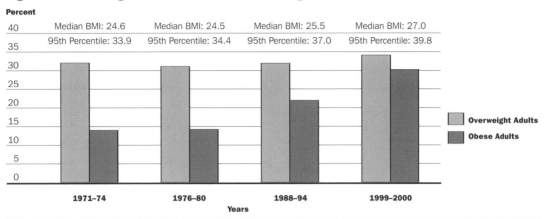

Figure 3. Percentage of Adults Who Are Overweight or Obese

Percent

Median BMI: 24.6   Median BMI: 24.5   Median BMI: 25.5   Median BMI: 27.0

95th Percentile: 33.9   95th Percentile: 34.4   95th Percentile: 37.0   95th Percentile: 39.8

- Overweight Adults
- Obese Adults

1971–74   1976–80   1988–94   1999–2000

Years

Source: Authors' calculations from National Health and Nutrition Examination Surveys (NHANES).

Figure 4. Percentage of Children Who Are Overweight or Obese

Percent

Median BMI: 17.7   Median BMI: 18.0   Median BMI: 18.2   Median BMI: 18.8

95th Percentile: 26.1   95th Percentile: 26.1   95th Percentile: 28.3   95th Percentile: 30.7

- Overweight Children
- Obese Children

1971–74   1976–80   1988–94   1999–2000

Years

Source: Authors' calculations from National Health and Nutrition Examination Surveys (NHANES).

twins raised apart, for example, have been found to have a correlation in BMI of about 0.7 (a correlation of 1 is perfect), only slightly lower than that of twins raised together.[13] Of course, the gene pool does not change nearly rapidly enough for a change in genes to explain the recent increase in childhood overweight and obesity. But it does appear that certain people may have a higher genetic susceptibility to weight gain. Thus, when identical twins are subjected to an overfeeding regimen, the correlation of the weight gain *within* twin pairs is significantly higher than that *between* twin pairs.[14] But as important as genes are, the primary focus in the search for the causes of rising obesity must be on changes in energy balance.

Maintaining a stable weight requires a delicate balance between energy intake and energy expenditures. Very young children seem capable of adjusting their intake to match their outflow, but as children grow up, they seem to lose this apparently innate ability.[15] Their food intake, rather than being based on energy needs, is influenced by external cues, such as the amount of food presented.[16] Much research on childhood obesity focuses on the role of energy intake, with most studies analyzing a particular source.

Studies of Energy Intake

Fast food is a common subject of such studies. Cross-sectional studies have established that individuals consuming fast-food meals

Patricia M. Anderson and Kristin F. Butcher

have higher energy intake with lower nutritional values than those not consuming fast food.[17] Such a finding, however, does not guarantee that children consuming more fast food will be more likely to be overweight. In fact, Cara Ebbeling and several colleagues find that although both overweight and lean adolescents consume more calories when eating fast food, the lean compensate for that energy intake, while the overweight do not.[18] A recent long-term study of eight- to twelve-year-old girls did find that those eating fast food two or more times a week at baseline, when 96 percent of study subjects were lean, had larger weight gains at a three-year follow-up.[19] But the study covers only middle-class, white females. And although its long-term design makes it more reliable than a cross-sectional study, it still does not conclusively prove a causal effect of fast food. Unobserved characteristics of the girls that may be correlated with both fast-food consumption and weight gain may be the true causal culprit.

Another frequently studied source of energy is sweet beverages, mainly soft drinks but also juice. As with fast food, studies generally establish that drinking these beverages results in higher overall energy intake. Several studies have also found a positive link between overweight and soft drink consumption.[20] Findings on juice consumption have been more mixed; cross-sectional studies find a link, but some long-term studies do not.[21] More recently, however, a long-term study of preschoolers has found a positive link between all sweet beverages (including soda, juice, and other fruit drinks) and overweight.[22] Another recent study looks at repeated cross-sections of fifth graders in one school and finds a positive, but not significant, relationship between sweetened beverage consumption and BMI.[23] Finally, another study uses a long-term design similar to that of

the fast-food study just noted. Children aged nine to fourteen in 1996 were followed annually through 1998. For both boys and girls, consumption of sugar-added beverages implied small increases in BMI over the years.[24]

Another much-studied source of energy intake is snacks. Although snack foods tend to be energy dense, implying that snacking may increase overall energy intake, snacking does not appear to contribute to childhood overweight. In a simple cross-sectional study comparing obese and non-obese adolescents, Linda Bandini and several colleagues find that energy intake from snacks is similar for both groups.[25] They conclude that obese adolescents eat no more "junk" food than non-obese adolescents, and thus the former's source of energy imbalance must lie elsewhere. A recent long-term study by Sarah Phillips and colleagues comes to a similar conclusion after collecting information from eight- to twelve-year-old girls annually for ten years.[26] The study finds no relationship between consuming snack foods (such as chips, baked goods, and candy) and BMI, although as in the beverage-specific studies just noted, it does find a relationship between BMI and soda.

Studies of Energy Expenditure
The other, equally important side of the energy balance equation is energy expenditures, both through physical activity and through dietary thermogenesis and the basal metabolic rate (BMR). Dietary thermogenesis refers to the energy required to digest meals, and the basal metabolic rate refers to the energy required to maintain the resting body's functions. For sedentary adults, physical activity is responsible for 30 percent of total energy expenditure, dietary thermogenesis for 10 percent, and BMR for the remaining 60 percent.[27] Several studies examine

whether a low BMR is responsible for overweight in children. For example, in a study of both obese and non-obese adolescents, Bandini, Dale Schoeller, and William Dietz find that obese teens do not have lower-than-average BMR, and thus lowered energy expenditure through BMR is not the cause of maintained obesity in adolescents.[28]

The lack of evidence that BMR affects childhood overweight and obesity argues for a research focus on physical activity—or the lack thereof. So far, though, studies of the link between physical activity and BMI have had mixed results.[29] One reason why researchers have difficulty proving that physical activity affects BMI may be that BMI is a potentially poor measure of adiposity in the presence of significant lean muscle mass. A study of twelve-year-old French children bears out this hypothesis. Looking at both BMI and waist circumference, researchers find that physical activity is linked with smaller waist circumference for both boys and girls but with lower BMI only for girls.[30] Although findings from cross-sectional studies have been somewhat mixed, long-term studies have associated increases in activity and decreases in BMI.[31]

Researchers have found much stronger links between sedentary activities, especially television viewing, and overweight and obesity. That said, at least one study that investigated the effect of television watching on physical activity found none.[32] Interestingly, it found computer use, reading, and homework time associated with higher levels of physical activity. The relationship, however, is just a cross-sectional correlation among these activities. It may be that the parents who encourage reading and homework and buy their children computers also encourage more physical activity.

William Dietz and Steven Gortmaker produced the canonical study on television's role in childhood obesity, finding that each additional hour of television per day increased the prevalence of obesity by 2 percent.[33] They note that television viewing may affect weight in several ways. First, it may squeeze out physical activity. Second, television advertising may increase children's desire for, and ultimately their consumption of, energy-dense snack foods. Third, watching television may

---

The lack of evidence that BMR affects childhood overweight and obesity argues for a research focus on physical activity—or the lack thereof.

---

go hand in hand with snacking, leading to higher energy intake among children watching television. Robert Klesges, Mary Shelton, and Lisa Klesges even concluded that children's metabolic rate was lower while watching television than while at rest.[34] That finding, however, has not been replicated, and later studies find no effect.[35]

Research on the relationship among television viewing and physical activity and overweight has mixed findings. Although many studies observe a positive relationship between television viewing and childhood obesity, Thomas Robinson and several colleagues find only a weak relationship (but William Dietz points out several potential methodological problems with this study), and Elizabeth Vandewater and colleagues find none at all.[36] These mixed findings, though, tend to come from observational or prospective studies. More rigorous experimental studies consistently find that reducing children's television watching lowers their BMI.[37] Because these experimental studies can establish causality while the others do not, it seems reasonable to conclude that watching television does contribute to childhood obesity, despite the overall mixed findings of past studies.

Studies of Other Correlates of Obesity

Overall, then, much research on childhood obesity's possible causes focuses on factors that are expected to affect either the child's energy intake or energy expenditure. Another line of research, however, simply documents childhood characteristics that are correlated with overweight, but it either does not or cannot determine their effects on the energy balance equation. Many studies, for example, document that children from certain demographic groups are more likely than other children to be overweight. As noted, data from the NHANES show that African American and lower-income children have a higher incidence of obesity than children overall. Using data from the National Longitudinal Survey of Youth, Richard Strauss and Harold Pollack demonstrate that both African American and Hispanic children are more likely to be overweight than white non-Hispanic children.[38] They also find a negative relationship between income and rates of overweight among whites only; the relationship for Hispanics is insignificant; and for African Americans, slightly positive. The study also documents regional differences, with children in the South and the West most likely to be overweight. It finds no significant difference between rural and urban children, although a recent study in Pennsylvania found nearly 20 percent of seventh graders from rural districts to be overweight compared to just 16 percent from urban districts.[39]

One other repeatedly analyzed characteristic—having been breast-fed as an infant—does not clearly line up with the energy balance equation. Beginning with Michael S. Kramer's work, many cross-sectional studies have found that older children are more likely to be lean if they were breast-fed.[40] But other studies have had somewhat more mixed findings.[41] More recently, though, Stephan Arenz and colleagues, in a comprehensive review of past studies, conclude that breast-feeding does seem to have a consistent negative effect on obesity, albeit a small one.[42] As William Dietz makes clear, the mechanism by which infant breast-feeding may affect weight at later ages is not certain.[43] One possibility is an endocrine response to breast milk. Another is that mothers have greater discretion over how much they feed their infants when they bottle-feed. Breast-feeding may even affect future food preferences. It is also possible that the relationship is purely an artifact of the cross-sectional study design. That is, the types of mothers who do and do not breast-feed may put into practice different nutritional and activity standards for their children as they grow up. Some evidence for this possibility can be found in a study by Melissa Nelson, Penny Gordon-Larsen, and Linda Adair, which confirms the cross-sectional finding of a link between breast-fed infants and normal-weight older children using long-term data from the National Longitudinal Study of Adolescent Health.[44] When using sibling pairs to control for unobserved maternal factors, however, they find no effect of breast-feeding on weight. In other words, a breast-fed child is no more likely to be thin than his or her sibling who was not breast-fed. Although this finding provides compelling evidence that breast-feeding does not affect children's weights, two considerations temper this conclusion. First, the sample of families in which one sibling is breast-fed and another is not is small, perhaps making it difficult to identify statistically significant effects of breast-feeding on weight. Second, with sibling pairs where only one is breast-fed, the issue is why the mother made different decisions. It may be that the decisions were related to factors that ultimately affected the children's weight.

Taken together, what do these studies on the energy balance have to say about the causes of increasing childhood overweight and obesity? Most studies do not determine clear causality, but rather they reveal only cross-sectional correlations. In the stronger long-term studies, many of the samples are relatively unrepresentative (for example, middle-class girls from a specific region), making it unclear whether the findings are broadly applicable. Even for studies replete with representative, long-term evidence (for example, the role of television), the question is whether the timing of the exposure matches the timing of childhood obesity trends.

Changes in the Determinants of Energy Balance

A range of environmental changes may have affected children's energy balance over the past several decades. Combined with a potential genetic susceptibility, these changes may have contributed to the increase in childhood overweight and obesity. In this section we consider four possible changes in the environment: the food market, the built environment, schools and day care, and parents. Subsequent articles in this volume discuss each in more detail.

Changes in the Food Market

Despite a lack of abundant, clearly causal evidence, researchers find many correlations between some types of energy intake and childhood obesity and overweight. As noted, probably the strongest evidence is for the role of soft drinks, followed by slightly mixed findings on the role of fast food. Very little evidence exists that snack foods have a specific effect. But even without a "smoking gun" in terms of energy intake, it is clear that more food, without a concomitant increase in energy expenditure, will result in weight gain. Could changes in the food market in the

One other repeatedly analyzed characteristic—having been breast-fed as an infant—does not clearly line up with the energy balance equation.

past several decades have caused the increase in childhood overweight and obesity? Judy Putnam and Shirley Gerrior analyze changes in the U.S. food supply and find a marked increase in overall consumption of carbonated soft drinks in the past several decades.[45] The consumption of regular (non-diet) sodas trended slightly upward in the 1970s, remained fairly stable in the early 1980s, and then exploded starting in 1987, continuing to rise steadily through the 1990s. Figure 5 illustrates this trend, superimposing children's obesity rates over the four periods for which NHANES data are available.

On first glance, the timing of the increase in soda consumption, which tracks closely the trends in increasing childhood obesity, suggests that soda consumption may well be a contributor. But the trend is for overall consumption and includes that of adults as well as

Figure 5. Annual Regular (Non-Diet) Soft Drink Consumption

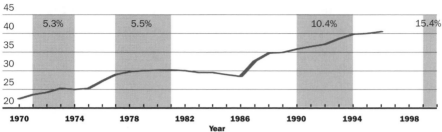

Sources: NHANES data; regular soft drink consumption data for the United States overall are from Judy Putnam and Shirley Gerrior, "Trends in the U.S. Food Supply, 1970–97," in *America's Eating Habits: Changes and Consequences,* edited by Elizabeth Frazao, USDA Agriculture Information Bulletin no. 750 (Washington: USDA, 1999), pp. 133–59 (www.ers.usda.gov/publications/aib750/ [September 26, 2005]).

Notes: Shaded areas represent years over which BMI measures are available. The percentage of children overweight in those data is shown.

children. Simone French, Bing-Hwan Lin, and Joanne Guthrie, however, document that children's consumption has risen, with the average intake more than doubling from five to twelve ounces a day.[46] Among those children who drink sodas (a share that increased from 37 to 56 percent), average consumption rose 50 percent, from 14 to 21 ounces. The two data points of this study, one from 1977–78 and one from 1994–98, make it impossible to pinpoint whether the increase occurred mainly in the late 1980s, as it did for overall soft drink consumption. But to the extent that children's consumption mirrored the overall trends, and given the significant effect on obesity that researchers have found for soft drinks, increased consumption may have contributed to the recent trends in obesity. The question then becomes, What led to an increase in soft drink consumption? Certainly, spending for advertising soft drinks has been on the rise—from $541 million in 1995 to $799 million in 1999, an almost 50 percent increase.[47] By contrast, overall food-related advertising over the period increased less than 20 percent, from $9.8 billion to $11.6 billion.

Although beverage advertising appears to have been growing disproportionately, the evidence on whether advertising increases overall con-

sumption of a product—or merely affects relative brand consumption—is somewhat mixed. Some evidence shows that advertising affects food preferences, even of children as young as two.[48] But Todd Zywicki, Debra Holt, and Maureen Ohlhausen argue that food advertising is not a cause of increasing childhood obesity and point out that children's exposure to advertising has increased little over time.[49] Howard Taras and Miriam Gage, however, note that commercials have grown shorter over time, thus exposing children to more advertisements. And children's programming had 11 percent more commercials per hour in 1993 than in 1987.[50] Throughout that period, about half of the ads were for foods and beverages, though only about 6 percent of the beverage advertising was for soft drinks. This study, however, like most studies on children and advertising, focuses only on children's programming. Many children are watching adult programming on television and are thus being exposed to the same advertisements as the general population.

Another possible source of the increase in soft drink consumption is the increase in food consumed away from home. French, Lin, and Guthrie note that the share of soft drinks consumed in restaurants (including fast-food restaurants) rose more than 50 percent while at the same time the share consumed at home fell almost 25 percent.[51] Consumption of soft drinks from every source has increased over this period, but there has been a shift away from consumption at home. This trend in soft drinks mirrors the overall trend in food consumed away from home. Lin and several colleagues document a jump in the share of calories from food consumed away from home from just 18 percent during 1977–78, to 27 percent by 1987–88, and to 34 percent by 1995.[52] The increase in food away from home is a major change in the food market. In fact, Shin-Yi Chou and colleagues claim that for adults, up to two-thirds of the increase in obesity since 1980 can be explained by the per capita increase in fast-food restaurants over the period.[53] Their methodology, however, does not rule out the possibility that the growth trends in both series are just coincidentally correlated.

Also looking at adults, David Cutler and colleagues argue that the mushrooming of fast-food restaurants is just part and parcel of an overall change in technology, with tastier treats becoming available at lower cost and greater convenience.[54] They point to snacking as the key source of increased energy intake for adults. As noted, though, there is little evidence for a direct effect of snacking on children's obesity. The change in the food market that remains in play, however, is portion size. As noted, all but the youngest children will eat more when offered larger portions.[55] Looking at convenience foods (both fast foods and other foods packaged for single-serving consumption), Lisa Young and Marion Nestle document increases in portion sizes.[56] For 181 products they can identify the date when portion sizes were increased. Throughout the 1970s portion sizes of those products increased rarely—fewer than ten

times every five years. That number doubled during the first half of the 1980s to about twenty and doubled again by the first half of the 1990s to more than forty. During the last half of the 1990s portion sizes increased more than sixty times. This timing too fits relatively closely with the timing of increases in childhood obesity. Thus the increase in childhood overweight may be driven not just by

---

Consumption of soft drinks from every source has increased over this period, but there has been a shift away from consumption at home. This trend in soft drinks mirrors the overall trend in food consumed away from home.

---

increased consumption of particular foods, such as sodas, but also by the change in the food market toward larger portion sizes.

No discussion of the food market would be complete without considering prices. Darius Lakdawalla and Tomas Philipson, for example, argue that declines in the relative price of food have led people to eat more—and hence to increased obesity.[57] They calculate that up to 40 percent of the adult increase in BMI since 1980 can be attributed to growing demand for calories resulting from lower prices. Within food groups, the consumer price index for food away from home rose only slightly more slowly than the index for food at home.[58] Starting with an index of 100 for 1982–84, the food-at-home index rose to

158.1 in 1997, while the food-away-from-home index rose to 157, making it unlikely that price was a primary cause of this shift in eating patterns. In general, it has been argued that energy-dense foods tend to be less costly than such foods as whole grains, fruits, and vegetables.[59] But based on scanner data, Jane Reed, Elizabeth Frazao, and Rachel Itskowitz conclude that it is possible to meet the daily

---

Thus the increase in childhood overweight may be driven not just by increased consumption of particular foods, such as sodas, but also by the change in the food market toward larger portion sizes.

---

recommendations of three servings of fruits and vegetables for just 64 cents.[60] They also note that although consumers may perceive fresh produce as more expensive than processed versions (such as canned, frozen, dried, or juiced), converted from a per-pound price to a per-serving price, 63 percent of fruits and 57 percent of vegetables were cheapest when purchased fresh. These prices, however, do not take into account the implicit time costs associated with preparing fresh foods. We will consider this idea below when we discuss the changing role of parents.

Changes in the Built Environment
We noted earlier the strong theoretical relationship between physical activity and overweight. Although the empirical studies establishing this link are comparatively weak,

changes in children's physical activity should nevertheless be investigated. Historically, physical activity was not something one set out to do; it was simply part of life. In fact, Tomas Philipson and Richard Posner argue that the long-run rise in adult obesity can be traced to technological changes that have made work much more sedentary.[61] Rather than being paid to undertake physical activity, modern Americans must pay, either explicitly in gym fees and equipment costs or implicitly in forgone leisure, to be physically active. Although attractive as a theory of historical trends and of differences between developing and developed countries, the argument provides little insight into the increase in childhood overweight and obesity over the past thirty years. Nonetheless, the basic insight that technological changes have made daily living less physically active can be applied to children. To do that, it is necessary to examine changes in the neighborhoods in which children are growing up.

Urban sprawl increases automobile travel.[62] Thus as sprawl has expanded, vehicle miles per person have increased. Daily vehicle miles traveled per household were fairly constant between 1977 and 1983, at about 33 and 32, respectively, and then jumped up to 41 in 1990.[63] Changes in methodology make it impossible to compare the data for these two periods with data for years after 1990, but the 1990 data can be adjusted to allow such comparisons. The adjusted data show about 50 vehicle miles traveled per household for 1990. The increase continued during the early 1990s, before slowing in the latter half of the decade. The 1995 measure is 57 miles; that for 2001, just 58. An increase in household vehicle miles traveled does not necessarily mean that children are spending more time in the car. But total miles traveled by those under age sixteen follows a pattern

...lina schools found that children ... much less likely to walk to a school ... en built more recently. More than ... of students in schools built during ... walked to school. For schools built ... s the share dropped below 15 per- ... for those built in the 1980s and ... below 5 percent.[66] Distance is not ... stacle, however. In the South Car- ... children living within 1.5 miles of ... were eligible for bus transportation ... ing route was deemed hazardous. ... built in the 1990s, more than 25 ... students received such transporta- ... ust a little more than 5 percent did ... built in the 1960s. The share in- ... sistently by the decade the school

...en, trends in the built environment ... ed in more car trips and in fewer ... t or by bicycle. Most notably, less ... rter of children walk or bike to ... y compared to more than two- ... eration ago. Today's lower-density development results in schools being further away from children's homes, and recent growth patterns do not provide safe walking routes. In addition to depriving children of an opportunity for physical activity, the change may have other effects on overall physical activity. Ashley Cooper and her colleagues find that at least for British boys, walking to school was correlated with higher levels of activity in other parts of the day.[67] Of course, this relationship may not be causal; it may simply reflect that boys who are naturally more active prefer to walk to school or that walking to school indicates that *other* opportunities for physical activity are also close by.

Changes in School and Child Care

Not only have children's methods of getting to school changed, but the environment once

"too much traffic and no safe walking route," "fear of child being abducted," and "not convenient for child to walk." "Crime in the neighborhood" and "your children do not want to walk" both tallied a 6 percent response. Interestingly, 1 percent said that there was a "school policy against children walking to school."

The 22 percent of children walking or riding bikes to school in 2002 represents a major decline from the share walking or biking when their parents were children, presumably about twenty to thirty years earlier. Just a little more than 70 percent of the parents reported walking or biking to school as children. Again, the increasing trend toward urban sprawl is presumably at least part of the explanation, with school being too far away. In fact, a study of they get there has evolved as well. In particular, the types of foods and beverages available at school have changed, as have physical education requirements. As noted, soft drink consumption has risen markedly over the past several decades, with some of the increase due to increased availability at school. Between 1977–78 and 1994–98, the share of overall soft drink consumption that took place in school cafeterias increased 3 percent.[68] Much of the food available at schools is sold not in the cafeteria, however, but in vending machines. Over that same period, the share of soft drink consumption from vending machines increased 48 percent. And between 1994 and 2000, student access to vending machines increased from 61 to 67 percent in middle schools and from 88 to 96 percent in high schools.[69] Schools have found it quite lucrative to enter into exclusive "pouring rights" contracts with soft drink companies. In 2000, 73 percent of high schools had such a contract, as did 58 percent of middle schools, and even 42 percent of elementary schools.[70] Many schools also allow these companies to advertise on school grounds—46 percent of high schools, 29 percent of middle schools, and 13 percent of elementary schools.

School vending machines dispense not only soft drinks, but also snacks, while school stores and snack bars also sell soft drinks and snacks. In fact, among elementary schools with such student access, more than 50 percent sell cookies, crackers, cakes, pastries, and salty snacks. The share grows to more than 60 percent for middle schools and more than 80 percent for high schools.[71] School cafeterias also sell these products à la carte, in competition with the National School Lunch Program. Sales of such competing foods are often an important part of the school budget, as most school food service programs must be self-supporting. These

sales often do more than subsidize the food service program, however. Increasingly, schools are using money raised through competitive food sales to supplement general budgets. One change in budgetary pressure on schools is the increased focus on academic accountability, which has also squeezed out other areas of study, such as nutrition and physical education, and even reduced the time available for lunch.[72]

Some observers have speculated that these changes in the school environment may have contributed to the increase in childhood overweight and obesity, though relatively few serious studies have been undertaken.[73] In a recent working paper we found that school financial pressures are linked to the availability of junk food in middle and high schools. We estimated that a 10 percentage point increase in the availability of junk food increases average BMI by 1 percent. For adolescents with an overweight parent the effect is double.[74] Effects of this size can explain about a quarter of the increase in average BMI of adolescents over the 1990s. Diane Schanzenbach focuses not on the competing foods in schools but on the National School Lunch Program.[75] She finds that for children who enter kindergarten with similar obesity rates, those who eat the school lunch are about 2 percentage points more likely to be overweight at the end of first grade. Changes in the school lunch program, however, could not clearly explain the increase in obesity over time, although between 1991–92 and 1998–99 the number of calories in an elementary school lunch increased a little, from 715 to 738. For secondary school lunches, on the other hand, calories have declined over this same period, from 820 to 798.[76]

As noted, it appears that physical activity has been squeezed out of schools to make room

Figure 6. Labor Force Participation Rate of Married Women with Children

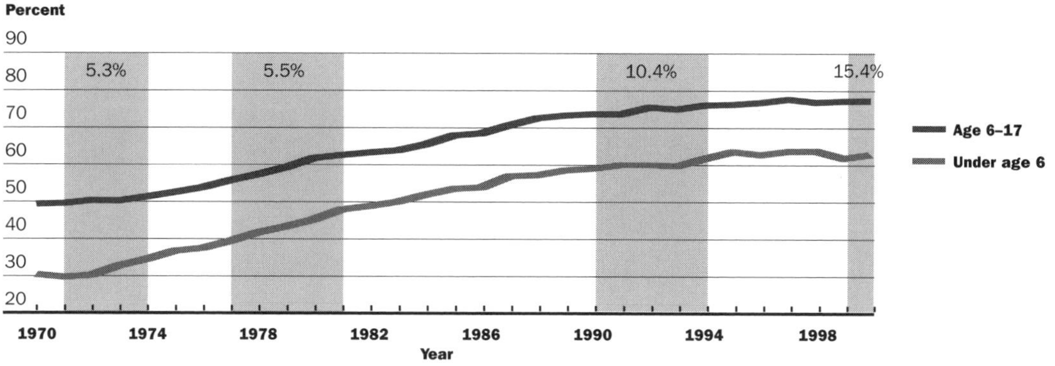

Sources: NHANES data; LFP rates are from various years of the Census Bureau's *Statistical Abstract of the United States*.

Notes: Shaded areas represent years over which BMI measures are available. The percentage of children overweight in those NHANES data is shown.

for more academics. The National Association of Early Childhood Specialists in State Departments of Education recently stressed the importance of recess and free play, observing that 40 percent of elementary schools have reduced, deleted, or are considering deleting recess since 1989, when 90 percent of schools had some form of recess.[77] Trends in physical education (PE) in high school are a bit less clear, with enrollment moving up and down during the 1990s. The trend for daily PE attendance is downward, though, with about 42 percent of schools reporting it in 1991 and just 29 percent by 2003.[78] More generally, Karen MacPherson notes that since the late 1970s, children have seen a 25 percent drop in play and a 50 percent drop in unstructured outdoor activities.[79] One potential culprit is an increase in homework between 1981 and 1997, especially for the youngest students. Sandra Hofferth and John Sandberg report that while time spent studying was up 20 percent overall, for children aged six to eight it rose 146 percent.[80]

Another source of a drop in unstructured play is the increase in the number of children in child care centers after school. Figure 6 il-

lustrates the basic trends in maternal employment for preschool-age and school-age children, again superimposing children's obesity rates over the four periods for which NHANES data are available. Note that the quality of child care used varies, so it is unclear whether being in child care per se affects children's obesity. Nonetheless, clearly the potential for less physical activity, more sedentary activities, more sweet drinks, and more energy-dense snacks exists when children move from parental care to a child care setting. It is worth noting, however, that the increase in labor force participation (LFP) appears fairly continuous from 1970 through about 1988 before flattening out in the 1990s, with no sudden increase between 1980 and 1988. Although the exact timing of the change is not entirely consistent with the timing of the increase in obesity, it remains worthwhile to investigate the changing role of parents more fully.

Changes in the Role of Parents

One major change over the past thirty years is the number of children with both parents (or their single parent) in the labor force. This change in the home environment may

Patricia M. Anderson and Kristin F. Butcher

explain the increase in consumption both of food away from home and of pre-prepared foods, as families value convenience more highly. That is, the food market may have changed because of consumer demand stemming from the increase in households with no full-time homemaker. Note, though, that studies of the effect of maternal employment on the quality of children's diets tend to find no relationship.[81] Nevertheless, a more recent study that directly examines how maternal employment affects childhood obesity concludes that a ten-hour increase in average hours worked each week over a child's lifetime increases the probability that the child is obese by about 1 percentage point.[82] The study finds that it is not the work per se that affects children's overweight and obesity, but rather the intensity of the mothers' work. This difference may explain why previous studies found no real effect of work on children's diets and is in line with the idea that more time at work takes away from time spent preparing nutritious meals.

With less intensive work hours, mothers may also spend more time supervising active play. Similarly, having two parents working full time may also discourage walking or biking to school, as it may fit parents' schedules better to drop the children off at school on the way to work. To the extent that maternal employment affects children's physical activity, rather than nutrition, both sets of studies may be reconciled.

Increasing maternal employment may also affect the incidence or length of breast-feeding. The labor force participation rate of married women with children under age one, about 31 percent in 1975, increased to 54 and 55 percent by 1990 and 2003, respectively.[83] Nevertheless, the share of children ever breast-fed has been increasing, as has the

fraction breast-fed at older ages. Based on NHANES data, about 25 percent of children aged two to six in 1971–74 were ever breast-fed, compared to 26 percent in 1976–80. By 1988–94 almost 54 percent were ever breast-fed, increasing again by 1999–2002 to 62 percent. Over this same period the share breast-fed for at least three months rose from 55 percent to 74 percent, and the share breast-fed for at least one year rose from 7 percent to almost 25 percent. The National Survey of Family Growth does not show quite as consistent a pattern. It finds that the share of babies who were breast-fed rose from about 30 percent in 1972–74 to 58 percent in 1993–94. At the same time, the share breast-fed for three months or longer fell from 62 percent to 56 percent, after having risen to 68 percent in 1981–83.[84] Overall, though, these trends do not appear to make breast-feeding a good candidate for explaining the increase in childhood overweight.

Another area where parental roles may be important in explaining childhood obesity is television. For example, school-age children of working parents may now increasingly spend their afternoon hours unsupervised, which may increase their screen time. More generally, parents make decisions about the number and placement of televisions in a home. In 1970, 35 percent of homes had more than one television, 6 percent had three or more, and just 6 percent of sixth graders had one in their bedroom. By 1999 fully 88 percent of homes had more than one, 60 percent had three or more, and a whopping 77 percent of sixth graders had a television in their bedroom.[85] Nonetheless, the Hofferth and Sandberg study finds that for children aged three to twelve, weekly television viewing dropped four hours between 1981 and 1997.[86] Reliable and representative data on people's television viewing are relatively diffi-

Figure 7. Average Daily Minutes of TV Watching, All Viewers

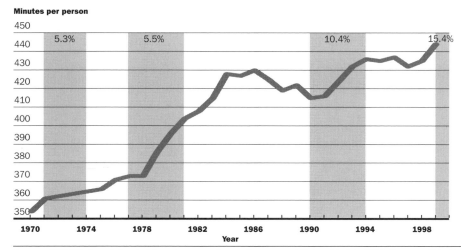

Sources: NHANES data; daily television minutes are from various years of Nielsen Media's 2000 *Report on Television*.

Notes: Shaded areas represent years over which BMI measures are available. The percentage of children overweight in those data is shown.

cult to come by because of the need for detailed diary keeping. But Nielsen Media Research is well known for its measurements of television audiences, which are used to set advertising rates.

Based on Nielsen data, overall daily minutes of television watching have climbed in recent decades.[87] Figure 7 shows the average daily minutes per person from 1970 to 1999, again superimposing children's obesity rates over the four periods for which NHANES data are available. The overall daily increase of almost an hour and a half is relatively concentrated in the early 1980s (perhaps because of increasing cable penetration), the same time when the increase in obesity began in earnest. And viewing appears to be continuing to increase, as is obesity. These data, however, are for all television viewers, not children specifically. In its annual reports, Nielsen presents weekly viewing for separate age groups. Although these subgroup numbers are fairly noisy and not consistently defined across all years, children's viewing appears to be between 70 and 90 percent of

overall viewing, but it also seems to have declined over time. For example, in 1982 overall weekly viewing was 28.4 hours, while for children aged six to eleven it was 24 hours. For teens it was about 21 hours for females and 24 hours for males. In 1999 overall weekly viewing was still just over 28 hours, but viewing time of both younger children and teens had fallen to 19.7 hours.[88]

Children may be substituting other forms of media, including videos, video games, and the Internet, for television watching. According to a 1999 study, children spent 19.3 hours a week watching television, another 2.3 hours playing video games, and 2.5 hours in front of the computer, implying just over one day (24.1 hours) of "screen time" a week.[89] Note that the television hours in this report are similar to the Nielsen numbers for that year. It may be reasonable to consider the overall Nielsen trend to be an approximation of children's screen time, with the decrease in children's television viewing relative to adults' resulting from the fact that children sometimes choose video games or play on the computer instead of watching television. Although precise evidence on children's total screen time is not easily obtainable, the available data generally support the possibility that changes in screen time may be an important contributor to the increase in childhood obesity.

Perhaps one of the biggest influences of parents on children's overweight and obesity is genetic. As noted, genetics alone cannot explain the increases in obesity in recent decades. But parents may pass along to their children a susceptibility to overweight in the presence of energy imbalance. Changes in the environment that affect energy intake or expenditure could then trigger weight gain in this susceptible population. Differentiating clearly between the extent to which nature or nurture is responsible for the strong correlation between parent and child BMI can be difficult, though. It is known, for example, that parents influence children's food selection.[90] Genetics and behavior can thus interact as both parents and children gain weight in households where more energy-dense foods are available. Similarly, children's physical activity can be affected by how active their parents are. Again, genes and behavior will interact as households engage in more sedentary behaviors, with both parents and children gaining weight.

Conclusion

The increase in childhood obesity seems to have begun between 1980 and 1988 and then continued during the 1990s. This period also saw children's environments change in multiple ways that research suggests might be contributing to the obesity epidemic.

Over the critical time period, calorie-dense convenience foods and soft drinks were both increasingly available to children at school and increasingly advertised to children. Children consumed more soda pop. They also consumed more pre-prepared food and consumed more food away from home, as increases in dual-career or single-parent working families may have driven up demand for convenience. A host of environmental changes also contributed to reducing children's activity levels over the period in question. In particular, children traveled more in cars and were less likely to walk to school than they were in the early 1970s. Changes in the built environment and in their parents' work lives also made it more difficult for children to engage in safe, unsupervised (or lightly supervised) physical activity. Finally, children spent more time in such sedentary activities as watching television, playing video games, and using computers.

Taken together, research on obesity singles out no one critical cause of the increase in children's obesity. Rather, many complementary developments seem to have upset the crucial energy balance by simultaneously increasing children's energy intake and decreasing their energy expenditure. The challenge in formulating policies to address children's obesity is not necessarily to determine what changed to create the current epidemic, but rather, what is the most effective way to change children's environment and restore their energy balance going forward.

Notes

1. In imperial measurements, BMI is calculated as (weight in pounds/[height in inches]^2) x 703.

2. National Institutes of Health, *Clinical Guidelines on the Identification, Evaluation, and Treatment of Overweight and Obesity in Adults: The Evidence Report*, NIH publication 98-4083 (September 1998).

3. William H. Dietz and Mary C. Bellizzi, "Introduction: The Use of Body Mass Index to Assess Obesity in Children," *American Journal of Clinical Nutrition* 70 (1999): 123S–125S.

4. In the medical literature the nomenclature used to describe children's and adults' weight is somewhat different. Adults with BMI above the cutoffs described above are either "overweight" or "obese." Children with BMIs above the 85th percentile are termed "at-risk-of-overweight," and those with BMIs above the 95th percentile are termed "overweight." To avoid confusion in comparisons between adults and children, we will term the former group of children "overweight" and the latter group "obese."

5. These percentile cutoffs are available at www.cdc.gov/nchs/about/major/nhanes/growthcharts/clinical_charts.htm#Clin%201 (September 26, 2005).

6. For more information on the National Health and Nutrition Examination Surveys, see the Centers for Disease Control website at www.cdc.gov/nchs/nhanes.htm (September 26, 2005).

7. These authors' calculations are based on the National Health and Nutrition Examination Surveys. The data include children aged two to nineteen and adults aged twenty to seventy. We exclude individuals with a BMI above 50, which drops a small number (fewer than 100) of individuals in each year. The data are weighted using the examination weight since we use the height and weight that are collected in the medical examination module to define BMI.

8. Obesity rates based on BMI cutoffs may understate obesity among adult women. The cutoff to define obese for both adult women and adult men is 30, but men likely have more lean muscle mass for a given BMI.

9. Robert C. Whitaker and others, "Predicting Obesity in Young Adulthood from Childhood and Parental Obesity," *New England Journal of Medicine* 337 (1997): 869–73.

10. Obesity rates are also higher among Hispanic children than among white non-Hispanic children. However, it is impossible to consistently define Hispanic across the different NHANES surveys. "Low income" roughly corresponds to children in families in the lowest quartile of family income. However, each NHANES survey reports family income in categories, and the categories do not always correspond to the level of family income that defines the lowest quartile. The income cutoffs used for each year and the mapping between NHANES income categories and income quartiles are available from the authors on request.

11. Gloria E. Zakus, "Obesity in Children and Adolescents: Understanding and Treating the Problem," *Social Work in Health Care* 8 (1982): 11–29.

12. World Health Organization, "Obesity: Preventing and Managing the Global Epidemic—Report of the WHO Consultation on Obesity" (Geneva: WHO, 1997).

13. Albert J. Stunkard and others, "The Body-Mass Index of Twins Who Have Been Reared Apart," *New England Journal of Medicine* 322 (1990): 1483–87.

14. Claude Bouchard and others, "The Response to Long-Term Overfeeding in Identical Twins," *New England Journal of Medicine* 322 (1990): 1477–82.

15. Leanne L. Birch and M. Deysher, "Caloric Compensation and Sensory Specific Satiety: Evidence for Self-Regulation of Food Intake by Young Children," *Appetite* 7 (1986): 323–31.

16. Jennifer O. Fisher, Barbara J. Rolls, and Leann L. Birch, "Children's Bite Size and Intake of an Entrée Are Greater with Larger Portions Than with Age-Appropriate or Self-Selected Portions," *American Journal of Clinical Nutrition* 77 (2003): 1164–70.

17. Sahasporn Paeratukul and others, "Fast-Food Consumption among U.S. Adults and Children: Dietary and Nutrient Intake Profile," *Journal of the American Dietetic Association* 103 (2003): 1332–38.

18. Cara B. Ebbeling and others, "Compensation for Energy Intake from Fast Food among Overweight and Lean Adolescents," *Journal of the American Medical Association* 291 (2004): 2828–33.

19. Olivia M. Thompson and others, "Food Purchased Away from Home as a Predictor of Change in BMI z-Score among Girls," *International Journal of Obesity* 28 (2004): 282–89.

20. David S. Ludwig, Karen E. Peterson, and Steven L. Gortmaker, "Relation between Consumption of Sugar-Sweetened Drinks and Childhood Obesity: A Prospective, Observational Analysis," *Lancet* 357 (2001): 505–08; Janet James and others, "Preventing Childhood Obesity by Reducing Consumption of Carbonated Drinks: Cluster Randomized Controlled Trial," *British Medical Journal* 328 (2004): 1237–40; Richard P. Troiano and others, "Energy and Fat Intakes of Children and Adolescents in the United States: Data from the National Health and Nutrition Examination Surveys," *American Journal of Clinical Nutrition* 72, supplement (2000): 1343–53S.

21. Barbara A. Dennison, Helen L. Rockwell, and Sharon L. Baker, "Excess Fruit Juice Consumption by Preschool-Aged Children Is Associated with Short Stature and Obesity," *Pediatrics* 99 (1997): 15–22; Jean D. Skinner and others, "Fruit Juice Intake Is Not Related to Children's Growth," *Pediatrics* 103 (1999): 58–64; Jean D. Skinner and Betty Ruth Carruth, "A Longitudinal Study of Children's Juice Intake and Growth: The Juice Controversy Revisited," *Journal of the American Dietetic Association* 101 (2001): 432–37.

22. Jean A. Welsh and others, "Overweight among Low-Income Preschool Children Associated with the Consumption of Sweet Drinks: Missouri, 1999–2002," *Pediatrics* 115 (2005): 223–29.

23. Ranganathan Rajeshwari and others, "Secular Trends in Children's Sweetened-Beverage Consumption (1973 to 1994): The Bogalusa Heart Study," *Journal of the American Dietetic Association* 105 (2005): 208–14.

24. Catherine S. Berkey and others, "Sugar-Added Beverages and Adolescent Weight Change," *Obesity Research* 12 (2004): 778–88.

25. Linda G. Bandini and others, "Comparison of High-Calorie, Low-Nutrient-Dense Food Consumption among Obese and Non-Obese Adolescents," *Obesity Research* 7 (2000): 438–43.

26. Sarah M. Phillips and others, "Energy-Dense Snack Food Intake in Adolescence: Longitudinal Relationship to Weight and Fatness," *Obesity Research* 12 (2004): 461–72.

27. World Health Organization, "Obesity: Preventing and Managing the Global Epidemic" (see note 12).

28. Linda G. Bandini, Dale A. Schoeller, and William H. Dietz, "Energy Expenditure in Obese and Nonobese Adolescents," *Pediatric Research* 27 (1990): 198–203.

29. James F. Sallis, Judith J. Prochaska, and Wendell C. Taylor, "A Review of Correlates of Physical Activity of Children and Adolescents," *Medicine & Science in Sports & Exercise* 32 (2003): 963–75.

30. C. Klein-Platat and others, "Physical Activity Is Inversely Related to Waist Circumference in 12-Year-Old French Adolescents," *International Journal of Obesity* 29 (2005): 9–14.

31. Catherine S. Berkey and others, "One-Year Changes in Activity and in Inactivity among 10- to 15-Year-Old Boys and Girls: Relationship to Change in Body Mass Index," *Pediatrics* 111 (2003): 836–43.

32. Jennifer Utter and others, "Couch Potatoes or French Fries: Are Sedentary Behaviors Associated with Body Mass Index, Physical Activity, and Dietary Behaviors among Adolescents?" *Journal of the American Dietetic Association* 103 (2003): 1298–1305.

33. William H. Dietz and Steven L. Gortmaker, "Do We Fatten Our Children at the Television Set? Obesity and Television Viewing in Children and Adolescents," *Pediatrics* 75 (1985): 807–12.

34. Robert C. Klesges, Mary L. Shelton, and Lisa M. Klesges, "Effects of Television on Metabolic Rate: Potential Implications for Childhood Obesity," *Pediatrics* 91 (1993): 281–86.

35. See, for example, William H. Dietz, "TV or Not TV: Fat Is the Question," *Pediatrics* 91 (1993): 499–501; Maciej S. Buchowski and Ming Sun, "Energy Expenditure, Television Viewing, and Obesity," *International Journal of Obesity* 20 (1996): 236–44.

36. Steven L. Gortmaker, Karen E. Peterson, and Jean Wiecha, "Reducing Obesity via a School-Based Interdisciplinary Intervention among Youth: Planet Health," *Archives of Pediatric and Adolescent Medicine* 153 (1999): 409–18; Carlos J. Crespo and others, "Television Watching, Energy Intake, and Obesity in U.S. Children: Results from the Third National Health Examination Survey, 1988–1994," *Archives of Pediatric and Adolescent Medicine* 155 (2001): 360–65; Thomas N. Robinson and others, "Does Television Viewing Increase Obesity and Reduce Physical Activity? Cross-Sectional and Longitudinal Analyses among Adolescent Girls," *Pediatrics* 91 (1993): 273–80; Elizabeth A. Vandewater, Mi-suk Shim, and Allison G. Caplovitz, "Linking Obesity and Activity Level with Children's Television and Video Game Use," *Journal of Adolescence* 27 (2004): 71–85.

37. Thomas N. Robinson, "Reducing Children's Television Viewing to Prevent Obesity: A Randomized Controlled Trial," *Journal of the American Medical Association* 282 (1999): 1561–67; Leonard H. Epstein and others, "Effects of Manipulating Sedentary Behavior on Physical Activity and Food Intake," *Journal of Pediatrics* 140 (2002): 334–39.

38. Richard S. Strauss and Harold A. Pollack, "Epidemic Increase in Childhood Overweight, 1986–1998," *Journal of the American Medical Association* 286 (2001): 2845–48.

39. Center for Rural Pennsylvania, *Overweight Children in Pennsylvania* (Harrisburg, Pa.: January 2005) (www.ruralpa.org/Overweight_child.pdf (September 26, 2005]).

40. Michael S. Kramer, "Do Breast-Feeding and Delayed Introduction of Solid Foods Protect against Subsequent Obesity?" *Journal of Pediatrics* 98 (1981): 883–87; Rüdiger von Kries and others, "Breast Feeding and Obesity: Cross-Sectional Study," *British Medical Journal* 319 (1999): 147–50; Matthew W. Gillman and others, "Risk of Overweight among Adolescents Who Were Breast-Fed as Infants," *Journal of the American Medical Association* 285 (2001): 2461–67; Karl E. Bergmann and others, "Early Determinants of Childhood Overweight and Adiposity in a Birth Cohort Study: Role of Breast-Feeding," *International Journal of Obesity* 27 (2003): 162–72.

41. Mary L. Hediger and others, "Association between Infant Breastfeeding and Overweight in Young Children," *Journal of the American Medical Association* 285 (2001): 2453–60.

42. Stephan Arenz and others, "Breast-Feeding and Childhood Obesity—a Systematic Review," *International Journal of Obesity* 28 (2004): 1247–56.

43. William H. Dietz, "Breastfeeding May Help Prevent Childhood Overweight," *Journal of the American Medical Association* 285 (2001): 2506–07.

44. Melissa C. Nelson, Penny Gordon-Larson, and Linda S. Adair, "Are Adolescents Who Were Breast-Fed Less Likely to Be Overweight? Analyses of Sibling Pairs to Reduce Confounding," *Epidemiology* 16 (2005): 247–53.

45. Judy Putnam and Shirley Gerrior, "Trends in the U.S. Food Supply, 1970–97," in *America's Eating Habits: Changes and Consequences,* edited by Elizabeth Frazao, USDA Agriculture Information Bulletin no. 750 (Washington: USDA, 1999), pp. 133–59 (www.ers.usda.gov/publications/aib750/ [September 26, 2005]).

46. Simone A. French, Bing-Hwan Lin, and Joanne Guthrie, "National Trends in Soft Drink Consumption among Children and Adolescents Age 6 to 17 Years: Prevalence, Amounts, and Sources, 1977/1978 to 1994/1998," *Journal of the American Dietetic Association* 103 (2003): 1326–31.

47. J. Michael Harris and others, "The U.S. Food Marketing System, 2002: Competition, Coordination, and Technological Innovations into the 21st Century," USDA Agricultural Economic Report no. 811 (Washington: USDA, 2002) (www.ers.usda.gov/publications/aer811/ [September 26, 2005]).

48. Dina L. G. Borzekowski and Thomas N. Robinson, "The 30-Second Effect: An Experiment Revealing the Impact of Television Commercials on Food Preferences of Preschoolers," *Journal of the American Dietetic Association* 101 (2001): 42–46.

49. Todd J. Zywicki, Debra Holt, and Maureen K. Ohlhausen, "Obesity and Advertising Policy" (Washington: Georgetown University Law Center mimeo, 2004) (contact author: tjz2@law.georgetown.edu).

50. Howard L. Taras and Miriam Gage, "Advertised Foods on Children's Television," *Archives of Pediatrics & Adolescent Medicine* 149 (1995): 649–52.

51. French, Lin, and Guthrie, "National Trends in Soft Drink Consumption" (see note 46).

52. Bing-Hwan Lin, Joanne Guthrie, and Elizabeth Frazao, "Nutrient Contribution of Food Away from Home," in *America's Eating Habits*, edited by Frazao, pp. 213–42.

53. Shin-Yi Chou, Michael Grossman, and Henry Saffer, "An Economic Analysis of Adult Obesity: Results from the Behavioral Risk Factor Surveillance System," *Journal of Health Economics* 23 (2004): 565–87.

54. David M. Cutler, Edward L. Glaeser, and Jesse M. Shapiro, "Why Have Americans Become More Obese?" *Journal of Economic Perspectives* 17 (2003): 93–118.

55. Barbara J. Rolls, Dianne Engell, and Leann L. Birch, "Serving Portion Size Influences 5-Year-Old but Not 3-Year-Old Children's Food Intakes," *Journal of the American Dietetic Association* 100 (2000): 232–34.

56. Lisa R. Young and Marion Nestle, "The Contribution of Expanding Portion Sizes to the U.S. Obesity Epidemic," *American Journal of Public Health* 92 (2002): 246–49.

57. Darius N. Lakdawalla and Tomas J. Philipson, "Technological Change and the Growth of Obesity," Working Paper 8946 (Cambridge, Mass.: National Bureau of Economic Research, 2002).

58. Howard Elitzak, *Food Cost Review, 1950–97*, USDA Agricultural Economic Report no. 780 (Washington: USDA, 1999) (www.ers.usda.gov/publications/aer780/ [September 26, 2005]).

59. Adam Drewnowski, "Obesity and the Food Environment: Dietary Energy Density and Diet Costs," *American Journal of Preventive Medicine* 27 (2004): 154–62; Adam Drewnowski, Nicole Damon, and André Brien, "Replacing Fats and Sweets with Vegetables and Fruits—A Question of Cost," *American Journal of Public Health* 94 (2004): 1555–59.

60. Jane Reed, Elizabeth Frazao, and Rachel Itskowitz, "How Much Do Americans Pay for Fruits and Vegetables?" USDA Agriculture Information Bulletin no. 790 (Washington: USDA, 1999).

61. Tomas J. Philipson and Richard A. Posner, "The Long-Run Growth in Obesity as a Function of Technological Change," *Perspectives in Biology and Medicine* 46 (2003): S87–S107.

62. Reid Ewing, Rolf Pendall, and Don Chen, *Measuring Sprawl and Its Impact*, Smart Growth America Report (Washington: Smart Growth America, 2002) (www.smartgrowthamerica.org/sprawlindex/sprawlreport.html [September 26, 2005]).

63. Patricia S. Hu and Timothy R. Reuscher, *Summary of Travel Trends: 2001 National Household Travel Survey*, USDOT Federal Highway Administration Report (Washington: USDOT, 2004) (http://nhts.ornl.gov/2001/reports.shtml [September 26, 2005]).

64. James Corless and Gloria Ohland, *Caught in the Crosswalk: Pedestrian Safety in California*, Surface Transportation Policy Project Report (San Francisco: Surface Transportation Policy Project, 1999) (www.transact.org/ca/caught99/caught.htm [September 26, 2005]).

65. Beldon Russonello and Stewart Research and Communications, *Americans' Attitudes toward Walking and Creating Better Walking Communities*, Surface Transportation Policy Project Report (Washington: Beldon Russonello & Stewart Research and Communications, 2003) (www.transact.org/report.asp?id=205/) [September 26, 2005]).

66. Christopher Kouri, "Wait for the Bus: How Low-Country School Site Selection and Design Deter Walking to School and Contribute to Urban Sprawl," Terry Sanford Institute of Public Policy at Duke University Report prepared for the South Carolina Coastal Conservation League, 1999 (www.scccl.org/pgm_over_reports.html [September 26, 2005]).

67. Ashley R. Cooper and others, "Commuting to School: Are Children Who Walk More Physically Active?" *American Journal of Preventive Medicine* 25 (2003): 273–76.

68. French, Lin, and Guthrie, "National Trends in Soft Drink Consumption" (see note 46).

69. Patricia M. Anderson, Kristin F. Butcher, and Philip B. Levine, "Economic Perspectives on Childhood Obesity," Federal Reserve Bank of Chicago, *Economic Perspectives* 3Q (2003): 30–48 (www.chicagofed.org/economic_research_and_data/economic_perspectives.cfm [September 26, 2005]).

70. Ibid.

71. Howell Weschler and others, "Food Service and Foods and Beverages Available at School: Results from the School Health Policies and Programs Study 2000," *Journal of School Health* 71 (2001): 313–24.

72. U.S. Department of Agriculture, "Foods Sold in Competition with USDA School Meal Programs," a Report to Congress, January 12, 2001; U.S. General Accounting Office, "School Lunch Program: Efforts Needed to Improve Nutrition and Encourage Healthy Eating," GAO-03-506, Report to Congressional Requesters, May 2003.

73. Robert Colin Carter, "The Impact of Public Schools on Childhood Obesity," *Journal of the American Medical Association* 17 (2002): 2180; Ellen J. Fried and Marion Nestle, "The Growing Political Movement against Soft Drinks in Schools," *Journal of the American Medical Association* 17 (2002): 2181.

74. Patricia M. Anderson and Kristin F. Butcher, "Reading, Writing, and Raisinets: Are School Finances Contributing to Children's Obesity?" Working Paper 11177 (Cambridge, Mass.: National Bureau of Economic Research, 2005).

75. Diane Whitmore Schanzenbach, "Do School Lunches Contribute to Childhood Obesity?" (University of Chicago, mimeo, 2005).

76. U.S. General Accounting Office, "School Lunch Program" (see note 72).

77. National Association of Early Childhood Development Specialists in State Departments of Education, "Recess and the Importance of Play," *A Position Statement on Young Children and Recess*, 2001 (www.eric.ed.gov [September 26, 2005]).

78. Centers for Disease Control, "Participation in High School Physical Education—United States, 1991–2003," *Morbidity and Mortality Weekly Report* 53 (2004): 844–47.

79. Karen MacPherson, "Development Experts Say Children Suffer due to Lack of Unstructured Fun," *Pittsburgh Post-Gazette*, October 1, 2002 (www.post-gazette.com/lifestyle/20021001childsplay1001fnp3.asp [September 26, 2005]).

80. Sandra L. Hofferth and John F. Sandberg, "Changes in American Children's Time, 1981–1997," in *Children at the Millennium: Where Have We Come From, Where Are We Going?* edited by Timothy Owens and Sandra Hofferth (New York: Elsevier Science, 2001), pp. 193–229.

81. Rachel K. Johnson, Helen Smiciklas-Wright, and Ann C. Crouter, "Effect of Maternal Employment on the Quality of Young Children's Diets: The CSFII Experience," *Journal of the American Dietetic Association* 92 (1992): 213–14; Rachel K. Johnson and others, "Maternal Employment and the Quality of Young Children's Diets: Empirical Evidence Based on the 1987–1988 Nationwide Food Consumption Survey," *Pediatrics* 90 (1992): 245–49.

82. Patricia M. Anderson, Kristin F. Butcher, and Philip B. Levine, "Maternal Employment and Overweight Children," *Journal of Health Economics* 22 (2003): 477–504.

83. U.S. Bureau of the Census, *Statistical Abstract of the United States, 2004–2005* (Washington, 2004) (www.census.gov/statab/www/ [September 26, 2005]).

84. National Center for Health Statistics, *Health, United States, 2004, with Chartbook on Trends in the Health of Americans* (Hyattsville, Md., 2004) (www.cdc.gov/nchs/hus.htm [September 26, 2005]).

85. Donald F. Roberts and others, *Kids & Media @ the New Millennium*, a Kaiser Family Foundation Report, November 1999 (www.kff.org/entmedia/1535-index.cfm [September 26, 2005]).

86. Hofferth and Sandberg, "Changes in American Children's Time, 1981–1997" (see note 80).

87. Nielsen Media Research, *2000 Report on Television: The First 50 Years* (New York: Nielsen Media Research, 2000).

88. A. C. Nielsen Company, *Report on Television* (Northbrook, Ill.: A. C. Nielsen Company, 1983); Nielsen Media Research, *2000 Report on Television* (see note 87).

89. Roberts and others, *Kids & Media @ the New Millennium* (see note 85).

90. Robert C. Klesges and others, "Parental Influence on Food Selection in Young Children and Its Relationships to Childhood Obesity," *American Journal of Clinical Nutrition* 53 (1991): 859–64.

The Consequences of Childhood Overweight and Obesity

Stephen R. Daniels

Summary

Researchers are only gradually becoming aware of the gravity of the risk that overweight and obesity pose for children's health. In this article Stephen Daniels documents the heavy toll that the obesity epidemic is taking on the health of the nation's children. He discusses both the immediate risks associated with childhood obesity and the longer-term risk that obese children and adolescents will become obese adults and suffer other health problems as a result.

Daniels notes that many obesity-related health conditions once thought applicable only to adults are now being seen in children and with increasing frequency. Examples include high blood pressure, early symptoms of hardening of the arteries, type 2 diabetes, nonalcoholic fatty liver disease, polycystic ovary disorder, and disordered breathing during sleep.

He systematically surveys the body's systems, showing how obesity in adulthood can damage each and how childhood obesity exacerbates the damage. He explains that obesity can harm the cardiovascular system and that being overweight during childhood can accelerate the development of heart disease. The processes that lead to a heart attack or stroke start in childhood and often take decades to progress to the point of overt disease. Obesity in childhood, adolescence, and young adulthood may accelerate these processes. Daniels shows how much the same generalization applies to other obesity-related disorders—metabolic, digestive, respiratory, skeletal, and psychosocial—that are appearing in children either for the first time or with greater severity or prevalence.

Daniels notes that the possibility has even been raised that the increasing prevalence and severity of childhood obesity may reverse the modern era's steady increase in life expectancy, with today's youth on average living less healthy and ultimately shorter lives than their parents—the first such reversal in lifespan in modern history. Such a possibility, he concludes, makes obesity in children an issue of utmost public health concern.

www.futureofchildren.org

Stephen R. Daniels is a professor of pediatrics and environmental health at the University of Cincinnati College of Medicine and Cincinnati Children's Hospital Medical Center.

Stephen R. Daniels

Health professionals have long known that being overweight carries many serious health risks for adults. Medical researchers have also investigated how obesity affects the health of children and adolescents, but work in this area has advanced more slowly. The epidemic of overweight and obesity in children and adolescents, however, has intensified the pace of research. In the face of this new epidemic, researchers are raising the question of whether children face the same set of health risks as adults—or whether their risks are unique. The answer, to a certain extent, is both. Many health conditions once thought applicable only to adults are now being seen in children and with increasing frequency. Even if the conditions do not appear as symptoms until adulthood, they may appear earlier than usual in a person's lifetime if the person had weight problems in childhood. Further, children are also more vulnerable to a unique set of obesity-related health problems because their bodies are growing and developing.

In this article, I will discuss both the adverse outcomes associated with childhood obesity and the risk that obese children and adolescents will become obese adults and be exposed to other health problems.

The obesity epidemic is taking a heavy toll on the nation's children. Some obesity-related conditions are having an immediate adverse effect on their health; others will have more chronic long-term effects. Because of overweight and obesity, today's young people may, on average, live less healthy and ultimately shorter lives than their parents. The epidemic is an issue of urgent public health concern.

Adverse Health Outcomes in Children

As the prevalence and severity of childhood obesity increase, concern about adverse health outcomes in childhood and adolescence is rising. Table 1 shows the prevalence in children and adolescents of various health problems associated with obesity. In what follows, I will provide details on how obesity affects various important body systems. Obesity can cause great damage to the cardiovascular system, for example, and being overweight or obese during childhood can accelerate the development of obesity-related cardiovascular disease. Likewise, obesity is linked with many disorders of the metabolic system. Such disorders, heretofore seen primarily in adulthood, are now appearing in children. Even when the disorders do not present themselves in childhood, childhood obesity or overweight increases the risk of their developing in adulthood. Much the same generalization applies to the obesity-related disorders in the other bodily systems.

Cardiovascular Problems

In the cardiovascular system, the heart pumps blood, which is carried back and forth between the heart and the body by blood vessels. Arteries, which move blood from the heart to the rest of the body, are not just simple tubes, but a dynamic series of conduits that control blood flow. They are vulnerable to many diseases that can ultimately lead, in the case of coronary arteries, to a heart attack or, in the case of cerebral arteries, to a stroke. The heart muscle is also vulnerable to processes that thicken it and diminish its function. The critical risk factors for heart attack or stroke—diabetes, high blood pressure, high blood cholesterol, and cigarette smoking—are well known.

Table 1. Disorders Related to Childhood Obesity, by Body System

System and disorder	Explanation	Estimated prevalence in pediatric populations
Cardiovascular		
Hypertension	High blood pressure	2–4%
Left ventricular hypertrophy	Increased thickness of the heart's main pumping chamber	Unknown
Atherosclerosis	Hardening of the arteries	50% (fatty streaks) 8% (fibrous plaques) 4% (>40 in those with stenosis)
Metabolic		
Insulin resistance	The process in which the action of insulin is retarded	Unknown
Dyslipidemia	Abnormal changes in cholesterol and triglycerides (fats) in the blood	5-10%
Metabolic syndrome	Constellation of risk factors including increased waist circumference, elevated blood pressure, increased triglyceride and decreased HDL-cholesterol concentrations, and raised plasma glucose	4% overall, 30% in obese
Type 2 diabetes	A condition in which the body either makes too little insulin or cannot properly use the insulin it makes, leading to elevated blood glucose	1–15 persons per 100,000 overall, almost all in obese
Pulmonary		
Asthma	A chronic inflammatory pulmonary disorder characterized by reversible obstruction of the airways	7–9%
Obstructive sleep apnea	A breathing disorder characterized by interruptions of breathing during sleep	1–5% overall, approx. 25% in obese
Gastrointestinal		
Nonalcoholic fatty liver disease	Fatty inflammation of the liver not caused by excessive alcohol use	3–8% overall, 50% in obese
Gastroesophageal reflux	Backward flow of stomach contents into the esophagus	2–20%
Skeletal		
Tibia vara (Blount disease)	Bowing of children's legs caused by a growth disturbance in the proximal tibial epiphysis	Uncommon
Slipped capital-femoral epiphysis	A disorder of the hip's growth plate	1–8 persons per 100,000
Psychosocial		
Depression	A mood disorder characterized by sadness and loss of interest in usually satisfying activities	1–2% in children, 3–5% in adolescents
Other		
Polycystic ovary syndrome	A constellation of abnormalities including abnormal menses, clinical manifestations of such androgen excess as acne and excessive growth of hair, elevated levels of circulatory androgens, and polycystic ovaries on ultrasound evaluation	Unknown in adolescents, 5–10% in adult women
Pseudotumor cerebri	Raised intracranial pressure	Rare

Source: Author's estimates based on various sources.

Until recently, most medical concerns about children's hearts involved birth defects. But as advances in noninvasive testing have made it possible to evaluate children's hearts and blood vessels, health professionals have discovered that some disease processes, such as hardening of the arteries, once thought to be predominantly adult health concerns can in fact begin in childhood.

One major risk factor for heart attack and stroke in adults is hypertension, or high blood pressure.[1] And obesity is an important contributor to developing high blood pressure not only in adults, but also in children and adolescents.[2] B. Rosner and several colleagues have demonstrated that the odds of elevated blood pressure are significantly higher for children whose body mass index (BMI) is at or above the 90th percentile than for those with BMI at or below the 10th percentile. The risk of elevated blood pressure ranges from 2.5 to 3.7 times higher for the overweight children, depending on their race and sex.[3]

Recent national epidemiological studies have suggested that today's children and adolescents have higher blood pressure than did their counterparts in past decades.

Recent national epidemiological studies have suggested that today's children and adolescents have higher blood pressure than did their counterparts in past decades.[4] P. Muntner and several colleagues have also found that a portion of this increase in blood pressure is due to population trends for increased overweight.[5] As children on average have become more overweight, their blood pressure on average has gone up. BMI during childhood and, to an even greater extent, the increase in BMI from childhood to adulthood have been linked significantly with blood pressure in adulthood.[6] Overweight and obese children and those who become even more overweight in adulthood are more likely than others to have high blood pressure as adults.

Left ventricular hypertrophy, or increased thickness of the heart's main pumping chamber, is an independent risk factor for cardiovascular disease in adults. Adults with high blood pressure and with a left ventricular mass index greater than 51 g/m have a fourfold increase in adverse cardiovascular outcomes.[7] Left ventricular hypertrophy has been associated with obesity and high blood pressure in adults.

As with high blood pressure, left ventricular hypertrophy has also been linked with increased BMI in children and adolescents.[8] The most important aspect of body composition that affects left ventricular mass is lean body mass, probably because the heart's development matches the development of the body's muscles to which it must supply blood.[9] This appears to be a physiologic— that is, normal—relationship. But fat mass and systolic blood pressure also have a significant relationship with left ventricular mass.[10] These more pathologic, or abnormal, relationships could lead to the increased heart thickness that raises the risk of a heart attack. In addition, among children with essential hypertension (the most common form of high blood pressure), increased BMI is linked with more severe left ventricular hypertrophy.[11] Left ventricular hypertrophy may thus be another important pathway by which obesity can increase the future risk of cardiovascular disease in children.

Ultimately the most important process for developing cardiovascular disease is hardening of the arteries, or atherosclerosis, which begins as a fatty streak on the artery's inner lining and progresses into a fibrous plaque (a raised lesion) that ultimately causes a heart attack or a stroke by blocking blood flow to the heart or to the brain. The well-known risk factors for this progression in adults include cigarette smoking, high blood pressure, elevated cholesterol, and diabetes.

Whether obesity directly influences the progression of atherosclerosis in adults is not clear.

Obesity's role in the earliest stages of atherosclerosis during childhood has been even less clear, in part because researchers lack noninvasive tools to evaluate the early atherosclerotic lesions. Two pathology studies, however, have helped to clarify these relationships. The Pathobiologic Determinants of Atherosclerosis in Youth (PDAY) and the Bogalusa studies used autopsy data on adolescents and young adults who died of accidental causes.[12] Pathologists working on these autopsies were able to observe directly the fatty streaks and fibrous plaques in these young people's arteries and to evaluate whether the presence of these lesions was related to the known risk factors for heart attack and stroke. In both studies, measures of adiposity (or fat) were significantly related to the presence of atherosclerotic lesions. In the Bogalusa study, an increase in the number of risk factors, including overweight, high blood pressure, and high cholesterol, was associated with a dramatically increased risk of atherosclerosis.[13] In another study L. T. Mahoney and several colleagues used electron beam computed tomography (EBCT) to evaluate calcium's presence in the coronary arteries of young adults.[14] Calcium deposits provide an important indication of the progression of the atherosclerotic process. Mahoney's team found coronary calcium in approximately 30 percent of healthy young adult males and approximately 10 percent of young adult females in a normal sample (that is, the sample did not consist only of overweight young people). They also found that increased weight during childhood and a high body mass index in young adulthood were linked with an increased risk of coronary artery calcium deposits in young adults.

All these studies provide important evidence that obesity is detrimental to the heart and blood vessels even in very young children. Doctors know that the processes that lead to a heart attack or stroke often take decades to progress to overt disease. It now appears, however, that these processes may be starting earlier than once thought and that becoming obese in childhood, adolescence, and young adulthood may accelerate them. The current generation of children may thus suffer the adverse effects of cardiovascular disease at a younger age than did previous generations, despite the advent of new drugs to treat such problems as high blood pressure and abnormal blood cholesterol.

Metabolic Disorders

The metabolic system is a complex set of interrelated processes that control how the body uses and stores energy. It includes the gastrointestinal tract, which governs absorption of nutrients and energy; the liver, which is the body's major metabolic organ; and a variety of hormonal systems that govern the ebb and flow of nutrients and energy. The system involves many overlapping components, each of which can, to some extent, compensate for an abnormality in another. But this compensation may often come at a price of an increased risk for other adverse health consequences.

Many metabolic disorders—among them insulin resistance, the metabolic syndrome, dyslipidemia (abnormal levels of fat in the blood), and type 2 diabetes mellitus—have been linked with obesity in adulthood.[15] In fact, many were long considered diseases of adulthood. Type 2 diabetes had even been called adult-onset diabetes. In the past fifteen years, however, much has changed in this field as the prevalence and severity of overweight have increased in children and adolescents, with type 2 diabetes now appearing in children as young as eight years old. Insulin resistance, for example, or the process in which the action of insulin is retarded, is a relatively new concern in the pediatric age range. The precise mechanism for insulin resistance is unknown, but it often occurs in the context of obesity and results in increased insulin secretion by the pancreas and increased circulating levels of insulin. The increased insulin helps keep the blood sugar in the normal

---

The metabolic syndrome is likely associated with an increased risk of cardiovascular disease and diabetes even in young people.

---

range but may cause other problems. J. Steinberger and several colleagues have shown that obesity in children is associated with decreased insulin sensitivity and increased circulating insulin and that these abnormalities persist into young adulthood.[16] Increased circulating insulin may in turn raise blood pressure and cholesterol levels.

The metabolic syndrome is a constellation of risk factors, including increased waist circumference, elevated blood pressure, increased triglyceride and decreased HDL-cholesterol concentrations, and raised blood sugar levels.[17] The underlying risk factors for the metabolic syndrome are abdominal obesity and insulin resistance. The metabolic syndrome is an important risk factor for cardiovascular disease and for the development of type 2 diabetes in adults.[18] It may also be

associated with other abnormalities, including fatty liver disease, polycystic ovary disease, and obstructive sleep apnea.

Defining the metabolic syndrome has been controversial in adults, so its definition has been even more complicated in pediatric populations. S. Cook and several colleagues evaluated the prevalence of the metabolic syndrome in children and adolescents using an adaptation of one adult definition. They found the metabolic syndrome in only 4 percent of all children but in 30 percent of children who are obese.[19] R. Weiss and colleagues reported that each half-unit increase in the BMI z score (equivalent to an increase of half a standard deviation in BMI) resulted in a roughly 50 percent increase in the risk of the metabolic syndrome among overweight children and adolescents.[20]

The metabolic syndrome is likely associated with an increased risk of cardiovascular disease and diabetes even in young people. The Bogalusa study noted above showed that young victims of accidental death who had a number of metabolic syndrome factors had increased atherosclerotic lesions. Such findings suggest that the risk associated with the metabolic syndrome begins early in life.[21]

Obesity is associated with cholesterol abnormalities, often referred to as atherogenic dyslipidemia, that involve abnormal changes in cholesterol and triglycerides (or fats) in the blood.[22] These abnormalities, which appear to accelerate atherosclerosis, also occur in obese children and adolescents.[23]

The prevalence of type 2 diabetes mellitus has increased dramatically in adolescents—in parallel with the increasing incidence and severity of obesity.[24] Type 2 diabetes is related to insulin resistance. Although the beta cells of the pancreas compensate for insulin resistance by making more insulin, they may not be able to keep up insulin production. When that happens, blood sugar starts to increase, first in response to meals and then ultimately even in the fasting state. At that point diabetes is present. In Cincinnati the prevalence of type 2 diabetes in adolescents increased tenfold between 1982 and 1994.[25] In the Bogalusa study 2.4 percent of overweight adolescents developed type 2 diabetes by age thirty while none of the lean adolescents did.[26] An American Diabetes Association review has suggested that as many as 45 percent of newly diagnosed cases of diabetes in children and adolescents are now type 2 diabetes.[27]

The increased prevalence of type 2 diabetes raises concern about cardiovascular disease risk. The National Cholesterol Education Program has identified diabetes as a coronary artery disease risk equivalent, meaning that patients with diabetes face a similar risk for a future adverse cardiovascular event as patients who have already had a heart attack or a stroke caused by an arterial blockage.[28] That finding suggests doctors should aggressively manage cardiovascular risk factors, such as high blood pressure and cholesterol in adults with diabetes, to prevent future illnesses and deaths from cardiovascular disease. If adolescents with type 2 diabetes have this same advanced risk, they may be more likely to have heart attacks, strokes, or heart failure at a very young age, perhaps even in their twenties and thirties. More research is needed to determine the likelihood of this happening and, if so, how best to prevent it.

Pulmonary Complications

The pulmonary system includes the lungs and associated blood vessels. The lungs take in air and exchange oxygen for carbon dioxide in the blood. The right side of the heart pumps blood through the pulmonary arteries to small capillaries in the lungs where this exchange occurs. The oxygenated blood then returns to the left side of the heart through the pulmonary veins to be pumped by the left ventricle to the body. Air is brought to the lungs by the trachea, which is connected to smaller and smaller airway branches, ultimately ending in the bronchioles where gas exchange occurs.

In asthma, one of the most common respiratory diseases of childhood, the airways in the lungs are constricted, either because inflammation causes the airways' lining to swell or because tightening of the smooth muscles that surround the airways can reduce their diameter. Asthma is generally thought to involve an allergic reaction, but much remains to be learned about the specific genetic and environmental factors that trigger the reaction. The prevalence and severity of childhood asthma have increased in the past two decades, again in parallel with the increasing prevalence and severity of childhood obesity.

Cross-sectional studies have demonstrated a link between overweight and asthma in children, though the link may be complicated by socioeconomic status, cigarette smoking, or other variables.[29] M. A. Rodriguez and colleagues found that children with a BMI above the 85th percentile had an increased risk of asthma independent of age, sex, ethnicity, socioeconomic status, and exposure to tobacco smoke. Their study also found socioeconomic status and cigarette smoking to be independent predictors of asthma.[30]

It is not clear why obesity may increase the risk of asthma. On the one hand, obesity has been associated with increased inflammation, which could contribute to asthma. On the other hand, children with asthma may have only limited physical activity and may be treated with corticosteroids, which may promote obesity development. Increased adipose mass could have a physical effect on lung function. And an excess of abdominal fat can alter lung function both through increasing the weight on the wall of muscle and bone that surrounds the lungs and through limiting the motion of the diaphragm. Stud-

Sleep-disordered breathing may be one of the most important but also most under-recognized medical complications in overweight children and adolescents.

ies in adults with asthma have shown that weight loss can improve pulmonary function, but such studies have not yet been done in children.[31]

Obesity and obstructive sleep apnea are clearly related, both in adults and in children. Obstructive sleep apnea, or an abnormal collapse of the airway during sleep, results in snoring, irregular breathing, and disrupted sleep patterns. Sleep disruption can lead to excessive daytime sleepiness, which may itself decrease physical activity and heighten the risk of further obesity. Daytime sleepiness may also harm school performance. Obstructive sleep apnea has also been associated with learning disabilities and memory defects.[32] G. B. Mallory and colleagues found that one-third of young severely overweight patients had symptoms associated with ob-

structive sleep apnea and 5 percent had severe obstructive sleep apnea.[33]

Obstructive sleep apnea can also have long-term adverse cardiovascular consequences. In the short term, episodes of low oxygen levels in the blood cause temporary increases in blood pressure in the pulmonary artery and decrease blood flow in areas in the heart.[34] Over the longer term, obstructive sleep apnea can lead to daytime elevated blood pressure, increased left ventricular mass, and diastolic dysfunction (or an inability of the heart to relax and fill with blood appropriately) of the left ventricle.[35] Treating obstructive sleep apnea improves left ventricular hypertrophy and cardiac function.[36] Sleep-disordered breathing may be one of the most important but also most under-recognized medical complications in overweight children and adolescents.

Gastrointestinal Disorders

The gastrointestinal (GI) system includes the mouth, esophagus, stomach, small and large intestines, and the anus. Often the liver is also considered part of the GI system. Although it has always been obvious that the GI system is involved in obesity because of its role in food intake, it has not always been clear that obesity can also affect the GI system. Recent research has verified that obesity can contribute to liver disease and gastroesophageal reflux disease, which causes the stomach's contents to flow back into the esophagus.

Nonalcoholic fatty liver disease (or fat deposition in the liver) and nonalcoholic steatohepatitis (or an inflammation of the liver related to fat deposits) are recognized as complications of obesity in adults. As obesity develops, fat can be deposited in the liver. In their early stages, the fat deposits are thought to be relatively innocuous, but the deposits lead to steatohepatitis, which can then progress to fibrosis, cirrhosis, and even to end-stage liver disease and liver failure, ultimately requiring a liver transplant.[37] No one knows why obesity-related nonalcoholic fatty liver disease progresses more rapidly to its more severe form in some people than in others.

Researchers now recognize that this same process of fat deposit and inflammation can afflict children and adolescents. The prevalence of nonalcoholic fatty liver disease is difficult to determine because it has no symptoms and requires a liver biopsy for confirmation. Some studies have attempted to estimate the prevalence, with one calculating that as many as 50 percent of obese children may have fat deposits in their livers while some 3 percent of obese children have the more advanced nonalcoholic steatohepatitis.[38] Another study has found that nonalcoholic fatty liver disease is the most common form of liver disease in children and adolescents.[39] Epidemiologic studies have shown that males and people of Hispanic ethnicity are at the highest risk for nonalcoholic fatty liver disease.[40] Most patients with nonalcoholic fatty liver disease also have insulin resistance. The degree of insulin resistance is associated with the severity of liver disease.[41] In adults with diabetes, the prevalence of fat deposits in the liver is high; approximately 50 percent have steatohepatitis and 19 percent have cirrhosis.[42] In adults, weight loss improves obesity-related fatty liver disease.[43] This and other potential treatments of nonalcoholic fatty liver disease have not been extensively studied in young patients.

Gastroesophageal reflux is a relatively common problem in adults that can cause acute symptoms of heartburn, long-term damage of the esophageal lining, and ultimately esophageal cancer. Several studies in adults have linked obesity with increased symptoms of gastroesophageal reflux. In a study of more than 10,000 adults aged twenty to fifty-nine in the United Kingdom, L. Murray and colleagues found that being above normal weight increased the likelihood of heartburn and acid regurgitation. Obese adults were almost three times as likely to have such symptoms as normal-weight individuals.[44] M. Nilsson and colleagues found a similar association, which was stronger among women, especially premenopausal women.[45] V. Di Francesco and colleagues reported that a vertical banded gastroplasty, an operation to decrease the stomach's size to produce weight loss, successfully reduced weight but not gastroesophageal acid reflux.[46] The disorder has not been studied extensively in obese children and adolescents, so researchers do not know whether it is linked with overweight in young people.

Skeletal Abnormalities

The skeletal system includes the bones and joints. In obesity, skeletal abnormalities, often referred to as orthopedic problems, can affect the lower extremities. Hip problems and abnormal growth of the tibia, or the main bone of the lower leg below the knee, are most common.

Some complications of obesity are physical—the effect of excess body weight—rather than metabolic, or the effect of increased adipose tissue. One such complication in adults is osteoarthritis, where excess weight results in wear and erosion of weight-bearing joints. Orthopedic problems also afflict obese children. Tibia vara, or Blount disease, is a mechanical deficiency in the medial tibial growth plate in adolescents that results in bowing of the tibia, a bowed appearance of the lower leg, and an abnormal gait. Adolescent tibia vara is not common but most often affects boys older than age nine who are overweight.[47]

Another orthopedic problem related to overweight in young patients is slipped capital femoral epiphysis, a disorder of the hip's growth plate that occurs around the age of skeletal maturity. In this disorder the femur (the bone in the upper leg and hip) is rotated

---

Although risk factors for depression in adolescents are not well known, one that has been studied, particularly in girls, is body dissatisfaction.

---

externally from under the growth plate, causing pain, making it impossible to walk, and requiring surgical repair. The pathophysiology is not completely known, but it seems to involve both mechanical and biological factors. The increased stress, which is mechanical, often results from excess weight. The bone's covering at this age, usually during the growth spurt, is thin and unable to resist the shearing forces. The abnormality is more common in overweight males and in African Americans. In about one-third to one-quarter of afflicted children, both legs are affected. Avoiding abnormal weight gain can prevent such orthopedic problems.[48]

Psychosocial Issues
Psychosocial issues involve psychological health and the ability to relate to family members and peers. Such issues may have many determinants, some of which are genetic and some, socioeconomic. Childhood

obesity is also linked with various psychosocial problems, the best studied of which is depression.

Depression is a common mental health problem in adolescents.[49] Adolescent-onset depression is often persistent and may be related to longer-term adverse mental health and health outcomes.[50] Although risk factors for depression in adolescents are not well known, one that has been studied, particularly in girls, is body dissatisfaction. In a long-term study, E. Stice and several colleagues found that body dissatisfaction, dietary restraint, and symptoms of bulimia are linked to depression.[51] Weight issues often cause body dissatisfaction, but they may affect girls of various ethnic groups differently. J. Siegel, for example, found that African American girls have a more positive body image than white, Hispanic, and Asian girls and that weight affects body image and satisfaction less in African American girls than in others.[52] The sample size in this study was small, however, so it is not conclusive.

Other studies have documented that obese adolescents seeking treatment for their obesity have more depressive symptoms than community-based obese or non-obese control groups.[53] In general, researchers have been unable to determine whether differences in depressive symptoms are based on the severity of obesity. Published studies have been based on relatively small samples, raising questions about the conclusions' validity. Nevertheless in a study by S. Erermis and several colleagues, more than half of their sample of obese adolescents had a clinically important diagnosis, often involving major depressive disorder.[54]

To discern the direction of the relationship between obesity and depression is difficult.

Depression itself is often associated with abnormal patterns of eating and physical activity that could result in future obesity; however, obesity may also result in psychosocial problems that can produce depression. Evidence supports both hypotheses. On the one hand, youths with depression are at greater risk to develop an increased body mass index.[55] E. Goodman and R. C. Whitaker found that increased BMI was associated with increased depression at a one-year follow-up, with depression scores highest among adolescents who had the greatest increase in body mass index.[56] On the other hand, in elementary school girls, higher BMI was linked with increasing symptoms of depression.[57] And overweight adolescents who had been teased by peers or family members were found to have increased suicidal thoughts and attempts.[58]

It appears that obese children and adolescents have difficulties with peer relationships. Overweight children, for example, tend to have few friends.[59] Mapping childhood social networks demonstrates that normal-weight children have more social relationships with a central network of children, while overweight children have more peripheral and isolated relationships in the network. In a contrary finding, however, a study of nine-year-old girls in the United Kingdom did not demonstrate that overweight girls were less popular and had fewer friends.[60]

An important psychosocial issue for overweight children and adolescents is quality of life. Research on this issue has not been extensive, and existing studies have focused on overall measures of quality of life rather than obesity-specific measures. J. S. Schwimmer and colleagues found that obese children and adolescents reported significantly lower health-related quality of life than their normal-weight counterparts, and they were five times more likely to have impaired quality of life.[61] In fact, the health-related quality of life for obese children and adolescents was similar to that of children diagnosed with cancer. And obese children and adolescents with obstructive sleep apnea reported even lower quality of life than those without it did, perhaps because of their increased daytime sleepiness. Ongoing research seeks to confirm the findings of Schwimmer's team and to refine the understanding of how, specifically, obesity affects children's quality of life.

Other Adverse Health Effects

Polycystic ovary syndrome consists of a constellation of abnormalities, including abnormal menses, such clinical manifestations of androgen excess as acne and excessive hair growth, elevated levels of circulatory androgens, and polycystic ovaries on ultrasound evaluation.[62] Among women with polycystic ovary syndrome, a substantial share is overweight or obese.[63] Although obesity is generally not considered the cause of the syndrome, it can exacerbate the associated metabolic derangements, including insulin resistance. The onset of polycystic ovary syndrome is often around the time of menarche, but it can occur after puberty, particularly after excess weight gain. The syndrome is one of the most common female hormonal disorders, with a reported prevalence of 5 to 10 percent.[64]

Women who suffer from polycystic ovary syndrome are at risk for infertility. Perhaps even more important, they are at substantial risk for type 2 diabetes and cardiovascular disease, as are those with metabolic syndrome.[65] Obesity is present in at least 35 percent of cases of polycystic ovary syndrome, with the share sometimes as high as 75 percent.[66] Weight loss or pharmacologic treatment improves insulin resistance and often improves metabolic abnormalities.[67]

Another important complication of obesity is pseudotumor cerebri, a condition in which increased intracranial pressure often results in headache and sometimes in vomiting or blurred vision.[68] Pseudotumor cerebri may have multiple causes, including obesity, though the precise relationship between obesity and increased intracranial pressure remains unknown. Pseudotumor cerebri may be difficult to treat and can call for aggressive weight-loss therapy, including bariatric surgery. The problem is uncommon in children and adolescents but may be more common in adults.

Economic Issues

Of all the economic issues related to obesity, perhaps the most important is the cost of its associated health problems. In an analysis of people younger than sixty-five, R. Sturm estimated that obese adults' medical expenses are 36 percent higher than those of their non-obese peers.[69] In preparing their estimate of obesity's medical costs, A. M. Wolf and G. A. Colditz began with the relative risk of disease for obese and non-obese adults for such conditions as type 2 diabetes, coronary heart disease, hypertension, and some types of cancer.[70] Based on estimates of disease costs, they projected spending on obesity to be about 6 percent of national health spending in 1995. Because their estimate is somewhat dated and because they used cost estimates from the 1980s, it likely underestimates current obesity-related health spending.

Using a nationally representative data set and complex statistical analysis to evaluate U.S. medical spending on overweight or obesity in 1998, E. A. Finkelstein and colleagues found that spending on obesity accounted for 5.3 percent of national health spending.[71] Spending on overweight and obesity together accounted for 9.1 percent of total annual U.S. medical spending, a total rivaling even the estimated medical costs attributable to smoking.[72] Also important, Medicaid and Medicare cover approximately half of these increased costs, so that increases in obesity will place further demands on public health care spending.

Evaluating the costs of overweight and obesity in childhood and adolescents is difficult because of a paucity of data. G. Wang and W. H. Dietz used hospital discharge diagnoses from 1997 through 1999 to estimate the cost of obesity-related disorders in childhood.[73] They used the most frequent principal diagnoses where obesity was listed as a secondary diagnosis and then compared hospital diagnosis figures with those in 1979–81 for children aged six to seventeen. Not surprisingly, they found increases in obesity-related diagnoses. Asthma associated with obesity increased from 6 to 8 percent; diabetes associated with obesity, from 1.4 to 2.4 percent. They also found that time spent as an inpatient was longer for children with obesity and estimated that obesity-related inpatient costs were about 1.7 percent of total annual U.S. hospital costs. Better understanding of childhood obesity's costs will help the health care system determine the best approach to preventing and treating childhood obesity. For example, A. M. Tershakovec and several colleagues estimated that payers covered only some 11 percent of costs in a pediatric weight-management program.[74]

Other obesity-related economic issues may begin in childhood and carry over into adulthood. Overweight people are stigmatized in many cultures, including the United States, where they are often characterized as lazy, sloppy, ugly, or stupid.[75] The degree of negative stereotyping increases with age and appears to affect girls more than it does boys.[76]

The implications of negative stereotyping in childhood carry into the experience of obese individuals as they enter adulthood. Women who are obese as adolescents become adults with less education, lower earning power, a higher likelihood of poverty, and a lower likelihood of marriage.[77] (These issues are substantially less pronounced for overweight adolescent males.) Obese individuals have more difficulty gaining admission to college.[78] Obese adults may also experience discrimination in renting apartments and houses.[79]

The indirect economic costs of adult obesity—reductions in economic opportunity or productivity—have been estimated at $23 billion a year in the United States.[80] One study of Swedish adult women estimated that 10 percent of all costs of sick leave and disability are obesity related.[81] The indirect costs of childhood obesity remain unknown. But if childhood obesity is causing an increased burden of disease, those costs may include time lost from work and day care costs for parents as well as time lost from school for the child.

Tracking Overweight and Obesity into Adulthood

With overweight and obesity such serious health risks for adults, an important question is whether overweight in children and adolescents predicts overweight in adulthood—in other words, whether children retain their relative ranking related to their peers as they age and become adults. That concept is known as "tracking."

Many studies have shown that overweight children are more likely than their normal-weight peers to become overweight adults. S. S. Guo and several colleagues evaluated how well BMI during childhood predicted overweight or obesity at age thirty-five in the Fels Longitudinal Study.[82] They found that for children and adolescents with BMI above the 95th percentile at any age during childhood, the probability of being obese at age thirty-five years ranged from 15 to 99 percent. The probability rises the older a child is when he or she becomes obese. Obese children, in other

The link between parental overweight and childhood obesity is likely to be both genetic and environmental, and untangling the two is often difficult.

words, are more likely to become obese adults the older they are obese as children.

Robert C. Whitaker and several colleagues investigated the relationship between obesity at various times during childhood and obesity in young adults aged twenty-one to twenty-nine.[83] Obesity in very young children (aged one to two) was not associated with adult obesity, but for obese children older than two and for obese adolescents, the odds of becoming an obese adult were higher. Those odds increased the higher their BMI was, and the older they were when they became obese as children. Finally, having obese parents made it more likely that an obese child would continue to be obese into adulthood. The probability that an obese child aged three to five would remain obese as a young adult was 24 percent if neither parent was obese at the time, but it rose to 62 percent if one parent was obese. The link between parental overweight and childhood obesity is likely to be both genetic and environmental, and untangling the two is often difficult. Researchers do not know which genes cause obesity to develop in children, though it is likely that many genes act together. And parents clearly create important aspects of the child's environment, including which foods are available and what opportunities the child has for physical activity or sedentary time. All of these factors may contribute to the tracking that makes it more likely that an obese child will become an obese adult.

Illness and Death Related to Obesity in Adults

Obesity in adulthood has long been associated with both increased illness and a greater chance of death. The Metropolitan Life Insurance Company's relative weight measure has been used for more than seventy-five years to assess mortality risks.[84] The most common adverse effects of adulthood obesity are cardiovascular disease and diabetes. Endometrial, colon, kidney, and post-menopausal breast cancer have also been associated with obesity. The Framingham Heart Study's consistent finding of a link between obesity and cardiovascular disease led the American Heart Association to recognize the emergence of obesity as one of the most important risk factors for heart disease and stroke in both men and women.[85] In the Nurses' Health Study, the heaviest subjects had fatal and nonfatal heart attacks three times more frequently than did the lightest subjects.[86] In addition to overweight and obesity in general, studies of adults have focused on the distribution of fat. For example in the Honolulu Heart Study, the risk of developing coronary artery disease was higher in men whose fat was concentrated around their abdomens, even after controlling for other risk factors.[87] The Framingham Heart Study found the same relationship for women.[88]

In adults obesity has been linked with cholesterol abnormalities, in particular lower HDL cholesterol (note that HDL is the "good" cholesterol, and higher values are better), elevation of triglycerides (fats), and high blood pressure.[89] In a review of population-based epidemiologic studies, B. N. Chiang and several colleagues reported increases in both systolic and diastolic blood pressure related to increasing weight.[90] Although these relationships between obesity and illness and death have long been well known in adults, relatively fewer data exist on the adverse health consequences of obesity in children and adolescents. Understanding these relationships in young people has become more urgent as the prevalence of overweight and obesity has increased in their age group.[91]

The cumulative effects of obesity-related diseases may be to cut short the lifespan of those affected. The question of how many people die because of obesity has been controversial. In 2004, A. H. Mokdad, of the Centers for Disease Control and Prevention (CDC), published a paper with several of his colleagues in the *Journal of the American Medical Association* that set the annual death toll at 400,000, an estimate that rivaled the toll of cigarette smoking.[92] Subsequent discussion led Mokdad's team to revise their estimate downward to 365,000.[93] A still later publication in the same journal used more recent data sets and lowered the estimated annual obesity-related death toll much further, to 112,000.[94] Part of the difficulty in estimating the obesity death toll is calculating a precise and valid estimate of obesity-related mortality. Each approach includes assumptions that are subject to question. For example, the analyses differed both in how they defined the normal weight used in the comparative calculations and in how they incorporated age into the analysis. That the analysis including more recent data sets found a lower overall obesity-related mortality is of interest. It seems counterintuitive because of obesity's increasing prevalence in recent years. But all heart disease risk factors except diabetes appear less likely to be present in overweight individuals in the more recent data, perhaps because of the medical profession's improved ability to treat these risk factors and heart disease. Unfortunately, the controversy over precisely what the death toll is has overshadowed the fact that both studies find obesity to be a major health threat. The focus on the death rate has also diverted attention from the illness and disability related to obesity.

A recent article in the *New England Journal of Medicine* raised the alarming possibility that the increasing prevalence of severe obesity in children may reverse the modern era's steady increase in life expectancy, with the youth of today on average living less healthy and ultimately shorter lives than their parents.[95] That claim too has been the subject of criticism. In an accompanying editorial in the same journal, S. H. Preston urged caution in accepting the claim, because many other factors continue to increase life expectancy in this and coming generations of children.[96] Methodological issues have also arisen regarding the calculations used to predict future longevity. Nevertheless, these data raise the possibility that the current generation of children could suffer greater illness or experience a shorter lifespan than that of their parents—the first such reversal in lifespan in modern history. That possibility makes childhood obesity an issue of utmost public health concern.

With the increasing prevalence of overweight and obesity in children and adolescents and the important tracking of overweight from childhood to adulthood, this generation of children could well have an even higher prevalence of obesity and adverse health consequences in adulthood than do their parents. Preventing childhood obesity is thus of urgent importance.

Notes

1. A. V. Chobanian and others, "The Seventh Report of the Joint National Committee on Prevention, Detection, Evaluation, and Treatment of High Blood Pressure: The JNC 7 Report," *Journal of the American Medical Association* 289 (2003): 2560–72.

2. B. Falkner and S. R. Daniels, "Summary of the Fourth Report on the Diagnosis, Evaluation, and Treatment of High Blood Pressure in Children and Adolescents," *Hypertension* 44 (2004): 387–88.

3. B. Rosner and others, "Blood Pressure Differences between Blacks and Whites in Relation to Body Size among U.S. Children and Adolescents," *American Journal of Epidemiology* 151 (2000): 1007–19.

4. P. Muntner and others, "Trends in Blood Pressure among Children and Adolescents," *Journal of the American Medical Association* 291 (2004): 2107–13.

5. Ibid.

6. R. M. Lauer and W. R. Clarke, "Childhood Risk Factors for High Adult Blood Pressure: The Muscatine Study," *Pediatrics* 84 (1989): 633–41.

7. G. de Simone and others, "Effect of Growth on Variability of Left Ventricular Mass: Assessment of Allometric Signals in Adults and Children and Their Capacity to Predict Cardiovascular Risk," *Journal of American College of Cardiology* 25 (1995): 1056–62.

8. M. Yoshinaga and others, "Effect of Total Adipose Weight and Systemic Hypertension on Left Ventricular Mass in Children," *American Journal of Cardiology* 76 (1995): 785–87.

9. S. R. Daniels and others, "Effect of Lean Body Mass, Fat Mass, Blood Pressure, and Sexual Maturation on Left Ventricular Mass in Children and Adolescents: Statistical, Biological, and Clinical Significance," *Circulation* 92 (1995): 3249–54.

10. Systolic blood pressure is the pressure that occurs each time the heart pushes blood into the vessels; diastolic pressure is pressure that occurs when the heart rests.

11. S. R. Daniels and others, "Left Ventricular Geometry and Severe Left Ventricular Hypertrophy in Children and Adolescents with Essential Hypertension," *Circulation* 97 (1998): 1907–11.

12. H. C. McGill Jr. and others, "Effects of Nonlipid Risk Factors on Atherosclerosis in Youth with a Favorable Lipoprotein Profile," *Circulation* 103 (2001): 1546–50; G. S. Berenson and others, "Association between Multiple Cardiovascular Risk Factors and Atherosclerosis in Children and Young Adults: The Bogalusa Heart Study," *New England Journal of Medicine* 338 (1998): 1650–56.

13. Berenson and others, "Association between Multiple Cardiovascular Risk Factors and Atherosclerosis" (see note 12).

14. L. T. Mahoney and others, "Coronary Risk Factors Measured in Childhood and Young Adult Life Are Associated with Coronary Artery Calcification in Young Adults: The Muscatine Study," *Journal of the American College of Cardiology* 27 (1996): 277–84.

15. S. Klein and others, "Clinical Implications of Obesity with Specific Focus on Cardiovascular Disease: A Statement for Professionals from the American Heart Association Council on Nutrition, Physical Activity, and Metabolism," *Circulation* 110 (2004): 2952–67.

16. J. Steinberger and others, "Adiposity in Childhood Predicts Obesity and Insulin Resistance in Young Adulthood," *Journal of Pediatrics* 138 (2001): 469–73.

17. "Third Report of the National Cholesterol Education Program (NCEP) Expert Panel on Detection, Evaluation, and Treatment of High Blood Cholesterol in Adults (Adult Treatment Panel III), Final Report," *Circulation* 106 (2002): 3143–421.

18. S. M. Grundy and others, "Diagnosis and Management of the Metabolic Syndrome: An American Heart Association/National Heart, Lung, and Blood Institute Scientific Statement," *Circulation* 112 (2005): 2735–52; A. J. Hanley and others, "Metabolic and Inflammation Variable Clusters and Prediction of Type 2 Diabetes: Factor Analysis Using Directly Measured Insulin Sensitivity," *Diabetes* 53 (2004): 1773–81.

19. S. Cook and others, "Prevalence of a Metabolic Syndrome Phenotype in Adolescents: Findings from the Third National Health and Nutrition Examination Survey, 1988–1994," *Archives of Pediatric and Adolescent Medicine* 157 (2003): 821–27.

20. R. Weiss and others, "Obesity and the Metabolic Syndrome in Children and Adolescents," *New England Journal of Medicine* 350 (2004): 2362–74.

21. Berenson and others, "Association between Multiple Cardiovascular Risk Factors and Atherosclerosis" (see note 12).

22. Atherogenic dyslipidemia includes an aggregation of lipid and lipoprotein abnormalities including an elevation of triglycerides and apolipoprotein B, a reduced level of HDL-cholesterol (the good cholesterol), and increased small LDL particles (a form of the bad cholesterol that predisposes to hardening of the arteries).

23. "Third Report of the National Cholesterol Education Program" (see note 17).

24. O. Pinhas-Hamiel, "Increased Incidence of Non-Insulin-Dependent Diabetes Mellitus among Adolescents," *Journal of Pediatrics* 128 (1996): 608–15.

25. Ibid.

26. S. R. Srinivasan and others, "Adolescent Overweight Is Associated with Adult Overweight and Related Multiple Cardiovascular Risk Factors: The Bogalusa Heart Study," *Metabolism* 45 (1996): 235–40.

27. American Diabetes Association, "Type 2 Diabetes in Children and Adolescents," *Diabetes Care* 23 (2000): 381–89.

28. Ibid.

29. E. Luder, T. A. Melnik, and M. DiMaio, "Association of Being Overweight with Greater Asthma Symptoms in Inner-City Black and Hispanic Children," *Journal of Pediatrics* 132 (1998): 699–703.

30. M. A. Rodriguez and others, "Identification of Population Subgroups of Children and Adolescents with High Asthma Prevalence: Findings from the Third National Health and Nutrition Examination Survey," *Archives of Pediatric and Adolescent Medicine* 156 (2002): 269–75.

31. B. Stenius-Aarniala and others, "Immediate and Long-Term Effects of Weight Reduction in Obese People with Asthma: Randomised Controlled Study," *British Medical Journal* 320 (2000): 827–32.

32. S. K. Rhodes and others, "Neurocognitive Deficits in Morbidly Obese Children with Obstructive Sleep Apnea," *Journal of Pediatrics* 127 (1995): 741–44.

33. G. B. Mallory Jr., D. H. Fiser, and R. Jackson, "Sleep-Associated Breathing Disorders in Morbidly Obese Children and Adolescents," *Journal of Pediatrics* 115 (1989): 892–97.

34. A. Orea-Tejeda and others, "SPECT Myocardial Perfusion Imaging during Periods of Obstructive Sleep Apnea in Morbidly Obese Patients without Known Heart Disease," *Rev Invest Clin.* 55 (2003): 18–25.

35. R. S. Amin and others, "Twenty-Four-Hour Ambulatory Blood Pressure in Children with Sleep-Disordered Breathing," *American Journal of Respiratory Critical Care Medicine* 169 (2004): 950–56; R. S. Amin and others, "Left Ventricular Hypertrophy and Abnormal Ventricular Geometry in Children and Adolescents with Obstructive Sleep Apnea," *American Journal of Respiratory Critical Care Medicine* 165 (2002): 1395–99; R. S. Amin and others, "Left Ventricular Function in Children with Sleep-Disordered Breathing," *American Journal of Cardiology* 95 (2005): 801–04.

36. Amin and others, "Left Ventricular Function" (see note 35); R. D. Ross and others, "Sleep Apnea-Associated Hypertension and Reversible Left Ventricular Hypertrophy," *Journal of Pediatrics* 111 (1987): 253–55.

37. B. A. Neuschwander-Tetri and S. H. Caldwell, "Nonalcoholic Steatohepatitis: Summary of an AASLD Single Topic Conference," *Hepatology* 37 (2003): 1202–19.

38. A. Kinugasa and others, "Fatty Liver and Its Fibrous Changes Found in Simple Obesity of Children," *Journal of Pediatric Gastroenterology and Nutrition* 3 (1984): 408–14.

39. J. E. Lavine and J. B. Schwimmer, "Nonalcoholic Fatty Liver Disease in the Pediatric Population," *Clinical Liver Disease* 8 (2004): viii–ix, 549–58.

40. J. B. Schwimmer and others, "Obesity, Insulin Resistance, and Other Clinicopathological Correlates of Pediatric Nonalcoholic Fatty Liver Disease," *Journal of Pediatrics* 142 (2003): 500–05.

41. Ibid.

42. J. F. Silverman, W. J. Pories, and J. F. Caro, "Liver Pathology in Diabetes Mellitus and Morbid Obesity: Clinical, Pathological, and Biochemical Considerations," *Pathology Annual* 24, pt. 1 (1989): 275–302.

43. M. L. Frelut and others, "Uneven Occurrence of Fatty Liver in Morbidly Obese Children: Impact of Weight Loss," *International Journal of Obesity* 22 (1995): 43.

44. L. Murray and others, "Relationship between Body Mass and Gastro-Esophageal Reflux Symptoms: The Bristol Helicobacter Project," *International Journal of Epidemiology* 32 (2003): 645–50.

45. M. Nilsson and others, "Obesity and Estrogen as Risk Factors for Gastroesophageal Reflux Symptoms," *Journal of the American Medical Association* 290 (2003): 66–72.

46. V. Di Francesco and others, "Obesity and Gastro-Esophageal Acid Reflux: Physiopathological Mechanisms and Role of Gastric Bariatric Surgery," *Obesity Surgery* 14 (2004): 1095–102.

47. T. F. Kling Jr. and R. N. Hensinger, "Angular and Torsional Deformities of the Lower Limbs in Children," *Clinical Orthopaedics and Related Research* (1983): 136–47.

48. R. T. Loder and others, "Acute Slipped Capital Femoral Epiphysis: The Importance of Physeal Stability," *Journal of Bone and Joint Surgery* 75 (1993): 1134–40.

49. R. G. Wight and others, "A Multilevel Analysis of Ethnic Variation in Depressive Symptoms among Adolescents in the United States," *Social Science and Medicine* 60 (2005): 2073–84.

50. B. Brimaher, C. Arbelaez, and D. Brent, "Course and Outcome of Child and Adolescent Major Depressive Disorder," *Journal of the American Academy of Child and Adolescent Psychiatry* 11 (2002): x, 619–37.

51. E. Stice and others, "Body Image and Eating Disturbances Predict Onset of Depression among Female Adolescents: A Longitudinal Study," *Journal of Abnormal Psychology* 109 (2000): 438–44.

52. J. Siegel, "Body Image Change and Adolescent Depressive Symptoms," *Journal of Adolescent Research* 17 (2002): 27–41.

53. B. Britz and others, "Rates of Psychiatric Disorders in a Clinical Study Group of Adolescents with Extreme Obesity and in Obese Adolescents Ascertained via a Population-Based Study," *International Journal of Obesity and Related Metabolic Disorders* 24 (2000): 1707–14; S. Erermis and others, "Is Obesity a Risk Factor for Psychopathology among Adolescents?" *Pediatrics International* 46 (2004): 296–301.

54. Ibid.

55. D. S. Pine and others, "The Association between Childhood Depression and Adulthood Body Mass Index," *Pediatrics* 107 (2001): 1049–56.

56. E. Goodman and R. C. Whitaker, "A Prospective Study of the Role of Depression in the Development and Persistence of Adolescent Obesity," *Pediatrics* 110 (2002): 497–504.

57. S. J. Erickson and others, "Are Overweight Children Unhappy? Body Mass Index, Depressive Symptoms, and Overweight Concerns in Elementary School Children," *Archives of Pediatrics and Adolescent Medicine* 154 (2000): 931–35.

58. M. E. Eisenberg, D. Neumark-Sztainer, and M. Story, "Associations of Weight-Based Teasing and Emotional Well-Being among Adolescents," *Archives of Pediatrics and Adolescent Medicine* 157 (2003): 733–38.

59. R. S. Strauss and H. A. Pollack, "Social Marginalization of Overweight Children," *Archives of Pediatrics and Adolescent Medicine* 157 (2003): 746–52.

60. R. G. Phillips and J. J. Hill, "Fat, Plain, but Not Friendless: Self-Esteem and Peer Acceptance of Obese Preadolescent Girls," *International Journal of Obesity and Related Metabolic Disorders* 22 (1998): 287–93.

61. J. S. Schwimmer, T. M. Burwinkle, and J. W. Varni, "Health-Related Quality of Life of Severely Obese Children and Adolescents," *Journal of the American Medical Association* 289 (2003): 1813–19.

62. "Revised 2003 Consensus on Diagnostic Criteria and Long-Term Health Risks Related to Polycystic Ovary Syndrome," *Fertility and Sterility* 81 (2004): 19–25.

63. D. A. Ehrmann and others, "Prevalence of Impaired Glucose Tolerance and Diabetes in Women with Polycystic Ovary Syndrome," *Diabetes Care* 22 (1999): 141–46.

64. M. Asuncion and others, "A Prospective Study of the Prevalence of the Polycystic Ovary Syndrome in Unselected Caucasian Women from Spain," *Journal of Clinical Endocrinology and Metabolism* 85 (2000): 2434–38.

65. C. J. Glueck and others, "Incidence and Treatment of Metabolic Syndrome in Newly Referred Women with Confirmed Polycystic Ovarian Syndrome," *Metabolism* 52 (2003): 908–15.

66. R. Azziz and others, "Troglitazone Improves Ovulation and Hirsutism in the Polycystic Ovary Syndrome: A Multicenter, Double Blind, Placebo-Controlled Trial," *Journal of Clinical Endocrinology and Metabolism* 86 (2001): 1626–32.

67. D. A. Ehrmann, "Polycystic Ovary Syndrome," *New England Journal of Medicine* 352 (2005): 1223–36.

68. S. D. Silberstein and J. Marcelis, "Headache Associated with Changes in Intracranial Pressure," *Headache* 32 (1992): 84–94.

69. R. Sturm, "The Effects of Obesity, Smoking, and Drinking on Medical Problems and Costs: Obesity Outranks Both Smoking and Drinking in Its Deleterious Effects on Health and Health Costs," *Health Affairs (Millwood)* 21 (2002): 245–53.

70. A. M. Wolf and G. A. Colditz, "Current Estimates of the Economic Cost of Obesity in the United States," *Obesity Research* 6 (1998): 97–106.

71. E. A. Finkelstein, I. C. Fiebelkorn, and G. Wang, "National Medical Spending Attributable to Overweight and Obesity: How Much, and Who's Paying?" *Health Affairs (Millwood)* Suppl. Web Exclusive (2003): W3-219-26. (http://content.healthaffairs.org/cgi/content/full/hlthaff.w3.219v1/DC1 [December 8, 2005]).

72. K. E. Warner, T. A. Hodgson, and C. E. Carroll, "Medical Costs of Smoking in the United States: Estimates, Their Validity, and Their Implications," *Tobacco Control* 8 (1999): 290–300.

73. G. Wang and W. H. Dietz, "Economic Burden of Obesity in Youths Aged 6 to 17 Years: 1979–1999," *Pediatrics* 109 (2002): e81.

74. A. M. Tershakovec and others, "Insurance Reimbursement for the Treatment of Obesity in Children," *Journal of Pediatrics* 134 (1999): 573–78.

75. J. R. Staffieri, "A Study of Social Stereotype of Body Image in Children," *Journal of Personality and Social Psychology* 7 (1967): 101–04.

76. J. A. Brylinsky and J. C. Moore, "The Identification of Body Build Stereotype in Young Children," *Journal of Research in Personality* 8 (1994): 170–181; N. H. Falkner and others, "Social, Educational, and Psychological Correlates of Weight Status in Adolescents," *Obesity Research* 9 (2001): 32–42.

77. S. L. Gortmaker and others, "Social and Economic Consequences of Overweight in Adolescence and Young Adulthood," *New England Journal of Medicine* 329 (1993): 1008–12.

78. H. Canning and J. Mayer, "Obesity: Its Possible Effect on College Acceptance," *New England Journal of Medicine* 275 (1966): 1172–74.

79. L. Karris, "Prejudice against Obese Renters," *Journal of Social Psychology* 101 (1977): 159–60.

80. "Obesity: Preventing and Managing the Global Epidemic—Report of a WHO Consultation," *World Health Organization Technical Report Series* 894 (2000): 1–253.

81. K. Narbro and others, "Economic Consequences of Sick Leave and Early Retirement in Obese Swedish Women," *International Journal of Obesity and Related Metabolic Disorders* 20 (1996): 895–903.

82. S. S. Guo and others, "Predicting Overweight and Obesity in Adulthood from Body Mass Index Values in Childhood and Adolescence," *American Journal of Clinical Nutrition* 76 (2002): 653–58.

83. Robert C. Whitaker and others, "Predicting Obesity in Young Adulthood from Childhood and Parental Obesity," *New England Journal of Medicine* 337 (1997): 869–73.

84. Metropolitan Life Insurance Company, "New Weight Standards for Men and Women" *Statistical Bulletin* 40 (1959): 1–4. The Metropolitan Life Insurance Company tables also take height into account.

85. H. B. Hubert and others, "Obesity as an Independent Risk Factor for Cardiovascular Disease: A 26-Year Follow-up of Participants in the Framingham Heart Study," *Circulation* 67 (1983): 968–77; R. H. Eckel and R. M. Krauss, "American Heart Association Call to Action: Obesity as a Major Risk Factor for Coronary Heart Disease—AHA Nutrition Committee," *Circulation* 97 (1998): 2099–100.

86. J. E. Manson and others, "A Prospective Study of Obesity and Risk of Coronary Heart Disease in Women," *New England Journal of Medicine* 322 (1990): 882–89.

87. R. P. Donahue and R. D. Abbott, "Central Obesity and Coronary Heart Disease in Men," *Lancet* 2 (1987): 1215.

88. W. B. Kannel, "Metabolic Risk Factors for Coronary Heart Disease in Women: Perspective from the Framingham Study," *American Heart Journal* 114 (1987): 413–19.

89. M. A. Berns, J. H. de Vries, and M. B. Katan, "Increase in Body Fatness as a Major Determinant of Changes in Serum Total Cholesterol and High-Density Lipoprotein Cholesterol in Young Men over a 10-Year Period," *American Journal of Epidemiology* 130 (1989): 1109–22.

90. B. N. Chiang, L. V. Perlman, and F. H. Epstein, "Overweight and Hypertension: A Review," *Circulation* 39 (1969): 403–21.

91. A. A. Hedley and others, "Prevalence of Overweight and Obesity among U.S. Children, Adolescents, and Adults, 1999–2002," *Journal of the American Medical Association* 291 (2004): 2847–50.

92. A. H. Mokdad and others, "Actual Causes of Death in the United States, 2000," *Journal of the American Medical Association* 291 (2004): 1238–45.

93. A. H. Mokdad, "Correction: Actual Causes of Death in the United States, 2000," *Journal of the American Medical Association* 293 (2005): 293–94.

94. K. M. Flegal and others, "Excess Deaths Associated with Underweight, Overweight, and Obesity," *Journal of the American Medical Association* 293 (2005): 1861–67.

95. S. J. Olshansky and others, "A Potential Decline in Life Expectancy in the United States in the 21st Century," *New England Journal of Medicine* 352 (2005): 1135–37.

96. S. H. Preston, "Deadweight? The Influence of Obesity on Longevity," *New England Journal of Medicine* 352 (2005): 1135-37.

Markets and Childhood Obesity Policy

John Cawley

Summary

In examining the childhood obesity epidemic from the perspective of economics, John Cawley looks at both possible causes and possible policy solutions that work through markets. The operation of markets, says Cawley, has contributed to the recent increase in childhood overweight in three main ways. First, the real price of food fell. In particular, energy-dense foods, such as those containing fats and sugars, became relatively cheaper than less energy-dense foods, such as fresh fruits and vegetables. Second, rising wages increased the "opportunity costs" of food preparation for college graduates, encouraging them to spend less time preparing meals. Third, technological changes created incentives to use prepackaged food rather than to prepare foods.

Several economic rationales justify government intervention in markets to address these problems. First, because free markets generally under-provide information, the government may intervene to provide consumers with nutrition information they need. Second, because society bears the soaring costs of obesity, the government may intervene to lower the costs to taxpayers. Third, because children are not what economists call "rational consumers"—they cannot evaluate information critically and weigh the future consequences of their actions—the government may step in to help them make better choices.

The government can easily disseminate information to consumers directly, but formulating policies to address the other two rationales is more difficult. In the absence of ideal policies to combat obesity, the government must turn to "second-best" policies. For example, it could protect children from advertisements for "junk food." It could implement taxes and subsidies that discourage the consumption of unhealthful foods or encourage physical activity. It could require schools to remove vending machines for soda and candy.

From the economic perspective, policymakers should evaluate these options on the basis of cost-effectiveness studies. Researchers, however, have as yet undertaken few such studies of obesity-related policy options. Such analyses, once available, will help policymakers achieve the greatest benefit from a fixed budget.

www.futureofchildren.org

John Cawley is an associate professor of policy analysis and management at Cornell University. The author thanks Elizabeth Donahue, J. A. Grisso, Barrett Kirwan, Philip Levine, Laura Leviton, Alan Mathios, Tracy Orleans, Christina Paxson, the Robert Wood Johnson Foundation working group on childhood obesity, and participants at the Future of Children conference on Childhood Obesity for their helpful comments and suggestions.

ince the early 1970s, the prevalence of overweight has more than doubled among children aged two to five, almost quadrupled for children aged six to eleven, and more than doubled among adolescents aged twelve to nineteen.[1] During 1999–2000, the prevalence of overweight was 11.6 percent among toddlers aged six months to twenty-three months, 10.4 percent among children aged two to five years, 15.3 percent among children aged six to eleven, and 15.5 percent among adolescents. The health risks associated with childhood obesity, including asthma, hypertension, type 2 diabetes, cardiovascular disease, and depression, have led medical authorities to declare the rise in childhood obesity a public health crisis.[2]

The epidemic of childhood obesity has many causes—cultural, economic, and genetic.[3] In this article, I focus on the causes and possible policy solutions that work through markets. I use economics to weigh and assess the evidence.[4]

How Markets May Have Contributed to the Rise in Childhood Overweight

Several strands of research investigate how markets may contribute to increased calorie consumption, sedentary lifestyles, or overweight and how changes in those markets may have contributed to the recent rise in childhood overweight. The problem for researchers is not figuring out what could have caused the rise in childhood obesity; the problem is that too many things could have caused it. James Hill and several colleagues calculate that the rise in obesity in the United States could have been caused by a daily surplus of just 15 calories for the median person, with 90 percent of the population increasing their intake by 50 or fewer calories a day.[5] To put this in perspective, the rise in weight for the median person could have been caused by consuming an extra three tablespoons of skim milk or walking 120 fewer yards each day. It will likely be impossible to determine which changes are responsible for such a small increase in daily calorie surplus, but I will consider several possible contributors.

Changes in the Cost of Food and Food Preparation

The most obvious contributor to the increasing calorie surplus is falling food prices. Between January 1980 and January 2005, the real price of food fell 13 percent.[6] One study attributes 40 percent of the recent rise in weight to lower food prices.[7]

Changes in the "opportunity cost" of time spent cooking may also have affected eating patterns. Strictly speaking, the opportunity cost of a person's time is the value of that time devoted to the next best available alternative, but in practice it is often measured by the wage rate. All else being equal, if someone's wage rate rises, he or she will likely spend less time cooking and will instead use prepackaged foods that require less preparation time or will eat food prepared by others, such as restaurant meals or "takeout." It is also possible that he or she would simply consume less food as a result of spending less time cooking.

How much wages have changed over the past twenty-five to thirty years varies by the wage earners' educational attainment. Real wages for high school dropouts have fallen, those for high school graduates have remained roughly constant, and those for college graduates have risen considerably.[8] These wage dynamics imply that the time cost of cooking rose for college graduates and fell for high school dropouts. To my knowledge, data on time spent cooking have not been sorted by education, but for the U.S. population as a whole, the number of minutes spent each day preparing meals fell from forty-four in 1965 to thirty-two in 1999.[9]

While changing wage rates affected the opportunity cost of time spent cooking, technological change may have reduced the time required to prepare some foods. David Cutler, Edward Glaeser, and Jesse Shapiro argue that innovations in food processing, preservation, and packaging made it possible for food to be mass prepared far from the place of consumption and to be consumed with less time cost. These innovations contributed to a shift away from home-cooked meals toward processed food, thus increasing obesity. In support of their argument, the researchers show that consumption of mass-produced foods increased the most, that people most able to take advantage of these technological changes had the greatest increases in weight, and that obesity is greatest in countries where people have the greatest access to processed food.[10]

Changes in the share of women who work also affected time spent cooking. Over the past three decades, the labor force participation rate of women with children younger than age eighteen rose from 47 to 72 percent, with the largest increase among mothers with children younger than age three.[11] The increased work time may have resulted in the increased use of prepackaged foods or of food consumed away from home. One study calculates that during the past three decades the increase in mothers' average weekly hours at work explains 12 to 35 percent of the increase in childhood obesity in families of high socioeconomic status.[12]

During this same period Congress reformed the nation's welfare system, in the process giving poor single mothers an economic incentive to spend less time cooking. With some exceptions, the 1996 welfare reform law required single mothers to work in the labor force to receive cash welfare benefits.[13] Thus even though falling real wages lowered the opportunity cost of cooking for high school dropouts, poor single mothers had

For the U.S. population as a whole, the number of minutes spent each day preparing meals fell from forty-four in 1965 to thirty-two in 1999.

good reason to spend more time in the labor force and less time in household production.

To better establish the link among changing costs of time, time spent cooking, eating out, and childhood obesity, researchers must answer several questions. First, they must find out how different groups of people responded to the changing costs of time. For example, do college graduates and welfare-eligible women spend less time cooking and high school dropouts spend more time cooking? Second, they must determine whether changes in cooking time led college graduates and welfare-eligible women to use more prepackaged foods or restaurant food and led high school dropouts to use less. And, third, they must prove the link between the consumption of prepackaged and restaurant foods and childhood obesity.

Another possible contributor to obesity is the price of energy-dense foods, such as those containing fats and sugars, relative to that of less energy-dense foods, such as fresh fruits and vegetables. Adam Drewnowski and S. E. Specter calculate that, on a per-calorie basis, energy-dense foods are cheap whereas foods low in energy density are much more expensive.[14] However, a Department of Agriculture (USDA) study suggests that less energy-dense foods can still be quite cheap in

Between 1977 and 1995, the share of total calories consumed away from home rose from 18 to 34 percent, the share of meals consumed away from home rose from 16 to 29 percent, and the total share of food dollars spent away from home rose from 26 to 39 percent.

absolute terms; it calculates that a person can satisfy the USDA's recommendation of three daily servings of fruit and four servings of vegetables for just 64 cents a day. The study also concludes that 63 percent of fruits and 57 percent of vegetables were cheapest in their fresh form.[15]

Further research must determine whether the relative price of energy-dense foods has fallen in the past several decades. A quick comparison of the various consumer price indexes indicates that between January 1989 and January 2005, the real price of fruits and vegetables rose 74.6 percent while that of fats and oils fell 26.5 percent and that of sugars and sweets fell 33.1 percent. Thus energy-

dense foods have become considerably cheaper, relative to less energy-dense foods, in the past fifteen years.[16]

Changes in Where Americans Eat Their Meals

Perhaps because of the increasing opportunity cost of time for college graduates or the movement of women into the labor force, Americans are eating more meals away from home today than they did thirty years ago. Between 1977 and 1995, the share of total calories consumed away from home rose from 18 to 34 percent, the share of meals consumed away from home rose from 16 to 29 percent, and the total share of food dollars spent away from home rose from 26 to 39 percent.[17] From 1994 through 1996, children consumed 32 percent of all their calories away from home: 10 percent in fast-food restaurants, 9 percent in schools, 4 percent in restaurants, and 9 percent from all other sources, such as vending machines and other people's houses.[18]

The move toward food away from home came just as this food itself (not the time costs of preparing it) was becoming more expensive relative to food at home. Between January 1980 and January 2005, the real price of food at home fell 16.2 percent while the real price of food away from home fell only 5.1 percent.[19] Eating out became more common even as it was becoming relatively more expensive.

The distinction between food at home and food away from home is important because consumers typically have less information about the calorie content of foods they eat away from home. Relative to food at home, food away from home has on average lower fiber and calcium density, similar sodium density, and higher cholesterol density.[20] Nutritional trends both for food at home and for food away from home are promising: in both, the densities of fat, saturated fat, and cholesterol have declined, and the density of fiber has increased slightly, though away-from-home foods have improved less than food at home.[21] Further research must explore whether the move toward consuming more food away from home and eating less at home has caused an increase in childhood obesity.

Changes in Portion Sizes

Portion sizes of certain foods have increased since the 1970s. One study of portion sizes looks at package labels and manufacturers' information and concludes that the portion sizes of "virtually all" the packaged foods and beverages it examines have increased during the past three decades.[22] Such a finding is important because several experiments have documented that when people are served larger portions, they consume more calories.[23] The portion size effect is first detectable in children five years old.[24]

The increase in portion sizes, combined with people's tendency to eat more when served larger portions, implies that the amount of food consumed at one sitting has increased. Smiciklas-Wright and her colleagues use the Continuing Survey of Food Intakes by Individuals to study the quantities consumed at one sitting and find significant increases for about a third of the 107 foods they examine. The study does not specify whether these items were ones packed in larger portions by manufacturers. They find significant decreases in amounts consumed for six other foods.[25]

One limit of the research on portion sizes and calorie intake is that the increases in portion sizes in experiments do not match the increased portion sizes in the market. For example, some studies experimentally increased portions of macaroni and cheese, but

the Smiciklas-Wright team found that the portions of macaroni and cheese that people reported consuming fell 17 percent between 1989–91 and 1994–96.

Whether people eat more when they are notified of the increase in portion size is unclear. In the market, some food manufacturers take pains to emphasize the increased size of their products—for example, the Big Gulp, Monster Thickburger, and "supersized" meals. Moreover, the increases in calorie consumption documented in these experiments (30 to 50 percent) are far larger than the small increase in daily calorie surplus that caused the rise in obesity. Because these experiments typically last no longer than a few meals or days, it is also unclear whether in the longer run people adapt to the larger portion sizes and return to consuming their normal amount. For example, suppose every day were Thanksgiving. You might eat large portions the first day, but you probably would not continue to eat "Thanksgiving-sized" meals every day. At some point you might return to your previous level of caloric consumption. Longer-term research is needed to determine the long-run effect of portion size, as well as what the effect is when consumers are notified of the larger portions.

Changes in Farm Policies

Agriculture policy may contribute to obesity by promoting lower prices and greater production of certain commodities. From 1933 to 1995, price supports kept the prices of wheat, corn, soybeans, oats, and other commodities above their free-market prices in the United States; the government purchased excess supplies to bolster prices. The 1995 Farm Bill, however, reformed the system. Rather than subsidizing farmers by keeping prices artificially high, the government now gives farmers a production subsidy, or a payment based on their historic production. In other words, the new law completely decoupled subsidies to farmers from production, and consumers switched from paying above-market to below-market prices for agricultural commodities.[26]

Trade policies still keep some commodities' prices high. A system of quotas and tariffs, for example, keeps the U.S. price of sugar above the world price.[27] Agriculture policy has lowered the prices of other sweeteners,

---

A system of quotas and tariffs keeps the U.S. price of sugar above the world price, while agriculture policy has lowered the prices of other sweeteners.

---

however. In particular, farm policy has been criticized for subsidizing the production of corn and, thereby, of high-fructose corn syrup, which is now common in soft drinks, fruit juices, jelly, and other foods.[28]

The USDA estimates that production subsidies increased the land under cultivation by 4 million acres and lowered the price of wheat by seven cents a bushel, of corn by nine cents a bushel, and of soybeans by forty-nine cents a bushel.[29] A second study figures that direct payments to farmers boost agricultural output 4.39 percent.[30] And a third calculates that policy changes in the 1995 Farm Bill and thereafter increased production of grains and soybeans 4 percent and lowered prices 5 to 8 percent.[31] Of course, consumers do not buy and consume bushels of wheat and soybeans directly; instead, they eat food manufactured from these crops. One study estimates that for every 1 percent decrease in commodity prices, food prices decline 0.25 percent.[32] Another study determines that agricultural subsidies explain about 1 percent of the increase in obesity over the past two decades.[33]

When price supports were still a mainstay of U.S. farm policy, Washington established "checkoff" programs to increase demand for covered commodities, thereby lessening the excess supply that it was obliged to purchase. The checkoff programs required producers to contribute a fixed amount per commodity unit sold to a nonprofit organization that used the money to increase consumer demand for that commodity by researching new uses for it and advertising those uses to consumers. Commodity checkoff programs, which have persisted even after price supports were removed, now spend $1 billion a year to increase demand for their products.[34]

Substantial checkoff resources go for advertising, and they have a considerable impact. Checkoff-funded advertising campaigns include "Ahh, the Power of Cheese," "Beef—It's What's for Dinner," "Pork—the Other White Meat," and "Got Milk?" Noel Blisard estimates that the generic advertising of milk totaled $29.8 million between October 1995 and September 1996, raising milk sales by 1.4 billion pounds, or 5.9 percent, while generic advertising of cheese funded by checkoff programs increased sales of cheese by 62.7 million pounds, or 2.8 percent.[35] Although advertising funded by checkoff dollars increases consumer demand, collecting checkoff funds from producers is a form of tax, which raises producers' costs and lowers the quantities sold. On net, however, the checkoff programs increase commodities' sales.[36]

Whether checkoff-funded advertising encourages consumers to spend more money overall on food or simply redirects their fixed food budget to the advertised products is unclear. Brenda Boetel and Donald Liu find that beef and pork advertising is "beggar thy neighbor" in the sense that beef advertising decreases the demand for pork and vice versa. They conclude that beef and pork producers would be better off if they agreed to reduce their generic checkoff-funded advertising campaigns.[37] Checkoff funds are also used to increase commodities' sales by developing new menu items for fast-food restaurants, such as the McRib pork sandwich for McDonald's and Insider Pizza (which used one pound of cheese per medium pizza) for Pizza Hut.[38]

Although analysts have linked various farm policies to the increased sales of certain crops and to the development of menu items for fast-food restaurants, documenting the effect these programs have on obesity itself requires more research.

Increased Food Advertising to Children

The food industry spent $7 billion on advertising in 1997, more than any other industry except automobiles. Two-thirds of that advertising was by food manufacturers, 28 percent by the food service industry (mostly fast-food restaurants), and 8 percent by food stores.[39] It is estimated that the number of television commercials viewed each year by the average American child doubled from about 20,000 in 1970 to 40,000 around the year 2000.[40] But although children are viewing more commercials, the length of the average commercial has fallen.[41] In addition, Roland Sturm finds that the average time children spent watching TV fell 23 percent, or four hours a week, between 1981 and 1997.[42]

One study, which analyzes the food advertisements aired during children's Saturday morning television programming, concludes that if a child consumed only the advertised food,

his diet would not be consistent with U.S. dietary recommendations.[43] Gerard Hastings and several colleagues conclude that over time advertisements for fruits and vegetables have disappeared and have been replaced by ads for fast-food restaurants, breakfast cereals, soft drinks, and snacks.[44]

Two broad reviews of the experimental research on food advertising and youth diets conclude that there is very mixed evidence on whether television advertising causally affects children's diets.[45]

Because of several limitations of this research, including the use of small, nonrepresentative samples, making it difficult to draw inferences about larger populations from their findings, the American Academy of Pediatrics and the Institute of Medicine have called for more research on whether food advertising affects the diets of American youth.[46]

Differences in Local Availability of Food and Exercise Opportunities

The prevalence of childhood obesity shows clear racial disparities. In 1998, 21.5 percent of African American children and 21.8 percent of Hispanic children but only 12.3 percent of white children were overweight.[47]

Whether there are also economic disparities in the prevalence of childhood obesity within race and ethnic groups is less clear. R. P. Troiano and K. M. Flegal find no significant correlation between income and childhood obesity for African Americans or Hispanics. They find weak evidence that higher-income white adolescents are less likely to be obese, but they warn this evidence must be interpreted cautiously because of small sample sizes.[48]

Some researchers have argued that racial and socioeconomic disparities in weight may be due in part to differences in the availability of food and exercise opportunities. One study finds that supermarkets are three times more common in census tracts with home values in the highest quintile than in tracts with homes in the lowest quintile and four times more common in predominantly white than in predominantly black neighborhoods.[49] Conversely, smaller grocery stores and convenience stores without gas stations are more common in lower-wealth and predominantly black neighborhoods. Another study finds that the probability of at least one supermarket located in an urban zip code is higher where income is high and the poverty rate is low. But it finds no link between that probability and the share of residents who had graduated from high school.[50]

Some researchers argue that these disparities are related to obesity because the proximity of such businesses is correlated with diet quality. Kimberly Morland, Steve Wing, and Ana Roux compare food consumption reported in questionnaires to food outlet availability in the census tract of residence and find that blacks living in census tracts with supermarkets are more likely to meet U.S. Dietary Guidelines for fruits and vegetables, total fat, and saturated fat. Findings for whites were generally not statistically significant.[51]

Joel Waldfogel finds that the population's educational and racial composition is correlated with restaurant density. Controlling for population size within a zip code (which may itself be correlated with both restaurant density and the educational and racial composition in an area), when the share of blacks and Hispanics is higher, there are fewer sit-down restaurants but more of certain fast-food restaurants.[52]

Analysts find similar patterns for active recreational facilities, such as public beaches, pools, youth centers, parks, YMCAs and YWCAs, dance studios, and athletic clubs. Penny Gordon-Larsen and several colleagues find that all major categories of such facilities are inequitably distributed across census block groups by socioeconomic status, minority population, and education. They find that the presence of just one such facility per census block group is associated with a 5 percent lower probability of overweight.[53]

These studies are observational, not based on randomized experiments, and thus include an unknown degree of what researchers term "selection bias." Supermarkets and health clubs may open outlets in places where people are most interested in them—where they can earn the highest profits—and not in areas with low demand. Likewise, when people choose where to live, they may consider the retail options available nearby. People who cook meals from scratch may find it more attractive to live near a full-service supermarket, and exercise buffs may want to live near parks and gyms. Because of such self-selection, correlations between diet and supermarket proximity and between physical activity and proximity to athletic facilities may arise even without a causal relationship. For this reason, these research findings cannot be interpreted as causal or evidence of discrimination.

A related research area claims that new suburbs and developments contribute to obesity because they lack sidewalks and places to which people could walk or because they require long commutes.[54] But children's physical activity appears uncorrelated with such neighborhood characteristics as the availability of local facilities and safety.[55]

Decreased Smoking

Over the same period that the prevalence of obesity has been on the rise, the prevalence of adult smoking has fallen—from 33.2 percent in 1980 to 21.6 percent in 2003.[56] The share of high school students who smoke has also declined, from 27.5 percent in 1991 to 21.9 percent in 2003.[57] The trends in smoking and obesity may be related. A surgeon general's report reviewed fifteen medical studies and found that between 58 percent and 87 percent of those who quit smoking gained, on average, four pounds.[58] One study finds adults' weight is positively correlated with the local price of cigarettes (the higher the price, the higher the weight); the correlation with weight is roughly the same as that of grocery prices. The study finds no correlation of weight with clean indoor air laws that restrict smoking.[59] A second study, however, faults the first for not taking into account time trends in smoking and for focusing on cigarette prices instead of cigarette taxes; after making the necessary corrections, that study finds that higher cigarette taxes are associated with *lower* weight.[60]

Economic Rationales for Market Intervention

If the government is to intervene in a market to reduce obesity, it should have an economic rationale to do so. Several such rationales exist. First, in free markets producers generally under-provide information. Governments can easily disseminate this information to help consumers make informed choices. The Nutrition Labeling and Education Act (NLEA) of 1990 requires producers to print nutrition labels on packaged foods, but no law requires the release of nutritional information for restaurant food or fountain drinks.

The second economic rationale for government intervention is that the costs of obesity are borne broadly by society. A 2003 study estimates that through Medicare and Medicaid, the government's medical care programs for the elderly and the indigent, taxpayers pay half the total costs of treating obesity-related illnesses—costs that in 1998 amounted to $92.6 billion (in 2002 dollars).[61] The government may seek to reduce obesity to lower these costs to taxpayers.

The third economic rationale for intervention, which applies specifically to childhood obesity, is that children are not what econo-

Over the same period that the prevalence of obesity has been on the rise, the prevalence of adult smoking has fallen—from 33.2 percent in 1980 to 21.6 percent in 2003.

mists call "rational consumers." They cannot evaluate information critically and weigh the future consequences of their actions. For much the same reason that the government bans sales of cigarettes and alcohol to minors—to protect them from making poor decisions that adversely affect their health—it may likewise seek to regulate sales of certain foods to youth.

How to Choose among the Policy Options

Given the three different economic rationales for government intervention, what policies are most appropriate? From an economic perspective, the primary goal is to repair the problem in the market. For example, the government can directly address the lack of information by requiring companies to provide it. One simple way to improve the food markets' efficiency is to expand the

NLEA to require that detailed nutritional information accompany all foods and menus. Adult consumers, at least, appear to respond to such information. One study finds that a media campaign urging people to shift from whole-fat to low-fat milk changed consumer purchases.[62] Another study documents a consumer shift from high-fat toward low-fat salad dressing after product labels were required to reveal fat content.[63] Another finds that the NLEA decreased weight gain for white females who read labels while shopping and estimates that the NLEA's benefits totaled $101 billion a year.[64]

It is not clear, however, how to present nutrition and calorie information so that consumers, especially children and adolescents, can use and understand it. Further research is needed on how to make nutritional information comprehensible to children.

When the government makes information available, it must be careful to put it in a proper context; failure to do so can lead to unfortunate unintended consequences. For example, in 2003, in an effort to inform parents, Arkansas passed a law requiring schools to weigh children and to notify parents of their child's body mass index. Although the law provides parents with information they may have lacked, it has had some unforeseen negative consequences. Some muscular children have been incorrectly classified as overweight, and concerns have arisen about privacy and self-esteem.[65] Failing to put the information into its proper context also raises a risk that parents may impose ineffective or harmful fad diets.

Although the government can correct the problem of incomplete information in a relatively straightforward manner, it cannot so easily fix the other two problems—societal costs of obesity and irrational consumers. The typical economic response to societal costs is to tax whatever imposes the cost or to subsidize behaviors that could decrease the societal costs. In this context, that would imply taxing obesity and subsidizing weight loss for the obese, but taxing people based on their weight or changes in weight would be difficult to implement and is politically unattractive. Subsidizing consumers who lose weight or maintain a healthy body weight would be similarly difficult to implement.

It is also hard to imagine how the government could implement a policy to enable children to become entirely rational consumers who take into account the future consequences of their actions. In the absence of an ideal policy to reduce societal costs and address children's "irrational" behavior, the question becomes whether other, "second-best" policies could both decrease obesity and do more good than harm for society overall.

Many possible second-best interventions exist. From the economic perspective, the correct way to choose among them is to analyze their cost-effectiveness. The first step in such analysis is to estimate all the costs and benefits associated with each intervention; the second is to rank the interventions according to how cheaply they achieve the policy goal, thus allowing policymakers to use a fixed budget most efficiently—to get, in other words, the most bang for the buck. Few anti-obesity interventions, however, especially those targeted to youth, have as yet been subjected to cost-effectiveness analysis. Nevertheless, I describe several possible second-best interventions.

Protecting Children from Advertising
If the government decides to protect children from advertising, one particular venue for in-

tervention is the public school system, where the government is solely responsible for the advertising environment. Under budgetary pressure, some school districts have signed contracts with Channel One, which gives them televisions, educational materials, and cash in exchange for allowing Channel One to advertise products such as candy, food, and soda pop directly to children in the classroom for two minutes each day.[66] The risk is that children who are a captive audience for such food advertising may increase both their consumption of the advertised foods and their risk of obesity. A cost-benefit analysis can determine whether the benefits of working with Channel One exceed the costs.

Some observers have advocated banning all food advertising to children in all venues.[67] Many developed countries, including Canada, Great Britain, and Australia, have banned all television advertising to children.[68] In the United States, however, Congress has historically tolerated little regulation of commercial speech. For example, the United States is one of only two industrialized countries (the other is New Zealand) to permit direct-to-consumer advertising of pharmaceuticals.[69] In 1979, the Federal Trade Commission (FTC) sought to regulate the television advertising of sugary cereals to children because of concerns about tooth decay. Congress, however, chose to recognize broad latitude for commercial speech and blocked the FTC from pursuing the case.[70]

The U.S. government has shielded children from advertising in some cases. The 1992 Telephone Disclosure and Dispute Resolution Act, for example, bans advertising of 1-900 phone numbers to children younger than age twelve and requires that advertising directed to children younger than age eighteen include the warning that children need their parents' permission to use the service. And in the mid-1990s the Food and Drug Administration adopted rules against advertising cigarettes near schools or in campaigns targeted to children.

Using Taxes and Subsidies to Change Behaviors That Cause Obesity

As noted, taxing or subsidizing people based on their weight or changes in weight would

---

It is also hard to imagine how the government could implement a policy to enable children to become entirely rational consumers who take into account the future consequences of their actions.

---

be politically unattractive and difficult to implement. However, some second-best tax and subsidy policies to alter behaviors may be feasible. For example, policymakers could implement taxes and subsidies that either discourage the consumption of certain foods or encourage physical activity. To evaluate whether such policies are worthwhile, policymakers must weigh their costs and benefits.

One could, for example, tax certain foods. Even though consuming food per se does not impose costs on society, a food tax might sufficiently decrease consumption that obesity would fall, cutting the costs imposed on society. Such taxes have been shown to affect food choices. A series of recent experiments confirms that even schoolchildren's purchases are sensitive to changes in the relative prices of foods.[71]

But taxing food involves several problems. The first is that although proponents often call for a "junk food" tax, it is not obvious which foods most contribute to obesity.[72] Any food, if consumed in sufficient quantity, can contribute to calorie surplus and weight gain. Second, food taxes would be regressive, falling more heavily on poor families who spend a larger share of their income on food than do wealthier families.

The other major option is to subsidize behavior that decreases obesity-related societal costs. In essence, local governments already do that when they subsidize public parks, pools, and athletic facilities and when they provide free physical education, nutrition education, and sports teams in public schools. Government subsidies for installing sidewalks or for full-service supermarkets that stock fresh fruits and vegetables to operate in low-income or minority neighborhoods are other possible interventions.

Before governments increase funding for these programs, though, they should subject them to cost-benefit analyses. So far, subsidies for youth physical activity appear to have little effect. Children's physical activity, for example, appears uncorrelated with the availability of local facilities or with neighborhood safety. Increased physical education requirements are associated with small changes in physical activity but have no detectable impact on weight or the probability of overweight.[73]

Regulating Food Markets in Schools

Again, a special venue for intervention is the public school, where the government is responsible for the food environment. For example, states could require all schools to remove vending machines for soda and candy. Because children are not generally capable of choosing foods to achieve energy balance, energy-dense foods such as sodas and candy may be the most likely to lead to energy imbalance and subsequent obesity (although, as noted, any food can cause obesity if consumed in sufficient quantity.) Schools could reconfigure meals to consist of low energy-dense foods that facilitate energy balance and serve portions that take into account the portion size effect observed in the research literature. A potential cost of removing vending machines and no longer selling energy-dense foods, however, is that schools may lose considerable revenue from "pouring rights" contracts with soft drink manufacturers and from cafeteria sales, revenue that may be used to advance the educational mission of the school.[74]

A 2005 Government Accountability Office report found that many schools generate considerable revenue by selling foods outside of their school lunch programs. The report estimates that about 30 percent of all high schools generated more than $125,000 per school through such sales, and that 30 percent of all elementary schools generated more than $5,000 per school. The study found that schools typically use these revenues to offset losses associated with their other food service programs and to fund student activities. Cost-benefit analyses should take into account the impact of any decrease in these revenues that would result from a ban on energy-dense foods.[75]

Mending or Ending Programs That May Inadvertently Contribute to Obesity

Government intervention could also take the form of modifying or canceling programs that contribute to obesity. For example, cost-benefit analyses could assess the net benefit of agricultural production subsidies and price supports. These programs clearly benefit farmers, and while some observers argue that uninsurable crop risks and weather uncertainty justify this agriculture policy, others counter that current policy is designed primarily to transfer wealth to farmers and processors.[76] Farm policy contributes to obesity by lowering food prices, but its effect on weight may be small.[77] A cost-benefit analysis could help determine whether society is better off with or without current agriculture policies.

Another existing policy that the government can reconsider is the ban on lawsuits against food companies by plaintiffs who allege that the company's products made them obese. In 2004 twelve states adopted laws that block consumers from filing such lawsuits; so far in 2005 seven more states have followed, and nineteen more states are considering such laws.[78] But such blanket liability waivers remove the food industry's incentives to disclose information about the food's content, to exercise restraint in advertising to children, and to ensure the food's safety. Legal scholars are generally skeptical that torts against the food industry will be as successful as recent ones against tobacco companies, in part because no subset of foods can be proven to be solely responsible for causing obesity and therefore no single food or restaurant company can be shown to be liable.[79] But to encourage the food industry to keep its customers' welfare in mind, consumers need to be able to pursue such legal cases, which can always be thrown out if frivolous.

Assessing Cost-Effectiveness

Although cost-effectiveness analysis of anti-obesity initiatives is in short supply, some evidence exists. Studies, for example, have calculated the cost of saving a quality-adjusted life year (QALY) associated with specific interventions. (A quality-adjusted life year attempts to take into account the quality of the extra lifespan; for example, an extra year of life in a persistent vegetative state receives a QALY score near zero whereas an extra year of life in perfect health receives a full QALY score of 1.) The decision rule for cost-effectiveness analysis is generally to implement the policy with the lowest cost per QALY and to continue implementing policies until either the initiative's budget is exhausted or the cost per QALY saved rises above some threshold. This threshold, historically $50,000 per QALY, has more recently been raised to $200,000, but other benchmarks are also used.[80] For example, Richard Hirth and several colleagues estimate that under various sets of circumstances, Americans are willing to pay from $150,000 per QALY to more than $425,000 per QALY.

The Centers for Disease Control and Prevention have conducted a multiyear project to assess the cost-effectiveness of seven "exemplary" interventions to increase physical activity. (None of the interventions was targeted at children and adolescents.) The study concludes that the lowest-cost exemplary intervention was Wheeling Walks, an eight-week, intensive community-wide intervention that promoted walking among sedentary fifty- to sixty-five-year-olds using paid media and public health activities at work sites, churches, and local organizations. That intervention cost $14,286 per QALY saved.[81] The other six interventions were estimated to cost between $27,373 and $68,557 per QALY saved. These estimates were for a forty-year analytic time horizon. For shorter time horizons the costs per QALY were considerably higher (more than $100,000 for a ten-year horizon), because many health benefits of weight loss are reaped only later in life while the intervention's costs are always paid up front.

In contrast, estimates show bariatric surgery for the severely obese costs between $5,400 and $16,100 per QALY for women and $10,700 to $35,600 per QALY for men.[82] Providing an anti-obesity drug to overweight patients with diabetes has been estimated to cost $8,327 per QALY.[83] These studies indicate that there may be available a variety of cost-effective anti-obesity interventions, some involving prevention and others involving treatment.

Conclusion

Researchers have concluded that the market has contributed to overweight in children in primarily three ways over the past several decades. First, the real price of food fell (perhaps in part because of changing agriculture policies). Second, the time cost of food preparation rose for college graduates. And, third, technological changes created incentives to use packaged food rather than to prepare foods. Given the few additional daily calories that caused the rise in obesity over the past two decades, it will likely be impossible to know which of these changes is most responsible for the increase in obesity.

Several economic rationales justify government intervention in markets to address childhood obesity: a lack of information, youthful irrationality, and the societal costs of obesity. The government can address the lack of information easily and directly, but formulating policies to address the other two rationales is more difficult. Several second-best policies to reduce obesity exist, but it is as yet impossible to choose among them without cost-effectiveness studies. Once such studies are available, they will help policymakers achieve the greatest benefit from a fixed budget.

Americans can be optimistic about policy interventions' effectiveness in addressing obesity because small changes in flows of calories can have enormous impacts on individuals. One calculation implies that if Americans had consumed 50 fewer calories per day over the past twenty years, 90 percent of Americans could have avoided recent weight gains.[84] Even small changes in behavior today can substantially decrease childhood obesity in future decades.

Notes

1. Cynthia Ogden and others, "Prevalence and Trends in Overweight among U.S. Children and Adolescents, 1999–2000," *Journal of the American Medical Association* 288, no. 14 (2002): 1728–32. To avoid stigmatizing children, the highest clinical weight classification for children is "overweight" rather than obesity. However, in this paper I use the terms "overweight" and "obesity" interchangeably for children.

2. Cara B. Ebbeling, Dorota B. Pawlak, and David S. Ludwig, "Childhood Obesity: Public Health Crisis, Common Sense Cure," *Lancet* 360 (2002): 473–82; S. Y. S. Kimm and E. Obarzanek, "Childhood Obesity: A New Pandemic of the New Millennium," *Pediatrics* 110, no. 5 (2002): 1003–07; Rebecca Puhl and Kelly D. Brownell, "Stigma, Discrimination, and Obesity," in *Eating Disorders and Obesity: A Comprehensive Handbook*, edited by C. G. Fairburn and K. D. Brownell (New York: Guilford Press, 2002); Richard S. Strauss, "Childhood Obesity and Self-Esteem," *Pediatrics* 105, no. 1 (2000): e15–e20.

3. Jeffrey P. Koplan, Catharyn T. Liverman, and Vivica I. Kraak, eds., *Preventing Childhood Obesity: Health in the Balance* (Washington: National Academies Press, 2004).

4. The economic framework or model of eating, physical activity, and obesity is provided in detail in John Cawley, "An Economic Framework for Understanding Physical Activity and Eating Behaviors," *American Journal of Preventive Medicine* 27, no. 3 (2004): 1–9; John Cawley, "The Economics of Childhood Obesity Policy," in *Obesity, Business, and Public Policy*, edited by Zoltan Acs and Alan Lyles (Northampton, Mass.: Edward Elgar, forthcoming); and Darius Lakdawalla and Tomas J. Philipson, "Economics of Obesity," in *The Elgar Companion to Health Economics*, edited by Andrew Jones (New York: Edward Elgar, 2006).

5. James Hill and others, "Obesity and the Environment: Where Do We Go from Here?" *Science* 299, no. 7 (2003): 853–55.

6. U.S. Bureau of Labor Statistics, "Consumer Price Index—All Urban Consumers" (http://data.bls.gov/PDQ/outside.jsp?survey=cu [November 15, 2005]).

7. D. Lakdawalla and T. Philipson, "The Growth of Obesity and Technological Change: A Theoretical and Empirical Examination," Working Paper 8946 (Cambridge, Mass.: National Bureau of Economic Research, 2002).

8. Daron Acemoglu, "Technical Change, Inequality, and the Labor Market," *Journal of Economic Literature* 40, no. 1 (2002): 7–72.

9. J. P. Robinson and G. Godbey, *Time for Life: The Surprising Ways That Americans Use Their Time* (Pennsylvania State University Press, 1999); Roland Sturm, "The Economics of Physical Activity: Societal Trends and Rationales for Interventions," *American Journal of Preventive Medicine* 27, no. 3S (2004): 126–35.

10. D. M. Cutler, E. L. Glaeser, and J. M. Shapiro, "Why Have Americans Become More Obese?" *Journal of Economic Perspectives* 17, no. 3 (2003): 93–118.

11. U.S. Department of Labor, *Women in the Labor Force: A Databook,* Report 973 (Bureau of Labor Statistics, 2004).

12. P. M. Anderson, K. F. Butcher, and P. B. Levine, "Maternal Employment and Overweight Children," *Journal of Health Economics* 22 (2003): 477–504.

13. R. M. Blank, "Evaluating Welfare Reform in the United States," *Journal of Economic Literature* 40, no. 4 (2002): 1105–66.

14. Adam Drewnowski and S. E. Specter, "Poverty and Obesity: The Role of Energy Density and Energy Costs," *American Journal of Clinical Nutrition* 79, no. 1 (2004): 6–16.

15. Jane Reed, Elizabeth Frazao, and Rachel Itskowitz, "How Much Do Americans Pay for Fruits and Vegetables?" U.S. Department of Agriculture, Economic Research Service, Agriculture Information Bulletin no. 790, July 2004.

16. Bureau of Labor Statistics, "Consumer Price Index" (see note 6).

17. Biing-Hwan Lin, Joanne Guthrie, and Elizabeth Frazao, "Away-from-Home Foods Increasingly Important to Quality of American Diet," U.S. Department of Agriculture, Economic Research Service, Agriculture Information Bulletin no. 749, 1999.

18. Biing-Hwan Lin, Joanne Guthrie, and Elizabeth Frazao, "Quality of Children's Diets at and away from Home: 1994–96," *Food Review* 22, no. 1 (1999): 2–10.

19. Bureau of Labor Statistics, "Consumer Price Index" (see note 6).

20. Lin, Guthrie, and Frazao, "Away-from-Home Foods" (see note 17).

21. Ibid.

22. Lisa R. Young and Marion Nestle, "The Contribution of Expanding Portion Sizes to the U.S. Obesity Epidemic," *American Journal of Public Health* 92, no. 2 (2002): 246–49.

23. Brian Wansink, "Environmental Factors That Increase the Food Intake and Consumption Volume of Unknowing Consumers," *Annual Review of Nutrition* 24 (2004): 455–79; Barbara J. Rolls, "The Supersizing of America: Portion Size and the Obesity Epidemic," *Nutrition Today* 38, no. 2 (2003): 42–53; Jenny H. Ledikwe, Julia Ello-Martin, and Barbara J. Rolls, "Portion Sizes and the Obesity Epidemic," *Journal of Nutrition* 135, no. 4 (2005): 905–09.

24. Barbara J. Rolls, Dianne Engell, and Leann L. Birch, "Serving Portion Size Increases 5-Year-Old but Not 3-Year-Old Children's Food Intakes," *Journal of the American Dietetic Association* 100 (2000): 232–34.

25. Helen Smiciklas-Wright and others, "Foods Commonly Eaten in the United States, 1989–1991 and 1994–1996: Are Portion Sizes Changing?" *Journal of the American Dietetic Association* 103 (2003): 41–47.

26. John Cawley and Barrett Kirwan, "U.S. Agricultural Policy and Obesity," unpublished manuscript, Cornell University, 2005.

27. U.S. Department of Agriculture, "Sugar and Sweeteners: Policy" (www.ers.usda.gov/Briefing/Sugar/policy.htm#trqs [November 15, 2005]).

28. G. A. Bray, S. J. Nielsen, and B. M. Popkin, "Consumption of High-Fructose Corn Syrup in Beverages May Play a Role in the Epidemic of Obesity," *American Journal of Clinical Nutrition* 79, no. 4 (2004): 537–43; Michael Pollan, "The (Agri)Cultural Contradictions of Obesity," *New York Times*, October 12, 2003; Greg Critser, *Fat Land: How Americans Became the Fattest People in the World* (New York: Houghton Mifflin, 2003).

29. P. C. Westcott and J. M. Price, "Analysis of the U.S. Commodity Loan Program with Marketing Loan Provisions," U.S. Department of Agriculture, Agricultural Economic Report 801, 2001.

30. E. Douglas Beach and others, "An Assessment of the Effect on Land Values of Eliminating Direct Payments to Farmers in the United States," *Journal of Economic Development* 22, no. 2 (1997): 1–27.

31. B. Gardner, "U.S. Agricultural Policies since 1995, with a Focus on Market Effects in Grains and Oilseeds," Working Paper 02-17 (Department of Agricultural and Resource Economics, University of Maryland, 2002).

32. C. J. M. Paul and J. M. MacDonald, "Tracing the Effects of Agricultural Commodity Prices and Food Costs," *American Journal of Agricultural Economics* 85, no. 3 (2003): 633–46.

33. Cawley and Kirwan, "U.S. Agricultural Policy" (see note 26).

34. Harry M. Kaiser, "Distribution of Benefits and Costs of Commodity Checkoff Programs: Introductory Remarks," *Agribusiness* 19, no. 3 (2003): 273–75.

35. Noel Blisard, "Advertising and What We Eat: The Case of Dairy Products," in *America's Eating Habits: Changes and Consequences,* edited by Elizabeth Frazao, Agriculture Information Bulletin no. 750 (Washington: U.S. Department of Agriculture, 1999).

36. Ibid.

37. Brenda L. Boetel and Donald J. Liu, "Evaluating the Effect of Generic Advertising and Food Health Information within a Meat Demand System," *Agribusiness* 19, no. 3 (2003): 345–54.

38. The Pork Board, "2003 Checkoff Timeline Brochure" (www.porkboard.org/docs/checkoff%20timeline%20bro2003.pdf [November 15, 2005]); Dairy Management, Inc., "February 2005 Dairy Checkoff Update," press release (www.dairycheckoff.com/DairyCheckoff/MediaCenter/CheckoffUpdate/Postings/February+2005.htm [October 28, 2005]).

39. Anthony E. Gallo, "Food Advertising in the United States," in *America's Eating Habits*: *Changes and Consequences,* edited by Elizabeth Frazao, Agriculture Information Bulletin no. 750 (Washington: U.S. Department of Agriculture, 1999).

40. D. Kunkel, "Children and Television Advertising," in *Handbook of Children and the Media,* edited by D. Singer and J. Singer (Thousand Oaks, Calif.: Sage Publications, 2001).

41. H. L. Taras and M. Gage, "Advertised Foods on Children's Television," *Archives of Pediatrics & Adolescent Medicine* 149, no. 6 (1995): 649–52.

42. Roland Sturm, "Childhood Obesity: What We Can Learn from Existing Data on Societal Trends, Part 1," *Preventing Chronic Disease* 2, no. 1 (2005): 1–9.

43. K. Kotz and M. Story, "Food Advertisements during Children's Saturday Morning Television Programming: Are They Consistent with Dietary Recommendations?" *Journal of the American Dietetic Association* 94, no. 11 (1994): 1296–1300.

44. Gerard Hastings and others, "Review of Research on the Effects of Food Promotion to Children" (Centre for Social Marketing, University of Strathclyde, Glasgow, U.K., 2003).

45. Hastings and others, "Review of Research" (see note 44); D. Borzekowski and T. Robinson, "The 30-Second Effect: An Experiment Revealing the Impact of Television Commercials on Food Preferences of Preschoolers," *Journal of the American Dietetic Association* 101, no. 1 (2001): 42–46.

46. American Academy of Pediatrics, "Children, Adolescents, and Advertising," *Pediatrics* 95, no. 2 (1995): 295–97; Koplan, Liverman, and Kraak, *Preventing Childhood Obesity* (see note 3).

47. Richard S. Strauss and Harold A. Pollack, "Epidemic Increase in Childhood Overweight, 1986–1998," *Journal of the American Medical Association* 286, no. 22 (2001): 2845–48.

48. R. P. Troiano and K. M. Flegal, "Overweight Children and Adolescents: Description, Epidemiology, and Demographics," *Pediatrics* 101, no. 3 (1998): 497–504.

49. Kimberly Morland and others, "Neighborhood Characteristics Associated with the Location of Food Stores and Food Service Places," *American Journal of Preventive Medicine* 22, no. 1 (2002): 23–29.

50. Diane Gibson, "Neighborhood Characteristics and the Local Food Environment: Supermarket Availability in the 50 Largest Cities in the United States," Working Paper (Baruch College, City University of New York, 2005).

51. Kimberly Morland, Steve Wing, and Ana Diez Roux, "The Contextual Effect of the Local Food Environment on Residents' Diets: The Atherosclerosis Risk in Communities Study," *American Journal of Public Health* 92, no. 11 (2002): 1761–67.

52. Joel Waldfogel, "The Median Voter and the Median Consumer: Local Private Goods and Residential Sorting," unpublished manuscript, University of Pennsylvania, 2004.

53. Penny Gordon-Larsen and others, "Inequality in the Built Environment Underlies Key Health Disparities in Physical Activity and Obesity," *Pediatrics* (forthcoming).

54. R. Ewing and others, "The Relationship between Urban Sprawl and Physical Activity, Obesity, and Morbidity," *American Journal of Health Promotion* 18, no. 1 (2003): 47–57; Lawrence Frank, Martin Andresen, and Tom Schmid, "Obesity Relationships with Community Design, Physical Activity, and Time Spent in Cars," *American Journal of Preventive Medicine* 27 (2004): 87–96.

55. J. M. Zakarian and others, "Correlates of Vigorous Exercise in a Predominantly Low SES and Minority High School Population," *Preventive Medicine* 23 (1994): 314–21; J. F. Sallis and others, "Predictors of Change in Children's Physical Activity over 20 Months: Variations by Gender and Level of Adiposity," *American Journal of Preventive Medicine* 16, no. 3 (1999): 222–29.

56. Centers for Disease Control and Prevention, "Smoking Prevalence among U.S. Adults" (www.cdc.gov/tobacco/research_data/adults_prev/prevali.htm [November 15, 2005]).

57. Centers for Disease Control and Prevention, "Cigarette Use among High School Students—United States, 1991–2003," *Morbidity and Mortality Weekly Report* 53, no. 23 (2004): 499–502.

58. U.S. Department of Health and Human Services, *The Health Benefits of Smoking Cessation: A Report of the Surgeon General* (Rockville, Md.: Centers for Disease Control and Prevention, 1990).

59. Shin-Yi Chou, Michael Grossman, and Henry Saffer, "An Economic Analysis of Adult Obesity: Results from the Behavioral Risk Factor Surveillance System," *Journal of Health Economics* 23, no. 3 (2004): 565–87.

60. Jonathan Gruber and Michael Frakes, "Does Falling Smoking Lead to Rising Obesity?" Working Paper 11483 (Cambridge, Mass.: National Bureau of Economic Research, 2005).

61. E. Finkelstein, I. Fiebelkorn, and G. Wang, "National Medical Spending Attributable to Overweight and Obesity: How Much and Who's Paying?" *Health Affairs Web Exclusive,* May 14, 2003.

62. B. Reger, M. G. Wootan, and S. Booth-Butterfield, "Using Mass Media to Promote Healthy Eating: A Community-Based Demonstration Project," *Preventive Medicine* 29 (1999): 414–21.

63. Alan Mathios, "The Impact of Mandatory Disclosure Laws on Product Choices: An Analysis of the Salad Dressing Market," *Journal of Law and Economics* 43, no. 2 (2000): 651–77.

64. Jayachandran N. Variyam and John Cawley, "Nutrition Labels and Obesity," paper presented at the 2005 Association for Public Policy Analysis and Management Conference, Washington, November 3, 2005.

65. Health Policy Tracking Service: A Thomson West Business, July 11, 2005.

66. Koplan, Liverman, and Kraak, *Preventing Childhood Obesity* (see note 3).

67. Marion Nestle, *Food Politics: How the Food Industry Influences Nutrition and Health* (University of California Press, 2002); E. Schlosser, *Fast Food Nation: The Dark Side of the All-American Meal* (New York: Houghton Mifflin, 2001).

68. Dale Kunkel and others, *Report of the APA Task Force on Advertising and Children* (Washington: American Psychological Association, 2004).

69. Ernst Berndt, "The United States' Experience with Direct-to-Consumer Advertising of Prescription Drugs: What Have We Learned?" Unpublished manuscript, Massachusetts Institute of Technology.

70. Ibid.; Mary Engle, testimony before the Institute of Medicine's Committee on Prevention of Obesity in Children and Youth, Washington, December 9, 2003.

71. S. A. French and others, "A Pricing Strategy to Promote Low-Fat Snack Choices through Vending Machines," *American Journal of Public Health* 87, no. 5 (1997): 849–51; S. A. French and others, "Pricing and Promotion Effects on Low-Fat Vending Snack Purchases: The CHIPS Study," *American Journal of Public Health* 91 (2001): 112–17; P. Hannan and others, "A Pricing Strategy to Promote Sales of Lower Fat Foods in High School Cafeterias: Acceptability and Sensitivity Analysis," *American Journal of Health Promotion* 17, no. 1 (2002): 1–6.

72. Koplan, Liverman, and Kraak, *Preventing Childhood Obesity* (see note 3).

73. Zakarian and others, "Correlates of Vigorous Exercise" (see note 55); Sallis and others, "Predictors of Change" (see note 57); John Cawley, Chad Meyerhoefer, and David Newhouse, "The Impact of State Physical Education Requirements on Youth Physical Activity and Overweight," Working Paper 11411 (Cambridge, Mass.: National Bureau of Economic Research, 2005).

74. Patricia M. Anderson and Kristin F. Butcher, "Reading, Writing, and Raisinets: Are School Finances Contributing to Children's Obesity?" Working Paper 11177 (Cambridge, Mass.: National Bureau of Economic Research, 2005).

75. U.S. Accountability Office, "School Meal Programs: Competitive Foods Are Widely Available and Generate Substantial Revenues for Schools," GAO-05-563 (Washington, GAO, 2005).

76. James E. Tillotson, "Pandemic Obesity: Agriculture's Cheap Food Policy Is a Bad Bargain," *Nutrition Today* 38, no. 5 (2003): 186–90.

77. Gardner, "U.S. Agricultural Policies since 1995" (see note 31); Paul and MacDonald, "Tracing the Effects" (see note 32); Cawley and Kirwan, "U.S. Agricultural Policy and Obesity" (see note 26).

78. Health Policy Tracking Service (see note 65).

79. Todd G. Buchholz, *Burger, Fries, and Lawyers: The Beef behind Obesity Lawsuits* (Washington: U.S. Chamber Institute for Legal Reform, 2003); Richard A. Daynard, Lauren E. Hash, and Anthony Robbins, "Food Litigation: Lessons from the Tobacco Wars," *Journal of the American Medical Association* 288, no. 17 (2002): 2179–81.

80. Larissa Roux, "Evaluation of Potential Solutions to the Health and Economic Problems Presented by Physical Activity: A Cost-Utility Analysis," unpublished manuscript, Centers for Disease Control and Prevention, 2005; R. A. Hirth and others, "Willingness to Pay for a QALY: In Search of a Standard," *Medical Decision Making* 20, no. 3 (2000): 332–42.

81. Roux, "Evaluation of Potential Solutions" (see note 80).

82. J. Fang, "The Cost-Effectiveness of Bariatric Surgery," *American Journal of Gastroenterology* 98, no. 9 (2003): 2097–98.

83. A. Maetzel and others, "Economic Evaluation of Orlistat in Overweight and Obese Patients with Type 2 Diabetes Mellitus," *Pharmacoeconomics* 21, no. 7 (2003): 501–12.

84. Hill and others, "Obesity and the Environment" (see note 5).

The Role of Built Environments in Physical Activity, Eating, and Obesity in Childhood

James F. Sallis and Karen Glanz

Summary

Over the past forty years various changes in the U.S. "built environment" have promoted sedentary lifestyles and less healthful diets. James Sallis and Karen Glanz investigate whether these changes have had a direct effect on childhood obesity and whether improvements to encourage more physical activity and more healthful diets are likely to lower rates of childhood obesity.

Researchers, say Sallis and Glanz, have found many links between the built environment and children's physical activity, but they have yet to find conclusive evidence that aspects of the built environment promote obesity. For example, certain development patterns, such as a lack of sidewalks, long distances to schools, and the need to cross busy streets, discourage walking and biking to school. Eliminating such barriers can increase rates of active commuting. But researchers cannot yet prove that more active commuting would reduce rates of obesity.

Sallis and Glanz note that recent changes in the nutrition environment, including greater reliance on convenience foods and fast foods, a lack of access to fruits and vegetables, and expanding portion sizes, are also widely believed to contribute to the epidemic of childhood obesity. But again, conclusive evidence that changes in the nutrition environment will reduce rates of obesity does not yet exist.

Research into the link between the built environment and childhood obesity is still in its infancy. Analysts do not know whether changes in the built environment have increased rates of obesity or whether improvements to the built environment will decrease them. Nevertheless, say Sallis and Glanz, the policy implications are clear. People who have access to safe places to be active, neighborhoods that are walkable, and local markets that offer healthful food are likely to be more active and to eat more healthful food—two types of behavior that can lead to good health and may help avoid obesity.

www.futureofchildren.org

James F. Sallis is a professor of psychology at San Diego State University and director of Active Living Research, a program of the Robert Wood Johnson Foundation. Karen Glanz is a professor of behavioral sciences, health education, and epidemiology at Emory University and the director of the Emory Prevention Research Center.

Any effort to understand or reduce obesity must consider the "built environment." Loosely defined, the built environment consists of the neighborhoods, roads, buildings, food sources, and recreational facilities in which people live, work, are educated, eat, and play. The way the built environment is created can affect many daily decisions. Whether people walk to work or school, eat frequently at fast-food restaurants, or take their children to parks may depend in part on how neighborhoods are built. When one studies the built environment in the context of the obesity epidemic, it is important to ask three questions. First, how does the built environment affect important lifestyle decisions? Second, would changing the infrastructure alter decisionmaking? And, third, would these changes affect Americans' weight and overall health? For example, although much of America's built environment has changed over the past forty years in ways that have promoted sedentary lifestyles, it is not known whether these changes have had a direct effect on obesity rates or whether changes in the built environment will lower these rates. In this paper, we attempt to shed some light on these issues.

Built environments affect children's weight by shaping both their eating habits and their physical activity. Research into the links between the physical places where children live and children's activity levels and eating habits, it must be said, is less conclusive than research in other areas covered in this volume. In the first place, research on youth is limited, though studies of adults can provide some insights for youth. A second important limitation of virtually all existing studies is the possibility of self-selection. A study may find that people who live near parks are more active than people who do not, but it cannot confidently conclude that proximity to parks is the cause of that activity. Perhaps, instead, active people choose to live near parks. A better study design would focus on the effect of environmental changes in a neighborhood on the people living there, but so far such studies have been limited to small changes such as building trails.[1] Tracking major environmental changes is extremely difficult because the changes are not under the control of investigators, and most such changes take far longer to be completed than the typical research study does. The "ideal" study, the randomized trial, is simply not possible because people cannot be randomly assigned to live in particular neighborhoods.

Despite the limits of research in this area, leaders in public health have stressed the need for changes in the built environment to improve health.[2] New reports by two authoritative panels recognize that consistent links between environmental factors and physical activity provide valuable evidence that should inform policy change.[3] Both available evidence and common sense support four obesity-related goals: ensuring that all children have access to safe and convenient places to be physically active, ensuring that the bulk of food available to children in most settings meets nutritional guidelines, reducing promotion of unhealthful food and sedentary behaviors, and making it easy to identify and affordable to buy healthful foods.

The Built Environment and Physical Activity

Children themselves know that characteristics of the built environment affect how active they can be: physical activity is welcome in certain places and is difficult, discouraged, or even prohibited in others. Buildings, transportation infrastructure, elements of land use and community design, and recreational facilities, such as parks and trails, all affect citizens' physical activity.

Active Recreation

Health and recreation researchers have focused on the link between access to recreation facilities and children's recreational physical activity. A handful of studies have shown what common sense would also suggest: children and adolescents with access to recreational facilities and programs, usually near their homes, are more active than those without such access.[4] Adolescent girls' physical activity is related to the proximity of recreational facilities.[5] The more often young adolescents use recreational facilities, the greater their total physical activity, with parks and the neighborhood most important for boys and with commercial facilities and the neighborhood most important for girls.[6] Preschool children are more active when there are more places nearby where vigorous play is welcome and when they spend more time in those places.[7] Three studies of preschool children using direct observation report that being outdoors is the strongest correlate of the children's physical activity.[8]

There are some contrary findings. Two studies, for example, reported no significant links between physical activity and such variables as environmental barriers, access to supervised programs, and distance to parks.[9] Both studies, however, were based on parental reports rather than direct observation. Another study of young children found no relation between their proximity to playgrounds and being overweight.[10]

To sum up, the broad conclusions of existing studies are consonant with a review of research on adults, which consistently linked physical activity with both access to and the attractiveness of recreational facilities and programs.[11]

If further research confirms the associations between access to facilities and youth physical activity, the policy implication is clear: all children need places where they can be physically active on a regular basis. The most important such places appear to be outdoors and in the neighborhood and include both public parks and commercial facilities. Because children

> *If further research confirms the associations between access to facilities and youth physical activity, the policy implication is clear: all children need places where they can be physically active on a regular basis.*

engage in such a variety of activities and because their recreational needs vary widely by age, providing many different types of facilities is a promising policy objective.

How accessible facilities are depends on how close they are to children's homes or schools, how costly they are to use, and how easily they can be reached. At least two U.S. studies found fewer parks, sports fields, fitness clubs, and trails in low-income neighborhoods than in more affluent ones, suggesting that low-income youth may face barriers to physical activity.[12] Interestingly, low-income neighborhoods had relatively fewer free than pay-for-use facilities, suggesting the possible influence of community tax bases and related spending policies. Because the distribution of facilities is likely to vary across cities, researchers should examine more locations, focusing on the quality of facilities as well as access.

Although market forces primarily govern the distribution of private recreational facilities, cities and states could enact tax-based incentives, similar to those often used to spur economic and business development, to locate private facilities in low-income neighbor-

Cities and states could enact tax-based incentives, similar to those often used to spur economic and business development, to locate private facilities in low-income neighborhoods.

hoods. Publicly funded parks and trails generally garner strong support.[13] Some 90 percent of a national sample of U.S. adults supported using local government funds for walking and jogging trails, recreation centers, and bicycle paths. People may support spending for recreational facilities because they believe public open space improves their quality of life, but building more and better public recreational facilities could also promote youth physical activity.[14] Also health care savings could conceivably offset the government's costs of building such facilities. Several cities have recently taken steps to improve their parks. Voters in Los Angeles have approved major bond issues in recent years to upgrade urban parks. Denver's public schools have approved converting school playgrounds to community parks. And pub-

lic-private partnerships in metropolitan Atlanta have accelerated the pace of building a regional network of mixed-use walking and cycling paths.[15]

Active Transportation

Transportation and urban planning researchers have for several decades been examining how a community's design encourages (or discourages) its citizens to walk and cycle for transportation (rather than for recreation), though until recently health professionals were unfamiliar with the researchers' work.[16] Though the original research focus was directed toward reducing traffic congestion and improving air quality, the findings have direct implications for physical activity.

Before the middle of the twentieth century, communities were designed to support convenient pedestrian travel for common activities, such as shopping and going to school. Indeed, many U.S. towns and cities developed before automobile use became widespread and were pedestrian oriented by necessity. These "traditional" neighborhoods are characterized by mixed land use, connected streets, and moderate to high density. Homes, stores, employment centers, and government services are located near one another, often with multiple uses in the same multistory building. Streets are laid out in a grid pattern that creates high levels of connectivity and offers pedestrians direct routes from place to place. High residential density, with a preponderance of multifamily dwellings, makes local stores financially viable. For obvious reasons, these traditional designs are termed "walkable."

As the twentieth century progressed and America's suburbs began to grow, however, a variety of policies were set in place to optimize automobile travel. Different forms of land use were separated by zoning codes, so homes and stores were no longer within walking distance. The street network within residential areas was disconnected, and long blocks and many cul-de-sacs made pedestrian travel all but impossible. Low-traffic residential streets fed into multilane, high-speed arterial streets that presented serious barriers and dangers to pedestrians. Because the design of suburbs essentially requires the use of automobiles for all trips, such communities are often described as "unwalkable," especially for transportation.

Many studies have examined components of walkability or compared walking and cycling for transportation in high- and low-walkable neighborhoods. They consistently show more walking and cycling for transportation in walkable neighborhoods.[17] Recent studies using objective measures of total physical activity have found that residents of high-walkable neighborhoods get one hour more of physical activity each week and are 2.4 times more likely to meet physical activity recommendations than residents of low-walkable neighborhoods.[18] Recent reports from the Transportation Research Board and Institute of Medicine and the Centers for Disease Control's "Guide to Community Preventive Services" conclude that the design of communities is linked with physical activity, though causality cannot be established because of the self-selection problem already noted.[19]

Though most such research has not focused on children, several studies suggest that young people would be more likely to walk to nearby destinations in traditional neighborhoods. Kevin Krizek, Amanda Birnbaum, and David Levinson have argued that community design is relevant to youth physical activity and have recommended that researchers examine the specific destinations, activities at those destinations, and travel modes that are most common for children.[20] An Australian study found that the way people perceive a neighborhood environment can affect the extent to which children in that neighborhood walk and cycle to destinations.[21] Perceptions of heavy traffic, a lack of public transit, a lack of street-crossing aids, the need to cross several roads, and a lack of nearby recreational facilities were all linked to lower rates of active transportation. One study of adolescents found that boys were more active when they lived near pedestrian-oriented shopping areas.[22] In an unexpected finding, girls were more active when streets were less connected, suggesting that low-traffic residential streets and cul-de-sacs may be play areas for some young people.[23] Researchers should also look into how community design variables may operate differently for children, adolescents, and adults.

Several investigators have examined how community design relates to the weight status of adults. Four studies have documented lower body mass index (BMI) or reduced risk of overweight and obesity in people living in more walkable areas.[24] The one study focusing on adolescents, however, found no link between neighborhood environment and BMI, so it would be premature to draw any final conclusions.[25]

Walking and cycling to school are of particular interest because both require substantial energy expenditures on a daily basis.[26] And, indeed, studies have found that children who walk to school are more physically active than those who travel to school by car, though we could locate none linking walking with weight status.[27] However, active commuting rates are low, ranging from only 5 to 14 percent.[28] Low-walkable suburban development patterns, such as the lack of sidewalks, long distances to schools, and the need to cross busy streets with fast-moving traffic, appear to create barriers to active commuting to school.[29]

The simple fact is that more children walk to school in neighborhoods with sidewalks.[30] An evaluation of the Marin County, California, Safe Routes to Schools program that combined promotional activities with built environment changes—more sidewalks and improved street crossings—found a 64 percent increase in walking and a 114 percent increase in cycling to school.[31] And an evaluation of statewide investments in sidewalks, crosswalks, and bike lanes in ten California schools found that 15 percent of parents of children who passed the improvements on their way to school reported their children walked or cycled more.[32] The Robert Wood Johnson Foundation's Active Living Leadership program has documented initiatives across the United States at the city, county, and state levels that are designed to create built environments that make it easy for people to be physically active for transportation and recreation purposes.[33]

With pedestrian injuries a major cause of childhood injuries and deaths, parents are understandably concerned about traffic safety.[34] Priority should thus be placed on designing roads, sidewalks, and crosswalks that make it safe for children to walk and cycle. The need for greater investment is clear. Rates of pedestrian death and injury are vastly higher in the United States than in Western European countries such as Germany and the Netherlands, where extensive networks of protected cycling and pedestrian lanes, along with laws that make drivers rather than pedestrians or cyclists liable in accidents, have dramatically improved pedestrian safety.[35] It is true that the development of safe sidewalks, crosswalks, and bike lanes

will not increase active commuting among children whose homes are too distant from their schools or who are driven to school to suit their parents' work schedules. However, the evidence suggests that rates of active commuting can be modified through environmental interventions.

Sedentary Behavior

Sedentary recreational behaviors, such as watching television and videos, using computers, and playing video games, are important parts of young people's daily lives. They are also risk factors for obesity in youth, and reducing such behaviors is another strategy for preventing childhood obesity.[36] Research is beginning to document connections between the built environment and sedentary behaviors. Without safe places to play near home, for example, children may spend more time being inactive indoors. Likewise, heavy traffic reduces the likelihood of children's walking and may thus keep children indoors, where they remain sedentary.[37] Time spent riding in a car is associated with a risk of overweight in adults, and residents of low-walkable neighborhoods spend more time driving, so community design is likely to have a similar effect on children.[38] These and other hypothesized associations between children's sedentary behavior and community design need to be more closely examined.

Strategies for Change

Making the multiple environmental changes supported most consistently by the limited but rapidly expanding evidence will require leadership from many sectors.[39] The strongest evidence links access to recreational facilities and programs with child and adolescent physical activity. Recreation departments in local and state governments are a primary interest group for intervention in this area. They could promote physical activity among youth of all ages by designing and outfitting parks to provide diverse opportunities for popular physical activities, ensuring equitable distribution of recreational facilities, and emphasizing physical activity over other programs. Because achieving these goals may require increased funding, government leaders could be targeted for advocacy. The Cleveland Parks Department could be a model for other cities. As another possible model, the National Recreation and Park Association has partnered with the National Heart, Lung, and Blood Institute to develop, evaluate, and disseminate the Hearts N' Parks program across the nation.[40]

Commercial groups, such as dance and martial arts studios, and community organizations, such as youth sports leagues, churches, and after-school programs, all manage or interact with places for youth physical activity. Such groups could boost physical activity in children of all skill and income levels. Youth groups could use these facilities for their social and recreational programs, using sliding-scale fees to increase access for low-income youth. Increasing physical activity opportunities for low-income youth is a priority, because these children have few options. Providing tax breaks for commercial physical activity providers, such as dance studios and health clubs, to build facilities in low-income areas is a strategy worth exploring.

Since 1990, the federal government has made transportation funds available for pedestrian and bicycling infrastructure. State and local transportation funds support sidewalks, trails, traffic calming, and crosswalks. Safe Routes to Schools construction funding is available from the U.S. Department of Transportation and from the transportation departments of California and a few other states. Organized advocacy, however, may be needed to shift priorities within transportation departments to ensure adequate funding of pedestrian and bicycle facilities.

Creating the mixed-use, highly connected communities found to be associated with more physical activity requires changes in zoning codes and development regulations. Such organizations as Congress for the New Urbanism and Smart Growth America are

Priority should thus be placed on designing roads, sidewalks, and crosswalks that make it safe for children to walk and cycle.

promoting these reforms.[41] To improve the comfort and safety of pedestrians and bicyclists, changes are needed to improve road design guidelines. The "complete streets" concept would make all streets suitable for pedestrians, cyclists, and motorists.[42] Subsequent research must determine whether walkable neighborhoods and complete streets are health-promoting for youth as well as adults. However, many initiatives are under way nationwide to advocate for policy changes that will make environments more supportive of physical activity. They should be carefully evaluated.

The Built Environment and Nutrition

The nutrition environment is widely believed to contribute to the epidemic of childhood and adult obesity in the United States and globally.[43] Research on nutrition environments is less advanced than that on physical activity environments, though several studies have examined schools as sources of food and found, for example, that the availability of fruits and vegetables in school lunches is linked with youngsters' overall consumption of fruits and vegetables.[44] (See the article in this volume by Mary Story, Karen Kaphingst, and Simone French for more details on nutrition in schools.) Few researchers have explored how other neighborhood environments may affect children's eating patterns, and even

---

The obesity epidemic makes it essential to improve our understanding of the effect of food environments on children as rapidly as possible.

---

fewer have looked into their possible links with childhood obesity. Thus we draw mainly from research on neighborhoods in relation to adults' dietary behaviors. The obesity epidemic makes it essential to improve our understanding of the effect of food environments on children as rapidly as possible.

Several aspects of the broad nutrition environment in the United States and other industrialized countries may help explain the increasing prevalence of childhood obesity. Cost concerns and time pressures often lead parents and their children to rely on convenience foods and fast foods. The increasing popularity of dining out over the past two decades has raised the proportion of nutrients consumed away from home. Because convenience foods and restaurant meals are typically higher in calories and fat and lower

in valuable nutrients than meals prepared at home, frequent consumption of such food increases the chances of obesity in children and adolescents as well as in adults.[45] A lack of access to and the high cost of fruits, vegetables, and other nutritious foods may keep children from consuming them. Expanding portion sizes also appear to be contributing to the obesity epidemic.[46]

Parents and school administrators are usually called on to provide more healthful foods to children. Evidence indicates, however, that there is a great deal of support for community-level policies that affect local food environments. In a recent survey in California, 50 percent of respondents rated their neighborhoods as being only fair, poor, or very poor in offering healthful food for children, with residents of large cities most likely to give negative ratings.[47] Eighty-seven percent of respondents favored requiring fast-food and chain restaurants to post nutritional information, and 46 percent favored limiting the number of fast-food restaurants in a community.[48] Respondents generally favored a community approach to reducing childhood obesity rather than leaving it to individual children and families. They rated parents, health care providers, and schools as more important than churches and faith-based organizations in helping to reduce childhood obesity, although relatively more African Americans and Latinos favored a major church role.[49]

Is the consumers' perception that childhood obesity can be altered through changes in the nutrition environment supported by evidence? Though the literature to date is limited, diverse studies support the principle that nutrition environments may be important influences on eating behavior and may help explain disparities in behavior and disease. The available research on nutrition environments outside schools and homes is based on concepts and empirical data from the fields of public health, health psychology, consumer psychology, and urban planning. It falls generally under two headings: *community* nutrition environments, which include the number, type, and location of food outlets, and *consumer* nutrition environments, which cover the availability and cost of, as well as information about, healthful and less healthful foods inside those food outlets. The distinction is important because each could have broad effects on child health, and the opportunities for modifying each can be quite different.

Community Nutrition Environments

In the community nutrition environment, stores and restaurants are the most numerous food outlets. Accessibility can include large issues, such as whether and to what extent these outlets are located in certain communities, as well as such smaller issues as whether they have drive-through windows and what their hours of operation are. Other food sources, such as cafeterias in schools, work sites, churches, and health care facilities, are considered "organizational nutrition environments," although the nonschool sources may be more influential for adults than for children and youth.

The community nutrition environment may explain some of the racial, ethnic, and socioeconomic disparities in nutrition and health, such as the increasing prevalence of overweight in low-income children.[50] Supermarkets, for example, are less common in lower-income and minority neighborhoods than in other neighborhoods.[51] And recent evidence links access to supermarkets with such indicators of healthful eating as fruit and vegetable intake among African American

adults, household fruit consumption, and a diet quality index for pregnancy.[52]

Evidence related to restaurants is intriguing but less consistent than that related to stores. A study in New Orleans found higher fast-food restaurant density in minority and lower-income neighborhoods, and a study in Australia found that people living in poorer areas had twice the exposure to these restaurants.[53] A state-level analysis in the United States found only a modest link between obesity and the prevalence of fast-food restaurants: the density of such restaurants accounted for only 6 percent of the variance in state obesity rates out of a total of 70 percent explained by a model that included many variables.[54] In another Australian study, the availability of take-away food and restaurants was not linked with obesity.[55] And in one of the only studies known to explore community nutrition environments and children, overweight was not linked with proximity to fast-food restaurants among urban low-income preschoolers.[56]

Consumer Nutrition Environments

Data on consumer nutrition environments, by contrast, reflect what consumers encounter within and around a store or restaurant, including the availability of healthful choices, price, promotions, placement, and nutritional information. Price is an influential feature of the nutrition environment. A study of why Americans eat what they do found that cost was the second most important factor, behind taste; convenience was ranked fourth, just after nutrition.[57]

The availability of healthful foods is also important. Some healthful foods, such as low-fat dairy products and fruits and vegetables, are less available and of poorer quality in minority and lower-income areas. Three studies have documented that disadvantaged neighborhoods have a proportionally lower availability of healthful options and produce of poorer quality than do more affluent and white neighborhoods.[58] A study in Los Angeles compared healthful food options and food preparation at restaurants in poorer neighborhoods and at restaurants in higher-income neighborhoods and found fewer healthful menu selections in the lower-income areas.[59]

Most low-income consumers had access to the healthier substitutes but at significantly greater cost than the less healthful options.

A recent study compared the availability and cost of a standard "market basket" of foods from the U.S. Department of Agriculture's Thrifty Food Plan for low-income consumers with a market basket of healthier foods, such as whole wheat bread and lean ground beef. Most low-income consumers had access to the healthier substitutes but at significantly greater cost than the less healthful options.[60]

Few studies have examined the connection between consumer nutrition environments and eating behaviors. Allen Cheadle and several colleagues found positive links between the availability of healthful (low-fat and high-fiber) products at the grocery store and individuals' consumption of these foods.[61] Follow-up surveys two years later, however, found that changes in food availability made relatively little difference to individuals' food consumption over time.[62] Researchers must develop better measures to use grocery store surveys to track community-level dietary changes over time.

Indeed, to better understand in general how the nutrition environment affects eating behavior, analysts must continue to improve their measures of how consumer nutrition environments vary. In a food availability study completed in 1990, Cheadle and his colleagues included calculations of the percentage of shelf space used for healthful food options, such as low-fat milk and cheese and lean meats, but such measures may be difficult to apply in contemporary grocery stores, which are now larger and more varied in layout than stores were only a decade ago.[63] Other opportunities for consumer measures in stores include assessing product promotion and placement related to children, such as displaying energy-dense foods and placing unhealthful products on lower shelves. The complexity of the research area is clear, but given the public health imperative to improve eating behaviors, it must be a high priority to enhance the public's understanding of the food environments' impact on their eating habits.

An important omission in these studies is that none makes it possible to evaluate the relative contribution of environmental and demographic, psychological, and social factors to diet and obesity. Such multilevel studies are critically necessary to better inform policymakers, researchers, and communities about the potential of environmental change strategies to make a genuine difference in the childhood obesity problem.

Strategies for Change

Although researchers are well informed about which eating patterns will help avoid or reduce obesity, they as yet know relatively little about how environmental change can affect eating patterns. Nevertheless, we can suggest promising strategies, many of which have already been shown to be feasible. Some of these strategies come from recent online and newspaper reports; although they are innovative, they have usually not been carefully evaluated. Others come from previously reported efforts to promote healthful eating, such as reducing fat intake or eating more fruits and vegetables. They provide interesting case examples, though, again, most have not been rigorously evaluated.[64]

At the community nutrition level, increasing the number of supermarkets (and the variety of fresh produce they sell) in low-income and minority neighborhoods could lead to healthier eating behaviors. Several cities have shown that it is feasible to increase the presence of supermarkets in disadvantaged areas through community advocacy and political action.[65] Providing transportation to food sources for poor families who do not own cars appears to be both feasible and popular with shoppers. Locating farmers' markets in low-income neighborhoods has also been well received, although whether the markets affect children's fruit and vegetable consumption or energy balance remains unclear.[66]

The Urban Nutrition Initiative in West Philadelphia combines the physical activity of gardening with the promotion of healthy eating. This university-community partnership has been recognized as a model health-promotion effort.[67] Similar grassroots efforts under the umbrella of community-supported agriculture connect local farmers and consumers to increase the production and consumption of fresh produce.[68]

Zoning and tax policies can also improve the types and quality of food sold at neighborhood stores. Some restaurant chains, includ-

ing fast-food restaurants, are increasing their menu of healthful foods by offering side orders of salad or vegetables as part of "combo meals."[69] A Produce for Better Health Foundation study is exploring opportunities to implement healthful menu changes in fast-food and fast-casual restaurant chains and family style restaurants.

Several metropolitan areas have convened forums to brainstorm ways to address their regional childhood obesity problems, with changes to the built environment among the options. Chicago leaders have come together in the Consortium to Lower Obesity in Chicago Children to identify local solutions with special attention to low-income communities and "urban re-design."[70] California health care organizations are promoting more healthful food environments in workplaces, hospitals, and clinics in models that might be adopted regionwide.[71] And in San Diego County, a community forum is planning to combat childhood obesity by, among other things, promoting better food labeling and by creating partnerships between the school system and farmers' markets.[72]

Common Issues for Physical Activity and Nutrition

Few studies simultaneously address both physical activity and nutrition within neighborhoods, though such work could advance understanding of how the built environment influences childhood obesity. Studies linking community design and adult weight raise the possibility that land use could work through both physical activity and eating.[73] Not only are people more physically active in traditional neighborhoods, such neighborhoods may also provide more convenient access to healthful foods or less dominance of fast-food restaurants.[74] Zoning laws can be used to require certain forms of destinations within walking distance of most residences, to limit the number of convenience stores and fast-food restaurants, or to encourage farmers' markets and family style, sit-down, or "slow-food," restaurants.

Because community design is related to walking for transportation and because food outlets are among the most common destinations for walkers, incentives for offering more healthful choices at food stores could affect both healthful eating and physical activity.[75] Neighborhoods that have community gardens can promote both physical activity and healthful eating.[76] Although urban planners are primarily motivated to reduce sprawl because of concerns about traffic congestion, air pollution, the cost of new infrastructure, and a lack of active transportation, reducing sprawl would also preserve agricultural areas near cities and thus maintain farmers' abilities to provide local produce.[77] In turn, more locally grown produce could reduce the cost of getting healthful foods to market and could support local economic development.

Drive-through windows at fast-food restaurants make food purchasing more convenient and may encourage consumers to eat while they drive. Drive-through windows are also symptomatic of the type of building design that discourages pedestrian activity. Restricting drive-through windows might improve both eating and physical activity. The politics of such restrictions could be complex, but demonstration projects could test how acceptable they are and what effects they might have.

Researchers hypothesize that social cohesion is higher in traditional neighborhoods, where people are more likely to see and talk with their neighbors while walking.[78] In socially cohesive neighborhoods, parents may also be more likely to feel comfortable letting their children play outdoors and walk or cycle to nearby stores for minor food-shopping errands. Socially cohesive communities may also be better advocates for more physical activity opportunities and for better access to healthful foods.

Problems with crime and traffic safety are likely to counter some of the benefits of traditional neighborhoods. Though we could locate no data on this topic, parental concerns about safety could keep children from taking advantage of walkable neighborhoods, recreational facilities, and healthful food sources such as community gardens and farmers' markets. Parents who are concerned about risks of violence or abduction are likely to act on those fears, regardless of real crime rates or an absolute risk of abduction. Likewise, parents who are concerned about heavy or fast vehicular traffic are likely to restrict a child's movements. Both types of concerns may be more prevalent and have greater impact among low-income families, who may not have cars to transport children to recreational and healthful eating opportunities. Researchers should focus on both objectively assessed and perceived safety issues as they relate to physical activity, eating, and built environments.

Lessons Learned and Challenges

Changing the built environment to increase children's physical activity for recreation and transportation, to improve access to healthful foods, and to reduce access to less healthful foods can help provide long-term solutions to the childhood obesity epidemic. Unlike the often-transitory effects of motivational and educational approaches to addressing obesity, changes in behavior prompted by changes in the built environment should be long lasting. Although research generally links aspects of the built environment with physical activity and eating behaviors, most data are from studies of adults, and findings to date are unable to pinpoint which specific variables would have the greatest effect on childhood eating, physical activity, and obesity. Nevertheless, we can draw some lessons from the studies to date and offer some tentative policy recommendations. Given the urgency of the childhood obesity epidemic, we cannot wait for optimal evidence and must instead base actions on the best available evidence.[79]

Children of all ages need and want places to play. To support the diversity of their physical activities, they need many types of recreational facilities, both public and private, near their homes and schools. To remedy the relative scarcity of such facilities in low-income neighborhoods, policymakers must ensure that these facilities are more equitably distributed.

Adults who live in walkable communities are more physically active and less likely to be overweight than those who do not. A few studies suggest that adolescents living in walkable neighborhoods may be more active and more likely to walk to school than their counterparts in unwalkable communities, but more studies of youth are needed. Combining physical improvements to enhance the safety of routes to school with activities that promote walking and cycling appears to increase active commuting to school. Improving the safety of roads, sidewalks, and crosswalks may reduce parental concerns about traffic danger and encourage more active transportation among children.

Low-income and minority neighborhoods not only have less access to healthful foods but also may face higher food costs. Evidence linking access to healthful foods with dietary intake in children is limited; more studies should be a high priority. But enough studies

document inequitable access to healthful foods to justify corrective efforts. With obesity rates among low-income children and adults much higher than those among well-to-do citizens, there is a strong rationale for grassroots efforts, public-private partnerships, and even public subsidies of healthful food sources in targeted areas.[80] Increasing the number of healthful, affordable food choices in a variety of food outlets is a complementary strategy that may be largely

Combining physical improvements to enhance the safety of routes to school with activities that promote walking and cycling appears to increase active commuting to school.

driven by commercial considerations. In this instance, public pressure and consumer demand can make a difference.

Challenges of Translating Research into Change

Conducting research on built environments and childhood obesity and implementing changes based on the findings will be challenging. Researchers will probably not find a single "smoking gun." It is more likely that many built environment variables will show a strong cumulative effect on diet, physical activity, and weight status in children than that any single variable will have a dominant influence. Further, different environmental variables are likely to be operating for children of different ages and genders as well as for those of different racial, ethnic, and cultural groups and socioeconomic backgrounds. Thus changing the built environment in all the ways needed to combat obesity may be a complex task. Research is further complicated by the paucity of reliable and valid measures of food and physical activity environmental factors. And changing the built environment alone is unlikely to induce large changes in eating habits and physical activity. Educational programs, promotional activities, incentives, and policies will all be necessary to support the physical changes.

Making so many changes in the built environment would affect not only many government departments at all levels, but also the food industry, the real estate industry, many transportation-related industries, recreation-related industries, and entertainment industries. Some of these industries will actively oppose policies that threaten their current operating practices.[81] Stimulating health-oriented policy change in government agencies not normally focused on health will require creative and sustained effort. Public support for changing the built environment to combat childhood obesity has seldom been studied but may be decisive in adopting and implementing both promising and evidence-based policies.[82]

Enhancements to encourage more active commuting in communities and potential subsidies for healthful foods may well be costly. Those costs must be better understood and balanced against the costs of continuing current policies that may be driving the youth obesity epidemic. Careful economic analyses must inform policy decisions.[83]

Making major changes in government policy and industry practice will require a substantial investment in advocacy that will in turn require people, organization, and funding. Although many organizations have interests consistent with the built environment's changes already noted, their capacity is not sufficient to achieve even the initial policy changes supported by existing data. Continuous evaluation will be required to learn whether the changes that are made lead to the expected outcomes and contribute to reducing the obesity epidemic.

Finally, there is an urgent need for the next generation of studies on how the built environment affects youth physical activity, eating, and obesity. Because simply identifying built environment risk factors is not sufficient to create change, advancing the science of policy change is also a high priority. A new research emphasis must be to improve the understanding of policy change processes of greatest relevance to youth physical activity, eating, and obesity.

Notes

1. Kelly R. Evenson, Amy H. Herring, and Sara L. Huston, "Evaluating Change in Physical Activity with the Building of a Multi-Use Trail," *American Journal of Preventive Medicine* 28 (2S2) (2005): 177–85.

2. U.S. Department of Health and Human Services, *Healthy People 2010* (2000); Jeffrey P. Koplan and William H. Dietz, "Caloric Imbalance and Public Health Policy," *Journal of the American Medical Association* 282 (2000): 1579–81; World Health Organization, *Obesity: Preventing and Managing the Global Epidemic* (Geneva,1998); Jeffrey P. Koplan, Catharyn T. Liverman, and Vivica I. Kraak, eds., *Preventing Childhood Obesity: Health in the Balance* (Washington: National Academies Press, 2004.)

3. Transportation Research Board–Institute of Medicine, *Does the Built Environment Influence Physical Activity? Examining the Evidence* (Washington: National Academies Press, 2005); Gregory W. Heath and others, "The Effectiveness of Urban Design and Land Use and Transport Policies and Practices to Increase Physical Activity: A Systematic Review," *Journal of Physical Activity and Health* (forthcoming).

4. James F. Sallis, Judith J. Prochaska, and Wendell C. Taylor, "A Review of Correlates of Physical Activity of Children and Adolescents," *Medicine and Science in Sports and Exercise* 32 (2000): 963–75.

5. Gregory J. Norman and others, "Community Design and Recreational Environmental Correlates of Adolescent Physical Activity and BMI," *Journal of Physical Activity and Health* (forthcoming).

6. Wendy R. Hoefer and others, "Parental Provision of Transportation for Adolescent Physical Activity," *American Journal of Preventive Medicine* 21 (2002): 48–51.

7. James F. Sallis and others, "Correlates of Physical Activity at Home in Mexican-American and Anglo-American Preschool Children," *Health Psychology* 12 (1993): 390–98.

8. Sallis, Prochaska, and Taylor, "A Review of Correlates" (see note 4).

9. James F. Sallis and others, "Correlates of Physical Activity in a National Sample of Girls and Boys in Grades Four through Twelve," *Health Psychology* 18 (1999): 410–15; James F. Sallis and others, "Correlates of Vigorous Physical Activity for Children in Grades 1 through 12: Comparing Parent-Reported and Objectively Measured Physical Activity," *Pediatric Exercise Science* 14 (2002): 30–44.

10. Hillary L. Burdette and Robert C. Whitaker, "Neighborhood Playgrounds, Fast-Food Restaurants, and Crime: Relationships to Overweight in Low-Income Preschool Children," *Preventive Medicine* 38 (2004): 57–63.

11. Nancy Humpel, Owen N. Neville, and Evie Leslie, "Environmental Factors Associated with Adults' Participation in Physical Activity: A Review," *American Journal of Preventive Medicine* 22 (2002): 188–99.

12. Paul A. Estabrooks, Rebecca E. Lee, and Nancy C. Gyurcsik, "Resources for Physical Activity Participation: Does Availability and Accessibility Differ by Neighborhood Socioeconomic Status?" *Annals of Behavioral Medicine* 25 (2004): 100–04; Linda M. Powell, S. Slater, and Frank J. Chaloupka, "The Relationship between Community Physical Activity Settings and Race, Ethnicity, and Socioeconomic Status," *Evidence-Based Preventive Medicine* 1 (2004): 135–44.

13. Ross C. Brownson and others, "Environmental and Policy Determinants of Physical Activity in the United States," *American Journal of Public Health* 91 (2001): 1995–2003.

14. Geoffrey C. Godbey and others, "Contributions of Leisure Studies and Recreation and Park Management Research to the Active Living Agenda," *American Journal of Preventive Medicine* 28 (2S2) (2005): 150–58.

15. Los Angeles park bond info: http://eng.lacity.org/projects/prop_k/aboutus.htm (accessed October 18, 2005); Denver school playground conversions: Lois Brink and Bambi Yost, "Transforming Inner-City School Grounds: Lessons from Learning Landscapes," *Children, Youth, and Environments* 14, no. 1 (2004).

16. Lawrence D. Frank, Peter O. Engelke, and Thomas L. Schmid, *Health and Community Design: The Impact of the Built Environment on Physical Activity* (Washington: Island, 2003); Brian E. Saelens, James F. Sallis, and Lawrence D. Frank, "Environmental Correlates of Walking and Cycling: Findings from the Transportation, Urban Design, and Planning Literatures," *Annals of Behavioral Medicine* 25 (2003): 80–91.

17. Saelens, Sallis, and Frank, "Environmental Correlates of Walking and Cycling" (see note 16).

18. Brian E. Saelens and others, "Neighborhood-Based Differences in Physical Activity: An Environment Scale Evaluation," *American Journal of Public Health* 93 (2003): 1552–58; Lawrence D. Frank and others, "Linking Objectively Measured Physical Activity with Objectively Measured Urban Form: Findings from SMARTRAQ," *American Journal of Preventive Medicine* 28 (2S2) (2005): 117–25.

19. Transportation Research Board–Institute of Medicine, *Does the Built Environment Influence Physical Activity?* (see note 3); Heath and others, "The Effectiveness of Urban Design" (see note 3).

20. Kevin J. Krizek, Amanda S. Birnbaum, and David M. Levinson, "A Schematic for Focusing on Youth in Investigations of Community Design and Physical Activity," *American Journal of Health Promotion* 19 (2004): 33–38.

21. Anna Timperio and others, "Perceptions about the Local Neighborhood and Walking and Cycling among Children," *Preventive Medicine* 38 (2004): 39–47.

22. Norman and others, "Community Design and Recreational Environmental Correlates" (see note 5).

23. Ibid.

24. Saelens and others, "Neighborhood-Based Differences" (see note 18); Billie Giles-Corti and others, "Environmental and Lifestyle Factors Associated with Overweight and Obesity in Perth, Australia," *American Journal of Health Promotion* 18 (2003): 93–102; Reid Ewing and others, "Relationship between Urban Sprawl and Physical Activity, Obesity, and Morbidity," *American Journal of Health Promotion* 18 (2003): 47–57; Lawrence D. Frank, Martin A. Andresen, and Thomas L. Schmid, "Obesity Relationships with Community Design, Physical Activity, and Time Spent in Cars," *American Journal of Preventive Medicine* 27 (2004): 87–96.

25. Norman and others, "Community Design and Recreational Environmental Correlates" (see note 5).

26. Catrine Tudor-Locke, Barbara E. Ainsworth, and Barry M. Popkin, "Active Commuting to School: An Overlooked Source of Children's Physical Activity?" *Sports Medicine* 31 (2001): 309–13.

27. Ashley R. Cooper and others, "Commuting to School: Are Children Who Walk More Physically Active?" *American Journal of Preventive Medicine* 25 (2003): 273–76.

28. John R. Sirard and others, "Prevalence of Active Commuting at Urban and Suburban Elementary Schools in Columbia, SC," *American Journal of Public Health* 95 (2005): 236–37; Centers for Disease Control and

Prevention, "Barriers to Children Walking and Biking to School—United States, 1999," *Journal of the American Medical Association* 288 (2002): 1343–44.

29. Howard Frumkin, Lawrence Frank, and Richard Jackson, *Urban Sprawl and Public Health: Designing, Planning, and Building for Healthy Communities* (Washington: Island, 2004).

30. Reid Ewing, W. Schroeer, and W. Greene, "School Location and Student Travel: Analysis of Factors Affecting Mode Choice," *Transportation Research Record* 1895 (2004): 55–63.

31. Catherine E. Staunton, Deb Hubsmith, and Wendi Kallins, "Promoting Safe Walking and Biking to School: The Marin County Success Story," *American Journal of Public Health* 93 (2003): 1431–34.

32. Marlon G. Boarnet and others, "Evaluation of the California Safe Routes to School Legislation: Urban Form Changes and Children's Active Transportation to School," *American Journal of Preventive Medicine* 28 (2S2) (2005): 134–40.

33. Robert Wood Johnson Foundation (www.activelivingleadership.org [accessed October 18, 2005]).

34. D. C. Grossman, "The History of Injury Control and the Epidemiology of Child and Adolescent Injuries," *Future of Children* 10, no. 1 (2000): 23–52; Transportation Research Board–Institute of Medicine, *Does the Built Environment Influence Physical Activity?* (see note 3).

35. John Pucher and Lewis Dijkstra, "Promoting Safe Walking and Cycling to Improve Public Health: Lessons from the Netherlands and Germany," *American Journal of Public Health* 93 (2003): 1509–16.

36. Brian E. Saelens, "Helping Individuals Reduce Sedentary Behavior," in *Obesity: Etiology, Assessment, Treatment, and Prevention,* edited by Ross E. Anderson (Champaign, Ill.: Human Kinetics, 2003), pp. 217–38.

37. Timperio and others, "Perceptions about the Local Neighborhood" (see note 21).

38. Frank, Andresen, and Schmid, "Obesity Relationships with Community Design" (see note 24).

39. James F. Sallis, Adrian Bauman, and Michael Pratt, "Environmental and Policy Interventions to Promote Physical Activity," *American Journal of Preventive Medicine* 15 (1998): 379–97.

40. www.nhlbi.nih.gov/health/prof/heart/obesity/hrt_n_pk/ (October 18, 2005).

41. The website for the Congress for the New Urbanism is www.cnu.org. The website for Smart Growth America is www.smartgrowthamerica.org.

42. See www.americabikes.org/bicycleaccommodation_factsheet_completestreets.asp. [October 18, 2005].

43. Karen Glanz and others, "Healthy Nutrition Environments: Concepts and Measures," *American Journal of Health Promotion* 19 (2005): 330–33.

44. Simone A. French and G. Stables, "Environmental Interventions to Promote Vegetable and Fruit Consumption among Youth in School Settings," *Preventive Medicine* 37 (2003): 593–610; Leslie A. Lytle and J. A. Fulkerson, "Assessing the Dietary Environment: Examples from School-Based Nutrition Interventions," *Public Health Nutrition* 5 (2002): 893–99; Mary Story, Diane Neumark-Sztainer, and Simone French, "Individual and Environmental Influences on Adolescent Eating Behaviors," *Journal of the American Dietetic Association* 102 (2002): S40–S51.

45. Bing-Hwan Lin, Elizabeth Frazao, and Joanne Guthrie, *Away-from-Home Foods Increasingly Important to Quality of American Diet,* Agriculture Information Bulletin no. 749 (Washington: U.S. Department of Agriculture, 1999); Eric A. Finkelstein, Christopher J. Ruhm, and Katherine A. Kosa, "Economic Causes and Consequences of Obesity," *Annual Review of Public Health* 26 (2005): 239–57.

46. Lisa R. Young and Marion Nestle, "The Contribution of Expanding Portion Sizes to the U.S. Obesity Epidemic," *American Journal of Public Health* 92 (2002): 246–49.

47. Field Research Corporation, "A Survey of Californians about the Problem of Childhood Obesity" (San Francisco: The California Endowment, 2003).

48. Ibid.

49. Ibid.

50. Bettylou Sherry and others, "Trends in State-Specific Prevalence of Overweight and Underweight in 2- through 4-Year-Old Children from Low-Income Families from 1989 through 2000," *Archives of Pediatric and Adolescent Medicine* 158 (2004): 1116–24.

51. Kimberly Morland and others, "Neighborhood Characteristics Associated with the Location of Food Stores and Food Service Places," *American Journal of Preventive Medicine* 22 (2002): 23–29; Shannon N. Zenk and others, "Neighborhood Racial Composition, Neighborhood Poverty, and the Spatial Accessibility of Supermarkets in Metropolitan Detroit," *American Journal of Public Health* 95 (2005): 660–67.

52. Kimberly Morland, Steve Wing, and Ana Diez Roux, "The Contextual Effect of the Local Food Environment on Residents' Diets: The Atherosclerosis Risk in Communities (ARIC) Study," *American Journal of Public Health* 92 (2002): 1761–67; Donald Rose and Rickelle Richards, "Food Store Access and Household Fruit and Vegetable Use among Participants in the U.S. Food Stamp Program," *Public Health Nutrition* 7 (2004): 1081–88; Barbara A. Laraia and others, "Proximity of Supermarkets Is Positively Associated with Diet Quality Index for Pregnancy," *Preventive Medicine* 39 (2004): 869–75.

53. Jason P. Block, Richard A. Scribner, and Karen B. DeSalvo, "Fast Food, Race/Ethnicity, and Income: A Geographic Analysis," *American Journal of Preventive Medicine* 27 (2004): 211–17; Daniel D. Reidpath and others, "An Ecological Study of the Relationship between Social and Environmental Determinants of Obesity," *Health and Place* 8 (2002): 141–45.

54. Jay Maddock, "The Relationship between Obesity and the Prevalence of Fast-Food Restaurants: State-Level Analysis," *American Journal of Health Promotion* 29 (2004): 137–43.

55. D. Simmons and others, "Choice and Availability of Takeaway and Restaurant Food Is Not Related to the Prevalence of Adult Obesity in Rural Communities in Australia," *International Journal of Obesity* 29 (2005): 703–10.

56. Burdette and Whitaker, "Neighborhood Playgrounds, Fast-Food Restaurants, and Crime" (see note 10).

57. Karen Glanz and others, "Why Americans Eat What They Do: Taste, Nutrition, Cost, Convenience, and Weight Control as Influences on Food Consumption," *Journal of the American Dietetic Association* 98 (1998): 1118–26.

58. Howell Wechsler and others, "The Availability of Low-Fat Milk in an Inner-City Latino Community: Implications for Nutrition Education," *American Journal of Public Health* 85 (1995): 1690–92; David C. Sloane

and others, "Improving the Nutritional Resource Environment for Healthy Living through Community-Based Participatory Research," *Journal of General Internal Medicine* 18 (2003): 568–75; Carol R. Horowitz and others, "Barriers to Buying Healthy Foods for People with Diabetes: Evidence of Environmental Disparities," *American Journal of Public Health* 94 (2004): 1549–54.

59. LaVonna B. Lewis and others, "African Americans' Access to Healthy Food Options in South Los Angeles Restaurants," *American Journal of Public Health* 95 (2005): 668–73.

60. Karen M. Jetter and Diana L. Cassady, "The Availability and Cost of Healthier Food Items," *AIC Issues Brief*, University of California Agricultural Issues Center 29 (2005): 1–6.

61. Allen Cheadle and others, "Community-Level Comparison between the Grocery Store Environment and Individual Dietary Practices," *Preventive Medicine* 20 (1991): 250–61.

62. Allen Cheadle and others, "Can Measures of the Grocery Store Environment Be Used to Track Community-Level Dietary Changes?" *Preventive Medicine* 22 (1993): 361–72.

63. Allen Cheadle and others, "Evaluating Community-Based Nutrition Programs: Assessing the Reliability of a Survey of Grocery Store Product Displays," *American Journal of Public Health* 80 (1990): 709–11.

64. Leslie Mikkelsen, "The Links between the Neighborhood Food Environment and Child Nutrition" (Oakland, Calif.: Issue paper for the Robert Wood Johnson Foundation, 2004); Karen Glanz and Amy Yaroch, "Strategies for Increasing Fruit and Vegetable Intake in Grocery Stores and Communities: Policy, Pricing, and Environmental Change," *Preventive Medicine* 39 (2004): S75–S80.

65. Karen Glanz and Deanna Hoelscher, "Increasing Fruit and Vegetable Intake by Changing Environments, Policy, and Pricing: Restaurant-Based Research, Strategies, and Recommendations," *Preventive Medicine* 39 (2004): S88–S93.

66. Mikkelsen, "The Links between the Neighborhood Food Environment" (see note 64).

67. Robert Wood Johnson Foundation News Digest: Childhood Obesity, July 15, 2005. (www.rwjf.org/obesity [August 7, 2005]).

68. www.umassvegetable.org/food_farming_systems/csa/index.html (August 7, 2005).

69. Glanz and Yaroch, "Strategies for Increasing Fruit and Vegetable Intake" (see note 64).

70. Robert Wood Johnson Foundation News Digest: Childhood Obesity, August 5, 2005 (rwjf.org/obesity).

71. Robert Wood Johnson Foundation News Digest: Childhood Obesity, July 15, 2005 (rwjf.org/obesity).

72. Robert Wood Johnson Foundation News Digest: Childhood Obesity, May 27, 2005 (rwjf.org/obesity).

73. Saelens and others, "Neighborhood-Based Differences in Physical Activity" (see note 18); Giles-Corti and others, "Environmental and Lifestyle Factors" (see note 24); Ewing and others, "Relationship between Urban Sprawl" (see note 24); Frank, Andresen, and Schmid, "Obesity Relationships with Community Design" (see note 24).

74. Saelens, Sallis, and Frank, "Environmental Correlates of Walking and Cycling" (see note 16).

75. Frank, Engelke, and Schmid, *Health and Community Design* (see note 16).

76. Mikkelsen, "The Links between the Neighborhood Food Environment" (see note 64).

77. Frumkin, Frank, and Jackson, *Urban Sprawl and Public Health* (see note 29).

78. Frank, Engelke, and Schmid, *Health and Community Design* (see note 16).

79. Koplan, Liverman, and Kraak, eds., *Preventing Childhood Obesity* (see note 2).

80. Ibid.

81. Gus Cannon, "Why the Bush Administration and the Global Sugar Industry Are Determined to Demolish the 2004 WHO Global Strategy on Diet, Physical Activity, and Health," *Public Health Nutrition* 7 (2004): 369–80.

82. Brownson and others, "Environmental and Policy Determinants" (see note 13).

83. Finkelstein, Ruhm, and Kosa, "Economic Causes and Consequences of Obesity" (see note 45).

The Role of Schools in Obesity Prevention

Mary Story, Karen M. Kaphingst, and Simone French

Summary

Mary Story, Karen Kaphingst, and Simone French argue that U.S. schools offer many opportunities for developing obesity-prevention strategies by providing more nutritious food, offering greater opportunities for physical activity, and providing obesity-related health services.

Meals at school are available both through the U.S. Department of Agriculture's school breakfast and lunch programs and through "competitive foods" sold à la carte in cafeterias, vending machines, and snack bars. School breakfasts and school lunches must meet federal nutrition standards, but competitive foods are exempt from such requirements. And budget pressures force schools to sell the popular but nutritionally poor foods à la carte. Public discomfort with the school food environment is growing. But can schools provide more healthful food options without losing money? Limited evidence shows that they can.

Although federal nutrition regulations are inadequate, they permit state and local authorities to impose additional restrictions. And many are doing so. Some states limit sales of nonnutritious foods, and many large school districts restrict competitive foods.

Several interventions have changed school food environments, for example, by reducing fat content of food in vending machines and making more fruits and vegetables available. Interventions are just beginning to target the availability of competitive foods.

Other pressures can also compromise schools' efforts to encourage physical activity. As states use standardized tests to hold schools and students academically accountable, physical education and recess have become a lower priority. But some states are now mandating and promoting more physical activity in schools. School health services can also help address obesity by providing screening, health information, and referrals to students, especially low-income students, who are at high risk of obesity, tend to be underinsured, and may not receive health services elsewhere.

www.futureofchildren.org

Mary Story is a professor in the Division of Epidemiology and Community Health, School of Public Health, University of Minnesota, and is the director of the Robert Wood Johnson Foundation (RWJF) Healthy Eating Research Program. Karen M. Kaphingst is in the Division of Epidemiology and Community Health, School of Public Health, University of Minnesota, and is the deputy director of the RWJF Healthy Eating Research Program. Simone French is a professor in the Division of Epidemiology and Community Health, School of Public Health, University of Minnesota.

Poor diets and physical inactivity are pushing rates of overweight and obesity among the nation's children to record levels.[1] Indeed, since 1960, U.S. childhood and adolescent overweight prevalence rates have more than tripled.[2] The health risks associated with childhood obesity pose a critical public health challenge for the twenty-first century.[3]

Schools can play an important part in a national effort to prevent childhood obesity. More than 95 percent of American youth aged five to seventeen are enrolled in school, and no other institution has as much continuous and intensive contact with children during their first two decades of life. Schools can promote good nutrition, physical activity, and healthy weights among children through healthful school meals and foods, physical education programs and recess, classroom health education, and school health services.

In this article we discuss the role of schools in preventing obesity. We analyze schools' food and physical activity environments and examine federal, state, and local policies related to food and physical activity standards in schools. We conclude by discussing promising and innovative obesity-prevention strategies.

Are Obesity, Nutrition, and Physical Activity Linked with School Performance?

Some observers have noted a worrisome correlation between weight problems and poor academic achievement.[4] One research study found that severely overweight children and adolescents are four times more likely than their healthy-weight peers to report "impaired school functioning." Overweight children are also more likely to have abnormal scores on the Child Behavior Checklist (a commonly used measure of children's behavior problems) and are twice as likely to be placed in special education and remedial classes than are children who are not overweight.[5] A study involving 11,192 kindergartners found that overweight children had significantly lower math and reading test scores at the beginning of the year than did their healthy-weight peers and that these differences persisted into first grade.[6] But such findings must be interpreted with caution. Because overweight is linked with poor academic performance does not mean that it causes poor performance. Low academic achievement can have many underlying causes, including low socioeconomic status, lower parental education, poor nutrition, and parental depression. Overweight should be considered a marker for poor academic performance and not the cause itself.

Overweight can impair school performance in many ways, including health-related absenteeism.[7] Among the medical conditions linked with overweight in school-aged children are asthma, joint problems, type 2 diabetes, depression and anxiety, and sleep apnea.[8] Social problems—such as being teased or bullied—loneliness, or low self-esteem can also affect how well children do in school.[9]

Although the evidence that child obesity affects school performance is limited, nutrition clearly affects academic performance. Poor nutritional status and hunger interfere with cognitive function and are associated with lower academic achievement. Iron deficiency is linked to shortened attention span, irritability, fatigue, and difficulty with concentration.[10] A recent review of studies of breakfast habits and nutritional status in children and adolescents found that breakfast consumption may improve cognitive function related to memory, test grades, and school attendance.[11] Studies have also found that children participating in the federal School Breakfast Program show increases in daily attendance, class participation, and academic test scores and decreases in tardiness.[12]

Research has also recently begun to elucidate the relationship between physical activity and student performance at school. Among the findings are that physical activity programs help school-aged children develop social skills, improve mental health, and reduce risk-taking behaviors.[13] Evidence also suggests that short-term cognitive benefits of physical activity during the school day adequately compensate for time spent away from other academic areas.[14] This evidence suggests that efforts to improve nutrition and increase physical activity in school may have the twin benefits of reducing obesity and improving the academic performance of all children, whether they are at risk of obesity or not.

The School Food Environment

Not only do most U.S. school-aged children attend school, they eat a large share of their daily food while they are there—estimates range from 19 to 50 percent or higher.[15] Food is typically available through the U.S. Department of Agriculture's (USDA) school breakfast and lunch programs and through "competitive foods" sold in vending machines, as à la carte offerings in the cafeteria, and at snack bars, school stores, and fundraisers.[16]

National School Breakfast and Lunch Programs

Ninety-nine percent of all public schools and 83 percent of all public and private schools participate in the National School Lunch Program.[17] The School Breakfast Program is

Table 1. Select Federal Child Nutrition Programs, 2003–04 School Year

School Breakfast Program	
Average daily student participation	8,680,178
Free and reduced-price	7,118,313
Paid	1,561,865
Increase in free and reduced-price participation in past 10 years	41.9 percent
Number of schools participating	78,118
Federal reimbursement	$1,740,181,232
School Lunch Program	
Average daily student participation	28,426,911
Free and reduced-price	16,508,440
Paid	11,918,471
Number of schools participating	98,375
Federal reimbursement	$6,527,731,630
Summer Food Service Program (July 2003)	
Average daily July participation	1,791,821
Number of sites	29,193
Federal funding	$215,805,038

Sources: Food Research and Action Center, "State of the States, 2005: A Profile of Food and Nutrition Programs across the Nation" (www.frac.org. [October 28, 2005]); USDA Food and Nutrition Service (FNS), "Nutrition Assistance Programs" (www.fns.usda.gov/fns/ [October 28, 2005]).

offered in 78 percent of the schools that offer the lunch program.[18] On an average school day, about 60 percent of children in schools offering the lunch program eat school lunch, and about 37 percent of children in schools in the breakfast program eat school breakfast (see table 1).

Meals in both programs must meet federally defined nutrition standards (see box) for schools to be eligible for federal subsidies, both cash and commodities. Federal school lunches must provide approximately one-third of the recommended dietary allowance (RDA) for key nutrients; school breakfasts offer one-fourth of the RDA. A 1998–99 national study found that federal school lunches generally meet standards for the key nutrients protein, vitamins A and C, calcium, and

Summary of Regulations and Funding for the National School Breakfast and National School Lunch Programs

Regulations

School meals must meet the applicable recommendations of the *Dietary Guidelines for Americans,* which recommend that no more than 30 percent of an individual's calories come from fat and less than 10 percent from saturated fat. School lunches must provide one-third of the recommended dietary allowance (RDA) for protein, calcium, iron, Vitamin A, Vitamin C, and calories. School breakfasts must provide one-fourth of these RDAs. Local school food authorities decide which specific foods to serve and how to prepare them.

"Foods of minimal nutritional value" as defined by federal regulations cannot be sold in school food service areas during the meal periods. Four categories of prohibited foods are soda pop, water ices, chewing gum, and certain candies, including hard candy, jellies and gums, marshmallow candies, fondant, licorice, spun candy, and candy-coated popcorn.

Funding

The National School Lunch and School Breakfast Programs are entitlement programs. As long as they follow regulations, enrolled public and nonprofit private schools are guaranteed funds to offer free or reduced-price meals. Both programs have a three-tiered system to determine the reimbursement rates. Children in families at or below 130 percent of the poverty line receive free meals. Children in families between 130 and 185 percent of the poverty line receive reduced-price meals. Children in families above 185 percent of the poverty line receive a small per-meal subsidy for full-price ("paid") meals, as set by the school.

The per-meal subsidies are indexed for inflation. For the 2005–06 school year, the per-meal reimbursement rate for school breakfasts is $1.27 for free breakfast, $0.97 for reduced-price breakfast, and $0.23 for the paid breakfast. Schools where at least 40 percent of the lunches served during the second preceding school year were free or reduced price may qualify for extra "severe need" school breakfast reimbursements if their costs exceed the standard federal reimbursement. For severe need, the reimbursement rate for free breakfast is $1.51, that for reduced-price breakfast is $1.21, and that for paid breakfast is $0.23.

For school lunches, the reimbursement rate for free lunch is $2.32, the rate for reduced-price lunch is $1.92, and the rate for paid lunch is $0.22. For schools where 60 percent or more lunches served during the second preceding school year were free or reduced price, the reimbursement rate for free lunch is $2.34, the rate for reduced-price lunch is $1.94, and the rate for paid lunch is $0.24. In addition to these rates, institutions may also receive 17.5 cents in commodities (or cash in lieu of commodities) as additional assistance for each lunch served.

Sources: *Code of Federal Regulations* 210.10; *Code of Federal Regulations* 220.8; *Code of Federal Regulations* appendix B to Part 210; *Federal Register* 70, no. 136 (July 18, 2005): 41196–200; Food Research and Action Center, Income Guidelines and Reimbursement Rates for the Federal Child Nutrition Programs (www.frac.org/pdf/rates.PDF [August 15, 2005]).

Note: Reimbursement rates are higher for Alaska and Hawaii.

iron.[19] The average calorie content of elementary school lunches was somewhat higher than the RDA while that of secondary school lunches was slightly lower.[20] Since 1995, federal school lunches and breakfasts have had to meet the requirements set in the *Dietary Guidelines for Americans*, which include limits on total and saturated fat (no more than 30 percent of calories from fat, with less than 10 percent from saturated fat). Schools reduced the average share of calories from fat in lunches from 38 percent in 1991–92 to 34 percent in 1998–99, but more than 75 percent of schools have not met the recommended share of 30 percent. Elementary schools are doing better than high schools.[21] The nutritional profile of school meals has improved over the past fifteen years but is not yet what it should be.

Impact of school meals on child nutrition. School meal programs significantly improve school-age children's diets.[22] Children who eat school lunches and breakfasts have higher mean intakes of micronutrients, both at mealtime and over twenty-four hours, than those who do not.[23] For the 59 percent of children eating school meals who come from low-income families, the meals provide a necessary safeguard against hunger.[24] Participation in the program declines drastically with age. It also declines as competing options to school meals become available.[25]

Commodity foods. Schools participating in the lunch program are eligible to receive commodity foods as well as bonus commodities. The commodity foods support American farmers by providing price supports and removing surpluses. Commodity foods must be of domestic origin, and 60 percent of the commodities purchased for schools must be from surplus stocks.[26] Commodities make up about 20 percent of the food schools use,

with local school districts buying the rest on the open market or through purchasing cooperatives.[27] During the 2005–06 school year, schools can receive donated commodity foods from the USDA, valued at 17.5 cents for each lunch served.[28] More than 94,000 schools receive commodities. During the 2004 school year, the USDA purchased more than $7.7 million worth of commodities for schools, totaling more than 1.1 billion pounds.[29] The states administer the commodities program, with each state selecting from a list of foods purchased by the USDA. Changes are needed in the commodity food program. The USDA should revise specifications to procure commodity foods that are consistent with those outlined in the *Dietary Guidelines.* The program should also offer more fresh produce and healthful lower-fat foods and make more connections with local farmers.

Financial issues. Budget pressures complicate schools' efforts to provide nutritious meals.[30] School food service programs, once regular line items in local school budgets, now must often be completely self-supporting and cover costs of food, labor, and other expenses, such as equipment, utilities, and trash removal.[31] Federal reimbursements and revenue from food sales are their principal sources of funds. In the 2005–06 school year, the USDA will reimburse participating schools $2.32 for every free lunch provided, $1.92 for every reduced-price lunch sold, and $0.22 for every other ("paid") lunch meal sold.[32] A recent analysis, however, found that expenses covered by federal reimbursements fell from 54 percent in 1996–97 to 51 percent in 2000–01.[33] Schools can enhance revenues in three ways: by increasing the number of students who eat federal meals, by increasing prices for full-price meals, and by expanding à la carte and catering sales.[34] The first two options—increasing school meal participation and raising prices of school meals—are difficult because many competing options are available from which students can purchase food at school. To try to break even, many food service directors thus choose the third option: selling popular but nutritionally poor foods à la carte.[35] In one analysis in 2000, total revenue from à la carte foods was 43 percent.[36] Not surprisingly, sales of à la carte items are inversely related to sales of school

---

Serving reimbursable meals that are more appealing to students and offering more healthful à la carte items would help students eat more healthfully.

---

lunch meals.[37] In states that restrict the sale of competitive foods, such as Mississippi, Louisiana, West Virginia, and Georgia, school meal participation rates exceed the national average.[38]

To encourage more students to participate in the school meal program, some schools are hiring culinary experts to develop healthful, tasty meals; are making cafeterias more youth friendly; and are enhancing the cafeteria's atmosphere. Indeed, the cafeteria itself can be a barrier to healthy eating. In some schools, lunch is served as early as 10:00 a.m. or as late as 1:30 p.m. Long cafeteria lines send students to vending machines or school stores. Insufficient time for lunch, cramped and unattractive cafeterias, and noise can also discourage participation in school meals. All these issues have financial implications, and structural issues, such as the cafeteria space

or time allowed for lunch, are not under the school food service's control.

School food services, facing difficult times, are using a variety of expense-containment and revenue-producing strategies to try to manage school food service finances. Serving reimbursable meals that are more appealing to students and offering more healthful à la carte items would help students eat more healthfully. For this change to happen, however, schools need to curtail foods sold outside the cafeteria that compete with school meals. Limiting competitive foods during school mealtimes could increase meal participation and increase revenues.

Full funding for the school meal programs could also relieve pressure on schools' food services to generate extra funding through competitive food sales. Schools that participate in the federal meal programs receive a fixed reimbursement for each meal served. Federal reimbursement rates are typically nine to ten times higher for free meals than for reduced-price or paid meals.[39] Although some states contribute supplemental funds and most schools receive donated USDA commodity foods, federal reimbursements are inadequate to cover the remainder of the meals' costs.

Competitive Foods

Competitive foods are all foods offered for sale at school except federal school meals.[40] They include à la carte foods offered in the school cafeteria as well as foods and beverages sold in snack bars, student stores, vending machines, and fund-raisers.[41] Current law tightly limits the Agriculture Department's authority to regulate competitive foods, which fall into two categories. The first category, called foods of minimal nutritional value, is defined in federal regulations as foods that provide less than 5 percent of the RDA per serving for each of eight key nutrients. They include soft drinks, water ices, chewing gum, and certain candies made largely from sweeteners, such as hard candy and jelly beans. These foods, which the USDA regulates, cannot be sold in food service areas during meal periods, but they may be sold anywhere else in the school at any time.[42] A vending machine with soft drinks and candy, for example, could be placed in the hall outside the cafeteria and be available to students all day. The second category of competitive foods, which is not under USDA authority, consists of all other foods offered for individual sale. This category, which includes candy bars, potato chips, cookies, and doughnuts, may be sold in the cafeteria during meal periods as well as anywhere else in the school. Although reimbursable school meals must meet federal nutrition and dietary guidelines, competitive foods have no such requirements. The federal definition of "foods of minimal nutritional value" is thirty years old and narrow in scope. It should be expanded to include additional foods with limited nutritional value. Further, although the federal school meal programs set appropriate portion sizes, competitive foods follow no size guidelines. Twenty ounces of soda, for example, is the standard size in many school vending machines.

Availability of competitive foods. The availability of high-fat, high-sugar foods and beverages in schools creates a food environment that invites excess energy intake and excess weight gain.[43] The national School Health Policies and Programs Study (SHPPS) 2000 found that 43 percent of elementary schools, 74 percent of middle schools, and 98 percent of high schools have vending machines, school snack bars, or other food sources outside of the school meal programs.[44] The most

common competitive foods are carbonated beverages, fruit drinks that are not 100 percent juice, salty snacks, and high-fat baked goods. Only 18 percent of the foods available through vending machines, school stores, or snack bars are fruits or vegetables. Most schools (58 percent of elementary schools, 84 percent of middle schools, and 94 percent of high schools) sell soft drinks, sports drinks, or fruit drinks.[45] In one study, the mean number of soft drink machines available to high school students was 5.3 (ranging from two to eleven).[46] Another study found that nearly nine out of ten schools offered competitive foods through à la carte cafeteria lines, vending machines, and school stores during the 2003–04 school year. The sale of competitive foods has increased over the past five years, with schools often selling them in or near the cafeteria and during lunch. High schools and middle schools were more likely to sell such foods than elementary schools.[47]

In the SHPPS 2000 survey, nearly all (83 percent) schools offered food à la carte.[48] And the wide availability of high-fat foods in cafeteria à la carte options has been documented.[49] In one study, Simone French and her colleagues found that only a third of foods in high school à la carte areas and in vending machines met the lower-fat guideline of less than 5.5 fat grams per serving.[50] The average number of à la carte food items typically available per school was 80 (ranging from 39 to 156), with chips and crackers making up the largest share of items. Fruits and vegetables were available à la carte in 85 percent of the schools, but they made up only 4 percent of total à la carte foods available.[51] School districts have also established contracts with fast-food vendors. In the 2003 California High School Fast Food Survey, roughly one-fourth of 173 districts reported selling brand-name products from Taco Bell,

Subway, Domino's, and Pizza Hut in high schools.[52]

School fundraisers often involve the sale of food or beverages. In the SHPPS 2000 survey, 82 percent of the schools reported that school clubs, sports teams, or the parent-teacher association (PTA) sold food at school or in the community to raise money.[53] According to the California fast-food survey, 74 percent of school food service directors re-

---

Competitive foods sold to students are displacing fruits and vegetables and other healthful foods and contributing to excessive fat and saturated fat intake.

---

ported that student clubs sell food during school mealtimes.[54] Other groups selling food at mealtimes in high schools are booster clubs (33 percent), the PTA (31 percent), and the physical education (PE) department (28 percent). Food fundraisers directly compete with the food service department and are subject to no nutritional standards. Student groups could instead raise funds by selling nonfood items, such as gift wrap, magazines, and plants, and by hosting walk-a-thons and auctions.

Impact of competitive foods on child nutrition. Competitive foods sold to students are displacing fruits and vegetables and other healthful foods and contributing to excessive fat and saturated fat intake. One study examined the diets of 598 seventh- and eighth-grade students and found that the greater the

availability at school of à la carte foods, the lower the daily intake of fruits and vegetables and the higher the intake of daily total fat and saturated fat. The greater the availability of snack vending machines, the lower the intake of fruit.[55] Karen Cullen and Issa Zakeri found that when elementary school students entered middle school and gained access to school snack bars, they consumed fewer fruits and non-starchy vegetables, less milk, and more sweetened beverages and high-fat vegetables than they did when they were in elementary school and had no option but the school lunch.[56] In a study of 743 sixth-grade students aged eleven to thirteen in three public middle schools in Kentucky, one-third who purchased the regular school lunch also bought competitive food items—mostly chips, fruitades or sport beverages, and cakes and cookies—in the lunchroom.[57] These students reduced their school lunch servings, resulting in lower intakes of minerals and vitamins and higher intakes of energy and fat. All these studies highlight the importance of school lunch program meals to fruit, vegetable, and milk consumption among children and adolescents.

School funding issues and competitive foods. As noted, competitive food sales generate an important revenue stream for schools in a climate of funding constraints. Many schools have come to rely on profits from competitive food sales to support food service operations, academic programs, cocurricular activities, and after-school activities.[58] Schools that are under financial pressure are more likely to make low-nutrition foods and beverages available to their students, have soft drink contracts, and allow food and beverage advertising to students.[59] A 2005 Government Accountability Office (GAO) report found that many schools, particularly high schools and middle schools, generated substantial revenues through competitive food sales—more than $125,000 apiece each year for the top 30 percent of high schools.[60] Food services generally spent their revenue on food service operations while school groups put theirs toward student activities.

School districts nationwide have also negotiated contracts for product sales, primarily soft drinks.[61] These "pouring rights" contracts typically involve substantial lump-sum payments to school districts and additional payments over five to ten years in return for exclusive sales of one company's products in vending machines and at all school events.[62] Companies also advertise on scoreboards, in hallways, on book covers, and elsewhere. Many contracts increase the share of profits schools receive when sales volume increases, further encouraging schools to promote consumption.

These practices contradict the nutrition and health messages students receive in the classroom and contribute to poor dietary habits. They also give soda companies unfettered access to youth and the chance to develop lifetime brand loyalty.[63] Despite increased public attention to food in schools and to the eroding quality of diets among youth, many schools hesitate to restrict competitive food for fear of losing income.

In August 2005, in response to growing pressure from parents and public health advocates, the American Beverage Association announced voluntary restrictions on sales of soft drinks in elementary and middle schools. The companies will encourage school districts and bottlers to provide only bottled water and 100 percent juice in elementary schools and to provide lower-calorie beverages in middle schools until after school. But because the new policy will apply only to new

contracts, it will take several years to phase high-calorie beverages out of elementary and middle schools.[64] And high schools, which have many more vending machines, will be unaffected.

Public discomfort with the school food environment is growing. The question is whether schools can provide more healthful food options without losing sales revenue.[65] Evidence about how reducing the sale of unhealthful foods and beverages or offering more healthful options would affect revenue is limited. But some studies have found that school food service staff reported no loss of revenue when they offered students more healthful à la carte choices.[66] And schools in Maine, California, Minnesota, and Pennsylvania replaced soft drinks with more healthful beverages without losing revenue.[67]

Surprisingly few national data are available on schools' income from vending machines.[68] A 2003 Texas Department of Agriculture survey found that total annual revenue from vending contracts for all 1,256 state schools was about $54 million.[69] It also found that food service departments lose $60 million a year in federal reimbursable meal sales to competitive foods, resulting in a net loss. During the 2001–02 school year, the total deficit for Texas school food service operations was $23.7 million, which had to be subsidized from other district sources.

Because many schools generate substantial revenue through competitive food sales, making changes entails financial risks.[70] Some school districts, however, have taken steps to mitigate potential revenue changes, such as substituting healthful foods for less healthful ones instead of removing all competitive foods, getting students involved in promoting healthful foods, using marketing approaches to encourage students to make healthful choices, offering alternate means for fundraising, and implementing changes gradually or at the beginning of the school year. Without support from the groups that use the revenue from competitive food sales, districts can see their policy changes curtailed.[71] Also, getting student suggestions about what types of nutritious foods would be offered will promote acceptance.

Policy implications. Federal rules governing the availability, content, and sale of competitive foods and setting schoolwide nutrition standards are inadequate.[72] Congress should grant the secretary of agriculture broader authority to regulate the availability, content, and sale of competitive foods during the school day and set nutrition standards for all foods and beverages sold. Such actions would not only enhance children's health and nutrition but also protect the federal investment in child nutrition through the national school meal programs.[73] Limiting the sale of competitive foods during school meals would increase participation in school meals and help ensure that children receive a nutritious meal.

Model School Nutrition Programs

Advocates, administrators, parents, educators, and health professionals across the country are promoting grassroots nutrition initiatives. *Making It Happen! School Nutrition Success Stories* showcases thirty-two schools that are offering and selling more nutritious foods and beverages. The schools carried out their reforms by setting nutrition standards for competitive foods, changing food and beverage contracts, making more healthful foods and beverages available, using marketing techniques to promote healthful choices, limiting access to competitive foods, and using fundraising activities and rewards that support rather than undermine student health.[74]

The message from *Making It Happen!* is that, given the opportunity, students will buy and consume healthy foods and beverages and, more important, that schools can maintain a profitable bottom line at the same time. Of the seventeen schools and school districts that reported income data, twelve increased revenue and four reported no change.

The School Physical Activity Environment

Schools are unique in their ability to promote physical activity and increase energy expenditure—and thereby help reduce childhood obesity.[75] A comprehensive school physical activity program should consist of PE, health education that includes information about physical activity, recess time for elementary school students, intramural sport programs and physical activity clubs, and interscholastic sports for high school students.[76] Schools can also encourage brief bouts of physical activity during classroom time—as in the Michigan Department of Education's "Brain Breaks" program and the International Life Sciences Institute's "Take 10!"—and walking and bicycling to school.[77]

Physical education—a formal, school-based educational program that uses physical activity to achieve fitness, skills, health, or educational goals—is at the center of a comprehensive school-based physical activity program.[78] It is an important but undervalued curricular area that aims to help all students develop the knowledge, skills, and confidence to be physically active both in and out of school and throughout their lives.[79]

Physical Activity Recommendations

Current guidelines recommend that children engage in at least sixty minutes of physical activity on most, preferably all, days of the week.[80] The Institute of Medicine's *Prevent-*

ing Childhood Obesity: Health in the Balance report recommends at least thirty minutes of activity during each school day.[81] The National Association for Sport and Physical Education recommends 150 minutes a week of PE for elementary school children and 225 minutes a week for middle- and secondary-school children.[82] Nationally, only 8 percent of elementary schools and 6 percent of middle schools and high schools meet these recommendations.[83]

Physical Education Classes and Barriers to Expanding PE

Physical education requirements decline drastically as a student's grade level increases. The share of schools requiring PE drops from around 50 percent for grades 1 through 5, to 25 percent in grade 8, to only 5 percent in grade 12.[84] Although the share of high school students enrolled in PE classes appears to have increased from 1991 to 2003 (49 percent to 56 percent), the share of students attending PE daily fell from 42 percent to 28 percent.[85] The quality of PE classes is also crucial to their effect on child and adolescent overweight. Only a third of adolescents were physically active in PE class for more than twenty minutes three to five days a week.[86]

Schools must fit many subjects and activities into the school day and must balance state and local resources, priorities, and needs for education. In recent years, however, the comprehensive curriculum has been eroding, especially in the wake of the federal No Child Left Behind Act of 2001, which focuses on student achievement in defined core academic subjects.[87] As states develop or select standardized tests to hold schools and students accountable, content that is not tested, such as physical education, has become a lower priority.[88] But, as noted, time devoted to physical education does not lessen performance in other areas and can in fact enhance both students' readiness to learn and academic achievement.[89]

Recess

Unstructured physical activity during recess allows children to have choices, develop rules for play, release energy and stress, and use skills developed in physical education.[90] It may also help in the classroom. Uninterrupted instructional time may cause attention spans to wane as restless children have difficulty concentrating on specific classroom tasks. One study found that fourth-graders had concentration problems on days without recess.[91]

The SHPPS 2000 survey found that 29 percent of elementary schools schedule no recess for students in kindergarten through fifth grade.[92] The National Association for Sport and Physical Education, by contrast, recommends that schools provide supervised, daily recess for students up to grades 5 or 6; that, if possible, recess not be scheduled back-to-back with physical education classes; that recess be viewed not as a reward but as a necessary educational support; that students not be denied recess to punish misbehavior or to make up work; and that recess complement, not substitute for, structured PE.[93]

Extracurricular Programs

Interscholastic sports programs, intramural activities, and physical activity clubs also keep children active in school. Intramural sports and clubs offer students with a wide range of abilities opportunities to engage in physical activity. But only 49 percent of schools offer intramural sports and sports clubs, and only 22 percent provide transportation home for students who participate in interscholastic sports, a problem for lower-income students who may need transportation.[94] To help prevent obesity, the Institute of Medicine calls for partnerships between schools and public and private sectors to enhance funding and opportunities for intramural sports and other activities in school and after-school programs.[95]

Health Curriculum

Health education is an essential part of a coordinated school health program, as recommended by the Centers for Disease Control and Prevention. By highlighting the importance of both nutrition and physical activity, health education can help students adopt and maintain physically active and healthful-eating lifestyles.[96] Key elements of health education include a planned and sequential educational program for students in grades K–12; behavioral skills development; instructional time at each grade level; instruction from qualified teachers; involvement of parents, health professionals, and other community members; and periodic curriculum evaluation and updating.[97] Research supports the effectiveness of behavioral-oriented curriculums in promoting healthful food choices and physical activity.[98] To maximize classroom time, nutrition and physical activity instruction could also be integrated into the lesson plans of other school subjects, such as math, biology, and the language arts.

Only six states do not require schools to provide health education.[99] Nearly 70 percent of states require health education curriculums to include instruction on nutrition and dietary behavior, and some 62 percent require content on physical activity and fitness.[100] But health education teachers at all levels average only about five hours a year teaching about the former and four hours a year about the latter—not nearly enough to affect children's behavior.[101] Competing time demands, a lack of resources, and the increased focus

on meeting state academic standards all chip away at teaching time.[102] Integrating health education into the existing curriculum is one way to overcome these problems.

School Health Services

School health services can play a central role in addressing obesity-related issues among students by providing screening, health information, and referrals to students. Services and settings vary widely, ranging from traditional, school-based basic core services to comprehensive primary care either in school-based health centers or in off-campus health centers.[103]

School-based health centers offer students primary care, including diagnostic and treatment services.[104] Their number is growing rapidly, from some 200 in 1990 to about 1,500 today.[105] A 2002 national survey found 61 percent of the centers in urban settings, 37 percent in elementary schools, and 36 percent in high schools. More than half of the students in schools with such health centers are African American or Hispanic.[106] The centers are typically open twenty-nine hours a week, and 39 percent are open during the summer. Survey participants cited nutrition as their most important prevention-related service.[107] The centers are an untapped resource for preventing obesity, because the students they serve are at high risk of obesity, tend to be underinsured, and may not receive health services elsewhere.[108]

Height, weight, and BMI screening and reporting. School health services are an ideal way to collect height, weight, or body mass index (BMI) information about children. These measurements are traditionally taken in a physician's office, and some observers think they should not be taken in schools.[109] But an estimated 9.2 million U.S. children and youth lack health insurance and therefore may not get regular medical care.[110] Because nearly all children attend school, these preventive screening measures would be available to all families at no cost. And collecting height and weight measures is already an established practice in schools. In 2000, 26 percent of states required schools to screen students for height and weight or body mass; of these, 61 percent required them to notify parents of the results. Among school districts, 38 percent required such screening, of which 81 percent required parental notification.[111] Taking these measures annually and converting them to an age- and gender-specific BMI percentile for each child makes it possible to monitor individual children over time. It also provides an opportunity for early intervention in obesity prevention.

A newer strategy is parental notification by health "report cards."[112] Family involvement in obesity interventions is considered integral, and sharing children's weight through report cards may help raise family awareness of children's weight status and health risk.[113] Concerns about this practice include privacy issues, the problem of labeling and stigmatizing certain children, risks that parents will place children on diets without consulting a physician, and risks of causing eating disorders.[114] Some also question whether BMI reporting can be effective if a school has an unhealthful food environment and lacks a good PE program.[115]

The Institute of Medicine endorses BMI reporting. It also recommends that schools measure each student's weight, height, and gender- and age-specific BMI percentile each year and make the information available to parents and also to the students when age-appropriate.[116] The institute acknowledges

concerns about BMI reporting and emphasizes that student data must be collected and reported validly and appropriately, with attention to privacy concerns and with information on referrals available if follow-up health services are needed.

Three school districts—Cambridge, Massachusetts; Allentown, Pennsylvania; and Citrus County, Florida—have adopted school-based BMI reporting measures.[117] They send

School health services can play a central role in addressing obesity-related issues among students by providing screening, health information, and referrals to students.

home each year a health report that includes the child's BMI percentage and a description of his or her risk category. The first study of this school-based practice, conducted with elementary school children and their parents in Cambridge, was promising.[118] Parents of overweight children who received health reports were more aware of their child's weight status and were more likely to consider looking into medical help, dieting, and physical activities for their child than parents who received general or no health information.

Arkansas also recently created a comprehensive program to combat childhood obesity. Major provisions include: conducting annual BMI screenings for all public school students, with results reported to parents; restricting access to vending machines in public elementary schools; disclosing schools' contracts with food and beverage companies; creating district advisory committees made up of parents, teachers, and local community leaders; and establishing a Child Health Advisory Committee to recommend additional physical activity and nutrition standards for public schools.[119] In 2004 Illinois required the state's Department of Health to collect height and weight measurements as part of the mandatory health exam for students. In 2005 West Virginia, Tennessee, and New York enacted legislation requiring student BMI reports.[120]

Schools as Work Sites

Schools are one of the nation's largest employers, with approximately 4 percent of the total U.S. workforce.[121] In 2001, nearly 6 million teachers and staff worked in the public school system.[122] The school setting thus holds great promise for their health promotion. Built-in advantages in this setting include fitness facilities, food service personnel, nursing and counseling staff, and health and physical education staff.[123] Work site health promotion could encourage staff and teachers to value nutrition and physical activity more highly and to heighten their commitment to adopting and implementing related programs for their students.[124] Faculty and staff who practice health-promoting behaviors could also be role models for students.[125]

Work site health promotion for faculty and staff is also part of the coordinated school health program recommended by the Centers for Disease Control and Prevention (CDC). It can include health screenings, health education, employee assistance programs, and health care.[126] But school districts lag behind other major employers in offering work site programs.[127] In schools, as in other work sites, successful programs require an involved, committed, and supportive administration.[128]

The SHPPS 2000 survey provides the first comprehensive data on work site programs.[129] Not one state requires districts or schools to fund or sponsor nutrition and dietary counseling, physical activity and fitness counseling, or programs such as walking or jogging clubs for teachers and staff. More districts and schools should implement or strengthen work site health promotion. And researchers should seek out interventions conducted in these settings to identify and replicate best practices.[130]

State and Local School Nutrition and Physical Activity Policies

While in many respects inadequate themselves, especially regarding competitive foods, USDA nutrition regulations permit state agencies and local school food authorities to impose additional restrictions on all food and beverage sales at any time in schools participating in the federal school meal programs. In recent years, many states, local school districts, and individual schools have taken up the challenge. States are also becoming more active in promoting physical activity.

Twenty-three states have adopted additional restrictions, including policies that limit the times or types of competitive foods available for sale in vending machines, cafeterias, and school stores and snack bars.[131] Most states restrict access to competitive foods when school meals are being served. Five restrict access all day long.[132] During the first six months of 2005, forty states introduced some 200 bills that provide nutritional guidance for schools. Eleven states—Arizona, California, Hawaii, Kansas, Kentucky, Louisiana, Maine,

New Mexico, South Carolina, Texas, and West Virginia—mandated nutritional standards for competitive foods.[133] See the legislative activity box for highlights of nutrition- and physical activity–related legislation enacted during the first half of 2005.

Several school districts have also taken action. More than half of the nation's ten largest school districts restrict competitive foods beyond federal and state regulations. The New York City Public School District, the nation's largest, eliminated candy, soda, and other snack foods from all vending machines starting in fall 2003. Vending machines on school grounds can sell only water, low-fat snacks, and 100 percent fruit juices.[134] The Los Angeles Unified School District passed a soda vending ban that went into effect in January 2004. A further ban on fried chips, candy, and other snack foods in school vending machines and stores went into effect in July 2004.[135] The Chicago public schools announced in 2004 a plan to ban soft drinks, candy, and high-fat snacks from school vending machines and to replace them with more healthful offerings. The Philadelphia School District recently passed a comprehensive school nutrition policy that includes nutrition education, guidelines for all foods and beverages sold in schools, family and community involvement, and program evaluation.

A 2005 report surveyed principals and found that 60 percent of schools in the 2003–04 school year had written policies in place that restricted competitive foods accessible to students, and most often school districts developed and enacted the policies. A recent study examined associations between high school students' lunch patterns and vending machine purchases and the schools' food environment and policies.[136] In schools with established policies, students reported making fewer

snack food purchases than students in schools without policies. Students at schools with open-campus policies during lunchtime were significantly more likely to eat lunch at a fast-food restaurant than students at schools with closed-campus policies. These findings suggest that school food policies that decrease access to foods high in fats and sugars are associated with less frequent consumption of these items during the school day.

A 2005 report surveyed principals and found that 60 percent of schools in the 2003–04 school year had written policies in place that restricted competitive foods accessible to students.

The Trust for America's Health recently examined state statutes and administrative codes for physical activity policies.[137] Only two states, South Dakota and Oklahoma, have no PE requirement for elementary and secondary schools. Twenty-seven states require PE in elementary, middle, and high school. Two states, Arizona and Mississippi, have no PE requirement for high school, and twenty-seven require only one-half credit or one credit of PE for graduation. Illinois is the only state that requires daily PE in every grade, although its duration is not specified. State requirements, however, are often not enforced. Amidst many other mandated curriculum requirements and tight school budgets, PE is often viewed as a low priority.[138]

Moreover, the SHPPS 2000 nationwide survey found that 17 percent of elementary

Highlights of 2005 State Legislative Activity

Nutrition-Related Legislation

Arizona has mandated the state Department of Education (DOE) to develop minimum nutrition standards that meet or exceed federal regulations for all foods and beverages sold or served at elementary and middle or junior high schools or at school-sponsored events. It also prohibits foods of minimal nutritional value from being sold or served during the school day at any elementary, middle, or junior high school campus. Finally the law forbids school administrators from signing food and beverage contracts that include the sale of sugared, carbonated beverages and all other foods of minimal nutritional value on elementary and middle or junior high school campuses.

In Kentucky the Board of Education must issue regulations that set minimum nutrition standards for all foods and beverages that are sold outside the National School Breakfast and National School Lunch Programs. State legislators also banned the sale of competitive foods and beverages, except those sold à la carte, from the first student's arrival at the school building until thirty minutes after the last lunch period. They allow only "school day–approved beverages"—defined as water, 100 percent fruit juice, low-fat milk, and any other beverage containing no more than 10 grams of sugar per serving—to be sold in elementary school vending machines, school stores, canteens, or fundraisers during the school day. The state will assess financial penalties for schools that violate the new state requirements.

Maine's legislators have asked the DOE to work with public schools to encourage nutrition education as part of a coordinated school health program. The law requires schools' food service programs to post caloric information for prepackaged à la carte items made available for purchase. In addition, the DOE must adopt policies that establish nutritional standards for food and beverage items sold outside the federal meal program. The standards must include maximum portion sizes that are consistent with the single-serving standards established by the Food and Drug Administration. It also establishes a pilot program to install vending machines that sell only flavored or unflavored milk, containing no more than 1 percent fat. Finally it mandates the DOE, in collaboration with the Department of Agriculture, Food and Rural Resources, to implement the National Farm to School Program. This program will provide locally grown fruits and vegetables to public schools.

West Virginia now prohibits the sale of soft drinks through vending machines, school stores, or on-site fundraisers during the school day in areas accessible to students in elementary and middle or junior high schools. During the school day, these schools are permitted to sell only "healthy beverages," defined as water, 100 percent fruit and vegetable juice, low-fat milk, and other juice beverages with at least 20 percent real juice. For high schools that permit the sale of soft drinks, the law also requires that "healthy beverages" must account for at least 50 percent of the total beverages offered and must be located near the vending machines containing soft drinks.

Physical Education and Physical Activity Legislation

In Kentucky each school council with grades K through 5 must develop and implement a wellness policy that includes moderate to vigorous physical activity each day. It may allow physical activity up to thirty minutes a day or 150 minutes a week to be part of instructional time. Legislators also mandated the state Board of Education to develop a physical activity environment assessment tool for school districts.

A new South Carolina law requires 150 minutes a week of physical education and physical activity for students in grades K through 5 beginning in the 2006–07 academic year. It sets student-to-certified physical education teacher ratios for elementary schools to be phased in from 700:1 for the 2006–07 academic year to 600:1 for the 2007–08 academic year and to 500:1 for the 2008–09 academic year. As the ratio is phased in, the amount of time in PE must increase from a minimum of sixty minutes a week to a minimum of ninety minutes a week, scheduled every day or on alternate days. Each elementary school must also appoint a physical education teacher to serve as its PE activity director to coordinate additional physical activity outside of PE instruction times. In addition, the DOE must provide each school district with a coordinated school health model while each school district must establish and maintain a Coordinated School Health Advisory Council to develop, implement, and evaluate a school wellness policy.

Texas legislators authorized the state Board of Education to extend its policy requiring elementary school students to engage in 30 minutes of physical activity a day or 135 minutes a week to apply to middle and junior high school students as well. Their legislation calls for health education to emphasize the importance of proper nutrition and exercise and adds reporting requirements for statistics and data related to student health and physical activity. It also establishes a state-level School Health Advisory Committee within the Department of State Health Services to provide assistance in developing and supporting coordinated school health programs and school health services.

In West Virginia each student in grades K through 5 must participate in at least thirty minutes of physical education, including physical exercise, at least three days a week. Students in grades 6 through 8 must participate in at least one full period of PE, including physical exercise, every day for one semester of the academic year. Those students in grades 9 through 12 must take at least one full PE course, including physical exercise, for high school graduation and be given the opportunity to enroll in an elective lifetime physical education course. In addition, the state Board of Education must establish a program within the existing health and PE program that incorporates fitness testing, reporting, recognition and fitness events, and incentive programs. The program will test cardiovascular fitness, muscular strength and endurance, flexibility, and body composition.

Source: Health Policy Tracking Service, a Thomson West Business, *State Actions to Promote Nutrition, Increase Physical Activity, and Prevent Obesity: A Legislative Overview*, July 11, 2005 (www.netscan.com/outside/HPTSServices.asp [August 22, 2005]).

schools, 25 percent of middle and junior high schools, and 40 percent of high schools exempt from required PE courses those students who participate in community or school sports or in other school activities or who have high physical competency test scores.[139] And few states and districts require skill performance tests, fitness tests, or written knowledge tests.

Recent legislative activity, however, as seen in the legislative activity box, demonstrates promising attention to this area of children's development. Several states are encouraging, not mandating, state and local education officials to enhance PE and physical activity in schools. During the first half of 2005, six states—North Dakota, Montana, Utah, Colorado, Tennessee, and Washington—adopted such resolutions.[140] In April 2005, the North Carolina State Board of Education voted to require thirty minutes of daily physical activity for all students in grades K–8 beginning in the 2006–07 school year.

Federal Policy Initiatives

The most recent federal policy initiatives for preventing childhood obesity are found in the Child Nutrition and Women, Infants, and Children (WIC) Reauthorization Act of 2004,

---

Several interventions have shown that the availability, promotion, and pricing of foods in schools can be changed to support more healthful food choices.

---

which requires each school district that participates in the federal school meal program to enact a wellness policy by the day the 2006–2007 school year opens. School districts must set goals for nutrition education and physical activity, write nutrition guidelines for all foods available at school, ensure that school meal guidelines are not less restrictive than federal requirements, and evaluate how well the new policy is implemented. Parents, students, the school food service, and school administrators must be involved in developing the new policy. The Food Research and Action Center and the National Alliance for Nutrition and Activity are developing information and guidelines to assist states and school districts.

The Child Nutrition and WIC Reauthorization Act also expanded a USDA pilot pro-

gram begun by the 2002 Farm Act that provided fresh fruits and vegetables at no cost to children in 107 elementary and secondary schools in four states and on one Indian reservation. A 2003 evaluation found that most participating schools considered the pilot program successful and felt strongly that it should continue.[141] The expanded program will serve children in four more states and two more Indian reservations, with special emphasis on low-income children.[142]

School-Based Obesity-Prevention Interventions

Many school-based interventions in recent years have promoted healthful eating and physical activity among children and adolescents, but relatively few interventions have specifically targeted obesity prevention. Several comprehensive reviews have summarized the research analyzing obesity-prevention, nutrition, and physical activity intervention.[143] Overall, the findings of studies that targeted eating and physical activity behaviors have been positive. School-based obesity-prevention interventions have also shown some success in changing eating and physical activity behaviors but have been less effective in changing body weight or body fatness.[144] A recent report by the Task Force on Community Preventive Services concluded that insufficient evidence existed to determine the effectiveness of combined nutrition and physical activity interventions to prevent or reduce obesity in school settings. The limited number of qualifying studies, for example, report noncomparable outcomes.[145]

In one such study, T. N. Robinson found that a school-based intervention to decrease television and video viewing reduced the prevalence of obesity among third and fourth graders.[146] Planet Health, a school-based intervention to decrease television viewing and increase physical activity and healthful eating among students, decreased obesity among girls but not boys.[147] A third intervention, which reduced soft drink consumption in England, lowered the number of overweight and obese children aged seven to eleven.[148]

Several interventions have changed food environments in schools, reducing the fat content of school lunches and modifying the prices of fruits and vegetables in the school cafeteria and in vending machines.[149] They have shown that the availability, promotion, and pricing of foods in schools can be changed to support more healthful food choices. Interventions are just beginning to target the availability of competitive foods and beverages. Little research has been done on the effects of school, district, or state policy changes regarding the school food environment or changes in student dietary outcomes or in body mass indexes.

Studies have also shown that school PE classes can be changed to make them much more active and increase the time spent in PE and in moderate to vigorous activity.[150] One recent analysis found that an extra hour of PE per week in first grade (compared with time spent in PE in kindergarten) lowered BMI in girls who had been overweight or at risk for overweight in kindergarten.[151] No effect was seen in boys. Interventions to increase energy expenditure through increased physical activity and decreased consumption of high-calorie, low-nutrition foods offer promising strategies for preventing obesity.

The few existing school-based obesity-prevention studies suggest that interventions hold promise.[152] For future studies, researchers should strengthen interventions and should target the school environment, the home environment, and student and par-

ent behaviors.[153] Interventions could modify the home environment by installing devices to monitor television time or by increasing the availability of healthful foods and limiting energy-dense, low-nutrition foods. School environment changes could include more frequent required PE classes, more interesting and fun physical education choices, and school-wide guidelines about food and beverage availability and sales.[154]

Research can also help reveal whether specific forms of interventions have different effects on children of different age, gender, or ethnic groups. For example, targeting particular behaviors may be more successful with one age group than with another. Younger children may respond better to reducing television viewing while adolescents may benefit from more structured and diverse PE opportunities. Changing à la carte and vending machine food and beverage availability may be more effective for high school students than for elementary school students. More research is also needed to identify obesity prevention's most potent behavioral targets, such as limiting screen time, sugar-sweetened beverages, and portion sizes.

School Links with Communities and Families

Although most physical activity and nutrition programs directed at youth are conducted in school, communities can also provide important resources. And family involvement is often crucial.

Farm-to-School Programs and School Gardens

Some schools are offering new farm-to-school programs that link local farmers with school cafeterias. The programs provide high-quality local produce, support locally based agriculture, and often directly connect farmers and children with reciprocal visits. Some schools also sponsor gardening programs. The Martin Luther King Junior Middle School in Berkeley, California, offers the Edible Schoolyard, a nonprofit program that allows students to participate in all aspects of organic gardening and cooking, from seed to table.[155] Such hands-on experience may encourage children to eat more healthfully. A recent study at three schools in California examined fourth graders' knowledge of nutrition and their preference for certain vegetables.[156] Students at one school received nutrition education, those at a second school received nutrition education and planted and harvested a vegetable garden, and those at a third served as a control group. Children who received nutrition education alone and those who received nutrition education combined with gardening had much higher scores than the control group. Children who gardened also increased their preferences for certain vegetables.

Walking and Biking to School

In recent decades, dramatically fewer children have been walking or biking to school. In 1969, 48 percent of students walked or biked to school. By 2001, less than 15 percent of students aged five to fifteen walked to or from school, and just 1 percent biked.[157] Today roughly one-third of students ride a school bus, and half are driven in a private vehicle.[158] Because the trip to and from school happens daily, active commuting (walking or biking) can provide substantial caloric expenditures over the school year.[159] One study used accelerometers, small electronic devices worn around the waist that capture minute-by-minute recordings of activity level, to measure physical activity among fourteen- to sixteen-year-old students. It found that boys who walked to school expended forty-four more calories a day and

girls expended thirty-three more calories a day than did their peers who were driven.[160] Projected over the course of a school year, or 200 days, this additional physical activity could account for a two- to three-pound difference between those who walk to school and those who do not, all other things held constant.

To examine why most children do not walk or bike to school, the CDC analyzed data from the annual national HealthStyles Survey.[161] Households with children aged five to eighteen were asked if their children walked or biked to school and about any barriers they faced in doing so. Reported barriers included long distances (55 percent), traffic danger (40 percent), bad weather (24 percent), crime (18 percent), opposing school policy (7 percent), and other reasons (26 percent). Sixteen percent of respondents reported no barriers; notably, within this group, 64 percent reported children walking and 21 percent reported children biking to or from school at least once a week in the preceding month.

One major cause of active commuting's decline is the trend toward constructing schools away from the center of communities.[162] Students with shorter walk and bike times to school are more likely to walk and bike. Recent nationwide trends toward bigger schools have also led to the decline of the "neighborhood" school. Since World War II, the number of schools has declined 70 percent, while the average size has grown fivefold. Today, however, communities are increasingly concerned about school siting decisions as they relate to children's health and overweight status. Communities, families, school districts, and governments at all levels have begun mobilizing to facilitate active commuting by improving pedestrian and biking safety, adding bike racks and crossing guards, mapping safe routes to schools, building new schools or renovating older schools in residential neighborhoods, and forming such programs as the Walking School Bus, Bike Trains, Safe Route to School, National Walk Our Children to School Day, and the federal Kids Walk-to-School Campaign.[163] Programs that involve adult volunteers—such as the Walking School Bus, which organizes neighborhood chaperones to supervise children as they walk to school—also increase physical activity among adults.[164]

After-School Programs

After-school programs in child care centers, schools, and community centers also offer opportunities to implement obesity-prevention strategies. The 1990s saw a substantial increase in after-school programs serving children of low-income families.[165] One of the best known is the federally funded 21st Century Community Learning Centers, a school-based after-school program providing academic enrichment and youth development opportunities. Federal funding grew from $40 million in 1997 to almost $1 billion in 2005. In 2001, 1.2 million elementary and middle school students in 3,600 schools participated.[166] Implementing obesity-prevention strategies in the 21st Century Community Learning Centers would not only reach many young people directly but also offer a model for other such programs.

A recent survey found that most after-school programs do not address physical activity and healthful eating, and that staff at many after-school programs are untrained.[167] But some programs are leading the way. For example, the Girls Health Enrichment Multi-Site Studies (GEMS) program aimed to prevent obesity among eight- to ten-year-old African American girls. In a set of four pilot interventions, girls and their parents were recruited through schools and other community channels to participate in after-school programs, such as ethnic dance, that targeted healthful eating, physical activity, and reduced television viewing.[168] The results of the GEMS pilot interventions were promising, demonstrating the feasibility and potential effectiveness of incorporating obesity-prevention efforts into after-school programs.

Federal funds are available to provide after-school snacks to children up to age eighteen

---

A recent survey found that most after-school programs do not address physical activity and healthful eating, and that staff at many after-school programs are untrained.

---

in after-school programs operated by schools, nonprofit organizations, and public agencies. Both the federal school lunch program and the Child and Adult Care Food Program (CACFP) offer cash reimbursements to after-school programs for snacks. Subsidies vary by the child's family income, as they do for breakfasts and lunches. Subsidies are provided with CACFP funds to provide free snacks in programs located in areas where 50 percent or more of the children enrolled in school are eligible for free or reduced-priced school meals. Participation in the after-school snack program has increased dramatically, from some 645,000 children in 1999 to about 1.2 million in 2003.[169] Reimbursable snacks must follow the CACFP's snack requirements, but more research is needed to assess the nutritional value of the snack foods being offered and to find ways to serve more fruits and vegetables.

Congress has recently allowed after-school programs in seven states—Delaware, Illinois, Michigan, Missouri, New York, Oregon, and Pennsylvania—to serve suppers as well as snacks to children in areas where more than 50 percent of the children qualify for free or reduced-price school meals.[170] Some low-income children may thus eat three meals and a snack every weekday during the school year from federal food programs—a fact that highlights both the growing importance of the federal child nutrition programs for children in low-income families and the need to ensure that the foods these programs serve are consistent with the recommendations in the *Dietary Guidelines for Americans.*

Family Involvement
Parents and caregivers provide the primary social environment in which children form attitudes and behaviors regarding eating and physical activity. Parents create an environment conducive to active or sedentary lifestyles, they select foods brought into the home, they determine how often and what types of meals are eaten outside the home, and they model eating and physical activity behaviors. Thus, to achieve maximal and sustained behavior change, parents and caregivers must be involved in obesity prevention.

Reviews of efforts to prevent youth high-risk behaviors, such as school failure, aggressive behaviors, and substance abuse, have found that combined school and family programs deliver more benefits than those managed separately.[171] Most obesity-prevention programs, however, have focused almost exclusively on school programs. Actively involving

parents is not always easy, but some programs that included families achieved high rates of recruitment and retention (around 80 percent) by using such incentives as food, child care, transportation, and rewards for homework completion or attendance.[172] Community organizations and other local resources can also help schools connect with low-income and minority parents.[173] One creative and effective way to involve parents is to make school gyms and swimming pools available to students and their families after school and on weekends.

Recommendations for Schools
Schools can become one of the nation's most effective weapons in the fight against obesity by creating an environment that is conducive to healthful eating and physical activity. Health and success in school are interrelated; schools cannot achieve their primary educational mission if their students and staff are not healthy and physically, mentally, and socially fit. Each school can follow ten key strategies, taken from CDC guidelines for its coordinated school health program, to promote lifelong physical activity and healthful eating for its population:

—address physical activity and nutrition through a Coordinated School Health Program approach,

—designate a school health coordinator and maintain an active school health council,

—assess the school's health policies and programs and develop a plan for improvement,

—strengthen the school's nutrition and physical activity policies,

—implement a high-quality health promotion program for school staff,

—carry out a high-quality course of study in health education,

—implement a high-quality PE course,

—increase opportunities for students to engage in physical activity,

—offer a quality school meals program, and

—ensure that students have appealing, healthful choices in foods and beverages offered outside of the school meals program.[174]

The Institute of Medicine report, *Preventing Childhood Obesity: Health in the Balance*, also offers comprehensive recommendations regarding school efforts to advance obesity prevention and outlines immediate steps schools can take to improve healthful eating and physical activity.[175] Among those steps are improving the nutritional quality of foods and beverages served and sold in schools and as part of school-related activities, increasing opportunities for physical activity during and after school, implementing school-based interventions to reduce children's screen time, and developing, implementing, and evaluating innovative pilot programs for both staffing and teaching about wellness, healthful eating, and physical activity.

Conclusion

Research consistently shows that the diets of most U.S. children fail to meet national nutrition guidelines. Nor do most U.S. children get the recommended levels of daily physical activity. As a result, today a larger share of the nation's children is overweight than at any time in history. The prevalence of obesity, having increased dramatically over the past forty years, now threatens the immediate and long-term health of children and youth.

With more than 54 million children in attendance daily, the nations' schools offer many opportunities for developing strategies to prevent childhood obesity. Children spend roughly a third of every weekday in school. While they are there, they can consume up to two meals, sometimes even three, plus snacks. They have many different avenues for recreation and physical activity. They also take courses in health education and receive health services of various kinds at school. If schools can work together with policymakers, advocates, parents, and communities to create an environment where children eat healthfully, become physically fit, and develop lifelong habits that contribute to wellness, the nation will be well on its way to preventing obesity.

Notes

1. U.S. Department of Health and Human Services (DHHS) and U.S. Department of Agriculture (USDA), *Dietary Guidelines for Americans, 2005* (Government Printing Office, 2005); U.S. Department of Health and Human Services, *Healthy People 2010: Understanding and Improving Health,* 2nd ed. (GPO, 2000).

2. Centers for Disease Control and Prevention, "Quickstats: Prevalence of Overweight among Children and Teenagers, by Age Group and Selected Period, U.S., 1963–2002," *Morbidity and Mortality Weekly Report* 54, no. 8 (2005): 203.

3. DHHS and USDA, *Dietary Guidelines for Americans* (see note 1); Jeffrey P. Koplan, Catharyn T. Liverman, and Vivica I. Kraak, eds., *Preventing Childhood Obesity: Health in the Balance* (Washington: National Academies Press, 2005).

4. Action for Healthy Kids, *The Learning Connection: The Value of Improving Nutrition and Physical Activity in Our Schools,* 2004 (www.ActionForHealthyKids.org [July 7, 2005]).

5. J. B. Schwimmer, T. M. Burwinkle, and J. W. Varni, "Health-Related Quality of Life of Severely Obese Children and Adolescents," *Journal of the American Medical Association* 289, no. 14 (2003): 1813–19; A. M. Tershakovec, S. C. Weller, and P. R. Gallagher, "Obesity, School Performance and Behaviour of Black, Urban Elementary School Children," *International Journal of Obesity & Related Metabolic Disorders* 18, no. 5 (1994): 323–27.

6. National Institute for Health Care Management Foundation, *Obesity in Young Children: Impact and Intervention,* Research Brief (Washington: August 2004) (www.nihcm.org [July 7, 2005]); A. Datar, R. Sturm, and J. L. Magnabosco, "Childhood Overweight and Academic Performance: National Study of Kindergartners and First-Graders," *Obesity Research* 12, no. 1 (2004): 58–68.

7. Action for Healthy Kids, *The Learning Connection* (see note 4).

8. National Institute for Health Care Management Foundation, *Obesity in Young Children* (see note 6); A. Must and others, "The Disease Burden Associated with Overweight and Obesity," *Journal of the American Medical Association* 282, no. 16 (1999): 1523–29; U.S. Department of Health and Human Services, *The Surgeon General's Call to Action to Prevent and Decrease Overweight and Obesity* (Rockville, Md.: 2001).

9. National Institute for Health Care Management Foundation, *Obesity in Young Children* (see note 6); I. Janssen and others, "Associations between Overweight and Obesity with Bullying Behaviors in School-Aged Children," *Pediatrics* 113, no. 5 (2004): 1187–94.

10. L. Parker, *The Relationship between Nutrition and Learning: A School Employee's Guide to Information and Action* (Washington: National Education Association, 1989).

11. G. C. Rampersaud and others, "Breakfast Habits, Nutritional Status, Body Weight, and Academic Performance in Children and Adolescents," *Journal of the American Dietetic Association* 105, no. 5 (2005): 743–60.

12. Action for Healthy Kids, *The Learning Connection* (see note 4).

13. H. Taras, "Physical Activity and Student Performance at School," *Journal of School Health* 75, no. 6 (2005): 214–18.

14. Ibid.

15. Phil Gleason, Carol Suitor, and U.S. Food and Nutrition Service, *Children's Diets in the Mid-1990s: Dietary Intake and Its Relationship with School Meal Participation*, Special Nutrition Programs, Report no. CN-01-CD1 (Alexandria, Va.: U.S. Dept of Agriculture, Food and Nutrition Service, 2001).

16. Trust for America's Health, "F as in Fat: How Obesity Policies Are Failing in America" (www.healthyamericans.org [March 22, 2005]).

17. M. K. Fox, W. Hamilton, and B. H. Lin, *Effects of Food Assistance and Nutrition Programs on Health and Nutrition*, vol. 3: *Literature Review,* Food Assistance and Nutrition Research Report no. 19-3 (Washington: U.S. Department of Agriculture, Economic Research Service, 2004).

18. Ibid.

19. M. K. Fox and others, *School Nutrition Dietary Assessment Study II: Summary of Findings* (Alexandria, Va.: U.S. Department of Agriculture, Food and Nutrition Service, Office of Analysis, Nutrition, and Evaluation, 2001).

20. Ibid.

21. Gleason, Suitor, and U.S. Food and Nutrition Service, *Children's Diets in the Mid-1990s* (see note 15); Fox and others, *School Nutrition Dietary Assessment Study* (see note 19).

22. Gleason, Suitor, and U.S. Food and Nutrition Service, *Children's Diets in the Mid-1990s* (see note 15).

23. Ibid.

24. Food Research and Action Center, "State of the States, 2005: A Profile of Food and Nutrition Programs across the Nation" (www.frac.org [March 22, 2005]).

25. Gleason, Suitor, and U.S. Food and Nutrition Service, *Children's Diets in the Mid-1990s* (see note 15).

26. U.S. Department of Agriculture, Food and Nutrition Service, "About the Child Nutrition Commodity Programs" (www.fns.usda.gov/fdd/programs/schcnp/about-cnp.htm [August 15, 2005]).

27. Josephine Martin, "Overview of Federal Child Nutrition Legislation," in *Managing Child Nutrition Programs: Leadership for Excellence*, edited by Josephine Martin and Martha T. Conklin (Gaithersburg, Md.: Aspen Publishers, 1999).

28. Food Research and Action Center, "Income Guidelines and Reimbursement Rates for the Federal Child Nutrition Programs Effective July 1, 2005–June 30, 2006," 2005 (www.frac.org [August 22, 2005]).

29. U.S. Department of Agriculture, Food and Nutrition Service, "About the Child Nutrition Commodity Programs" (see note 26).

30. U.S. General Accounting Office, *School Lunch Program: Efforts Needed to Improve Nutrition and Encourage Healthy Eating*, Report no. GAO-03-506 (May 2003).

31. U.S. Department of Agriculture, *Foods Sold in Competition with USDA School Meal Programs: A Report to Congress* (2001) (www.fns.usda.gov/cnd/Lunch/CompetitiveFoods/report_congress.htm [May 25, 2005]).

32. *Federal Register* 70, no. 136 (January 18, 2005): 41196–99.

33. U.S. General Accounting Office, *School Meal Programs: Revenue and Expense Information from Selected States*, Report no. GAO-03-569 (2003).

34. Ibid.

35. Robert Wood Johnson Foundation, *Healthy Schools for Healthy Kids* (Princeton, N.J.: 2003).

36. U.S. General Accounting Office, *School Meal Programs* (see note 33).

37. Fox and others, *School Nutrition Dietary Assessment Study* (see note 19).

38. U.S. Department of Agriculture, *Foods Sold in Competition with USDA School Meal Programs* (see note 31).

39. Koplan, Liverman, and Kraak, *Preventing Childhood Obesity* (see note 3).

40. U.S. General Accounting Office, *School Meal Programs: Competitive Foods Are Available in Many Schools; Actions Taken to Restrict Them Differ by State and Locality*, Report no. GAO-04-673 (2004).

41. Food Research and Action Center, *Competitive Foods in Schools: Child Nutrition Policy Brief*, 2004 (www.frac.org [March 22, 2005]).

42. Ibid.

43. U.S. General Accounting Office, *School Meal Programs: Competitive Foods* (see note 40); H. Wechsler and others, "Using the School Environment to Promote Physical Activity and Healthy Eating," *Preventive Medicine* 31, suppl. (2000): S121–37; Simone A. French and others, "Food Environment in Secondary Schools: A la Carte, Vending Machines, and Food Policies and Practices," *American Journal of Public Health* 93, no. 7 (2003): 1161–67; Lisa Harnack and others, "Availability of à la Carte Food Items in Junior and Senior High Schools: A Needs Assessment," *Journal of the American Dietetic Association* 100, no. 6 (2000): 701–03; Marianne B. Wildey and others, "Fat and Sugar Levels Are High in Snacks Purchased from Student Stores in Middle Schools," *Journal of the American Dietetic Association* 100, no. 3 (2000): 319–22.

44. H. Wechsler and others, "Food Service and Foods and Beverages Available at School: Results from the School Health Policies and Programs Study 2000," *Journal of School Health* 71, no. 7 (2001): 313–24.

45. Ibid.

46. French and others, "Food Environment in Secondary Schools" (see note 43).

47. U.S. Government Accountability Office, *School Meal Programs: Competitive Foods Are Widely Available and Generate Substantial Revenues for Schools*, Report no. GA0-05-563 (August 2005).

48. Wechsler and others, "Food Service and Foods and Beverages Available at School" (see note 44).

49. U.S. General Accounting Office, *School Meal Programs: Competitive Foods* (see note 40); French and others, "Food Environment in Secondary Schools" (see note 43); Harnack and others, "Availability of à la Carte Food Items in Junior and Senior High Schools" (see note 43); Lisa Craypo and others, "Fast Food Sales on High School Campuses: Results from the 2000 California High School Fast Food Survey," *Journal of School Health* 72, no. 2 (2002): 78–82; Lisa Craypo, Sarah E. Samuels, and Amanda Purcell, *The 2003 California High School Fast Food Survey* (Oakland, Calif.: Public Health Institute, 2004) (www.phi.org [August 22, 2005]).

50. French and others, "Food Environment in Secondary Schools" (see note 43).

51. Ibid.

52. Craypo, Samuels, and Purcell, *The 2003 California High School Fast Food Survey* (see note 49).

53. Wechsler and others, "Food Service and Foods and Beverages Available at School" (see note 44).

54. Craypo, Samuels, and Purcell, *The 2003 California High School Fast Food Survey* (see note 49).

55. Martha Y. Kubik and others, "The Association of the School Food Environment with Dietary Behaviors of Young Adolescents," *American Journal of Public Health* 93, no. 7 (2003): 1168–73.

56. Karen Weber Cullen and Issa Zakeri, "Fruits, Vegetables, Milk, and Sweetened Beverages Consumption and Access to à la Carte/Snack Bar Meals at School," *American Journal of Public Health* 94, no. 3 (2004): 463–67.

57. S. B. Templeton, M. A. Marlette, and M. Panemangalore, "Competitive Foods Increase the Intake of Energy and Decrease the Intake of Certain Nutrients by Adolescents Consuming School Lunch," *Journal of the American Dietetic Association* 105, no. 2 (2005): 215–20.

58. U.S. General Accounting Office, *Commercial Activities in Schools*, Report no. GAO/HEHS-00-156 (September 2000).

59. Patricia M. Anderson and Kristin F. Butcher, "Reading, Writing, and Raisinets: Are School Finances Contributing to Children's Obesity?" (Cambridge, Mass.: National Bureau of Economic Research, March 2005) (www.nber.org/papers/w11177 [June 21, 2005]).

60. U.S. Government Accountability Office, *School Meal Programs* (see note 47).

61. U.S. General Accounting Office, *Commercial Activities in Schools* (see note 58).

62. M. Nestle, "Soft Drink 'Pouring Rights': Marketing Empty Calories to Children," *Public Health Reports* 115, no. 4 (2000): 308–19.

63. M. Nestle, *Food Politics: How the Food Industry Influences Nutrition and Health* (Los Angeles: University of California Press, 2002).

64. American Beverage Association, Press Release: "Beverage Industry Announces New School Vending Policy" (www.ameribev.org/pressroom/2005_vending.asp [August 16, 2005]).

65. U.S. Senate Committee on Agriculture, Nutrition, and Forestry, "Food Choices at School: Risks to Child Nutrition and Health Call for Action," prepared by the Democratic Staff of the Senate Committee on Agriculture, Nutrition, and Forestry, May 18, 2004.

66. L. A. Lytle and others, "Environmental Outcomes from the Teens Study: Influencing Healthful Food Choices in School and Home Environments," *Health Education & Behavior* (forthcoming); Simone A. French and others, "An Environmental Intervention to Promote Lower-Fat Food Choices in Secondary Schools: Outcomes of the TACOS Study," *American Journal of Public Health* 94, no. 9 (2004): 1507–12.

67. Center for Science in the Public Interest, *Dispensing Junk: How School Vending Undermines Efforts to Feed Children Well*, 2004 (www.cspinet.org/schoolfoods [March 22, 2005]).

68. U.S. Department of Agriculture, Food and Nutrition Service, Centers for Disease Control and Prevention, U.S. Department of Health and Human Services, and U.S. Department of Education, *Making It Happen! School Nutrition Success Stories* (Alexandria, Va.: January 2005) (www.fns.usda.gov/tn/Resources/ makingithappen. html [June 30, 2005]).

69. Texas Department of Agriculture, "School District Vending Contract Survey, 2003" (www.squaremeals.org [March 24, 2005]).

70. U.S. Government Accountability Office, *School Meal Programs* (see note 47).

71. Ibid.

72. U.S. Senate Committee on Agriculture, Nutrition, and Forestry, "Food Choices at School" (see note 65).

73. Ibid.

74. U.S. Department of Agriculture and others, *Making It Happen!* (see note 68).

75. Centers for Disease Control and Prevention, "Guidelines for School and Community Programs to Promote Lifelong Physical Activity among Young People," *Morbidity and Mortality Weekly Report* 46 (1997): 1–36; C. R. Burgeson, "Physical Education's Critical Role in Educating the Whole Child and Reducing Childhood Obesity," *State Education Standard* 5, no. 2 (2004): 27–32.

76. Ibid.

77. Michigan Department of Education, "Brain Breaks: A Physical Activity Idea Book for Elementary Classroom Teachers" (www.emc.cmich.edu/BrainBreaks/default.htm [July 7, 2005]); International Life Sciences Institute, "Take 10!" (www.take10.net [August 18, 2005]).

78. J. F. Sallis, "Behavioral and Environmental Interventions to Promote Youth Physical Activity and Prevent Obesity," June 22, 2003 (www-rohan.sdsu.edu/faculty/sallis/Sallis_PA_interventions_for_Georgia_6.03.pdf [May 30, 2005]).

79. Burgeson, "Physical Education's Critical Role" (see note 75).

80. DHHS and Department of Agriculture, *Dietary Guidelines for Americans, 2005* (see note 1); National Association for Sport and Physical Education, *Physical Activity for Children: A Statement of Guidelines for Children 5–12*, 2nd ed. (Reston, Va.: 2004).

81. Koplan, Liverman, and Kraak, *Preventing Childhood Obesity* (see note 3).

82. National Association for Sport and Physical Education, *Physical Activity for Children* (see note 80).

83. C. R. Burgeson and others, "Physical Education and Activity: Results from the School Health Policies and Programs Study 2000," *Journal of School Health* 71, no. 7 (2001): 279–93.

84. Ibid.

85. J. A. Grunbaum and others, "Youth Risk Behavior Surveillance—United States, 2003," *Morbidity and Mortality Weekly Report* 53, no. 2 (2004): 1–96.

86. DHHS, *Healthy People 2010* (see note 1).

87. Burgeson, "Physical Education's Critical Role" (see note 75).

88. National Association for Sport and Physical Education, *Shape of the Nation: Executive Summary* (Reston, Va.: 2001).

89. President's Council on Physical Fitness and Sports Research Digest, *Physical Activity Promotion and School Physical Education* (Washington: September 1999) (www.fitness.gov/digest_sep1999.htm [July 7, 2005]); C. W. Symons and others, "Bridging Student Health Risks and Academic Achievement through Comprehensive School Health Programs," *Journal of School Health* 67, no. 6 (1997): 220–27; R. J. Shephard, "Curricular Physical Activity and Academic Performance," *Pediatric Exercise Science* 9 (1997): 113–26; J. F. Sallis and others, "Effects of Health-Related Physical Education on Academic Achievement: Project Spark," *Research Quarterly for Exercise & Sport* 70, no. 2 (1999): 127–34.

90. National Association for Sport and Physical Education and Council on Physical Education for Children, *Position Paper: Recess in Elementary Schools*, 2001 (www.aahperd.org/naspe/pdf_files/pos_papers/current_res.pdf [July 7, 2005]).

91. O. S. Jarrett, "Effect of Recess on Classroom Behavior: Group Effects and Individual Differences," *Journal of Education Research* 92, no. 2 (1998): 121–26.

92. Burgeson and others, "Physical Education and Activity" (see note 83).

93. National Association for Sport and Physical Education and Council on Physical Education for Children, *Position Paper* (see note 90).

94. Burgeson and others, "Physical Education and Activity" (see note 83).

95. Symons and others, "Bridging Student Health Risks and Academic Achievement" (see note 89).

96. Centers for Disease Control and Prevention, "Coordinated School Health Program" (www.cdc.gov/HealthyYouth/CSHP/ [July 15, 2005]).

97. L. Kann, N. D. Brener, and D. D. Allensworth, "Health Education: Results from the School Health Policies and Programs Study 2000," *Journal of School Health* 71, no. 7 (2001): 266–78; National Association of State Boards of Education, *National Commission on the Role of the School and Community in Improving Adolescent Health, Code Blue: Uniting for Healthier Youth* (Alexandria, Va.: 1990).

98. Koplan, Liverman, and Kraak, *Preventing Childhood Obesity* (see note 3).

99. Trust for America's Health, "F as in Fat" (see note 16).

100. Kann, Brener, and Allensworth, "Health Education" (see note 97).

101. Ibid.; L. A. Lytle and C. Achterberg, "Changing the Diet of America's Children: What Works and Why?" *Journal of Nutrition Education* 27, no. 5 (1995): 250–60.

102. U.S. General Accounting Office, *School Lunch Program* (see note 30).

103. N. D. Brener and others, "Health Services: Results from the School Health Policies and Programs Study 2000," *Journal of School Health* 71, no. 7 (2001): 294–304; D. D. Allensworth, "School Health Services: Issues and Challenges," in *The Comprehensive School Health Challenge: Promoting Health through Education,* vol. 1, edited by P. Cortese and K. Middleton (Santa Cruz, Calif.: ETR Associates, 1994).

104. Brener and others, "Health Services" (see note 103).

105. The Center for Health and Health Care in Schools, George Washington University, "2002 State Survey of School-Based Health Center Initiatives" (www.healthinschools.org/sbhcs/survey02.htm [July 5, 2005]).

106. Ibid.

107. Ibid.

108. The Center for Health and Health Care in Schools, George Washington University, "School-Based Health Centers: Background" (www.healthinschools.org/sbhcs/sbhc.asp [July 5, 2005]).

109. L. M. Scheier, "School Health Report Cards Attempt to Address the Obesity Epidemic," *Journal of the American Dietetic Association* 104, no. 3 (2004): 341–44.

110. S. Bhandari and E. Gifford, *Children with Health Insurance: 2001*, Current Population Report P60-224 (U.S. Census Bureau, 2003).

111. Brener and others, "Health Services" (see note 103).

112. Scheier, "School Health Report Cards" (see note 109).

113. Ibid.

114. Koplan, Liverman, and Kraak, *Preventing Childhood Obesity* (see note 3); Scheier, "School Health Report Cards" (see note 109).

115. Scheier, "School Health Report Cards" (see note 109); B. R. Morris, "Letters on Students' Weight Ruffle Parents," *New York Times*, March 26 2002, p. F7.

116. Koplan, Liverman, and Kraak, *Preventing Childhood Obesity* (see note 3).

117. Scheier, "School Health Report Cards" (see note 109).

118. Ibid.

119. James Raczynski and others, "Establishing a Baseline to Evaluate Act 1220 of 2003: An Act of the Arkansas General Assembly to Combat Childhood Obesity" (University of Arkansas for Medical Sciences College of Public Health, 2005).

120. Health Policy Tracking Service, a Thomson West Business, *State Actions to Promote Nutrition, Increase Physical Activity, and Prevent Obesity: A Legislative Overview*, July 11, 2005 (www.netscan.com/outside/HPTSServices.asp [August 22, 2005]).

121. J. A. Grunbaum, S. J. Rutman, and P. R. Sathrum, "Faculty and Staff Health Promotion: Results from the School Health Policies and Programs Study 2000," *Journal of School Health* 71, no. 7 (2001): 335–39.

122. U.S. Department of Education and National Center for Education Statistics, "Elementary and Secondary Education—Table 82: Staff and Teachers in Public Elementary and Secondary School Systems, by State or Jurisdiction, Fall 1995 to Fall 2001," *Digest of Education Statistics*, 2003 (nces.ed.gov/programs/digest/d03/tables/dt082.asp [July 5, 2005]).

123. D. J. Ballard, P. M. Kingery, and B. E. Pruitt, "School Worksite Health Promotion: An Interdependent Process," *Journal of Health Education* 22 (1991): 111–15.

124. Mary Story and Dianne Neumark-Sztainer, "School-Based Nutrition Education Programs and Services for Adolescents," *Adolescent Medicine: State of the Art Reviews* 7 (1996): 287–302.

125. Grunbaum, Rutman, and Sathrum, "Faculty and Staff Health Promotion" (see note 121).

126. Centers for Disease Control and Prevention, "Coordinated School Health Program" (see note 96); Grunbaum, Rutman, and Sathrum, "Faculty and Staff Health Promotion" (see note 121).

127. C. A. Galemore, "Worksite Wellness in the School Setting," *Journal of School Nursing* 16, no. 2 (2000): 42–45.

128. C. C. Cox, R. Misra, and S. Aguillion, "Superintendents' Perceptions of School-Site Health Promotion in Missouri," *Journal of School Health* 67, no. 2 (1997): 50–55.

129. Grunbaum, Rutman, and Sathrum, "Faculty and Staff Health Promotion" (see note 121).

130. A. Fiske and K. W. Cullen, "Effects of Promotional Materials on Vending Sales of Low-Fat Items in Teachers' Lounges," *Journal of the American Dietetic Association* 104, no. 1 (2004): 90–93; K. Resnicow and others, "Results of the Teachwell Worksite Wellness Program," *American Journal of Public Health* 88, no. 2 (1998): 250–57.

131. Trust for America's Health, "F as in Fat" (see note 16); Health Policy Tracking Service, *State Actions to Promote Nutrition* (see note 120).

132. U.S. General Accounting Office, *School Meal Programs* (see note 40).

133. Health Policy Tracking Service, *State Actions to Promote Nutrition* (see note 120).

134. U.S. General Accounting Office, *School Meal Programs: Competitive Foods Are Available in Many Schools* (see note 40).

135. Ibid.

136. U.S. Government Accountability Office, *School Meal Programs* (see note 47); Dianne Neumark-Sztainer and others, "School Lunch and Snacking Patterns among High School Students: Associations with School Food Environment and Policies," *International Journal of Behavioral Nutrition and Physical Activity* 2, no. 14 (2005) (www.ijbnpa.org/content/2/1/14 [October 6, 2005]).

137. Trust for America's Health, "F as in Fat" (see note 16).

138. Ibid.

139. Burgeson and others, "Physical Education and Activity" (see note 83).

140. Health Policy Tracking Service, *State Actions to Promote Nutrition* (see note 120).

141. J. C. Buzby, J. F. Guthrie, and L. S. Kantor, *Evaluation of the USDA Fruit and Vegetable Pilot Program: Report to Congress*, Report no. E-FAN-03-006 (U.S. Department of Agriculture, May 2003).

142. Ibid.

143. Koplan, Liverman, and Kraak, *Preventing Childhood Obesity* (see note 3); Simone French and Mary Story, "Obesity Prevention in Schools," in *Handbook of Pediatric Obesity: Etiology, Pathophysiology, and Prevention*, edited by M. I. Goran (Boca Raton, Fla.: CRC Press, forthcoming); T. Lobstein, L. Baur, and

R. Uauy, "Obesity in Children and Young People: A Crisis in Public Health," *Obesity Reviews* 5, suppl. 1 (2004): 4–104; K. Resnicow and T. N. Robinson, "School-Based Cardiovascular Disease Prevention Studies: Review and Synthesis," *Annals of Epidemiology* S7, no. 1997 (1997): S14–31; K. Campbell and others, "Interventions for Preventing Obesity in Childhood: A Systematic Review," *Obesity Reviews* 2, no. 3 (2001): 149–57; Mary Story, "School-Based Approaches for Preventing and Treating Obesity," *International Journal of Obesity and Related Metabolic Disorders* 23, suppl. 2 (1999): S43–51.

144. Campbell and others, "Interventions for Preventing Obesity in Childhood" (see note 143).

145. D. L. Katz and others, "Public Health Strategies for Preventing and Controlling Overweight and Obesity in School and Worksite Settings," *Morbidity and Mortality Weekly Report* 54, no. RR-10 (2005): 1–8.

146. T. N. Robinson, "Reducing Children's Television Viewing to Prevent Obesity: A Randomized Controlled Trial," *Journal of the American Medical Association* 282, no. 16 (1999): 1561–67.

147. S. L. Gortmaker and others, "Reducing Obesity via a School-Based Interdisciplinary Intervention among Youth: Planet Health," *Archives of Pediatrics and Adolescent Medicine* 153, no. 4 (1999): 409–18.

148. J. James and others, "Preventing Childhood Obesity by Reducing Consumption of Carbonated Drinks: Cluster Randomised Controlled Trial," *British Medical Journal* 328, no. 7450 (2004): 1237 (erratum appears in *British Medical Journal* 328, no. 7450 [May 22, 2004]: 1236).

149. French and others, "An Environmental Intervention to Promote Lower-Fat Food Choices" (see note 66); S. A. French and G. Stables, "Environmental Interventions to Promote Vegetable and Fruit Consumption among Youth in School Settings," *Preventive Medicine* 37, no. 6, pt. 1 (2003): 593–610; Cheryl L. Perry and others, "A Randomized School Trial of Environmental Strategies to Encourage Fruit and Vegetable Consumption among Children," *Health Education and Behavior* 31, no. 1 (2004): 65–76; Simone A. French and others, "Pricing Strategy to Promote Fruit and Vegetable Purchase in High School Cafeterias," *Journal of the American Dietetic Association* 97, no. 9 (1997): 1008–10; Simone A. French and others, "Pricing and Promotion Effects on Low-Fat Vending Snack Purchases: The CHIPS Study," *American Journal of Public Health* 91, no. 1 (2001): 112–17.

150. James F. Sallis and others, "Environmental Interventions for Eating and Physical Activity: A Randomized Controlled Trial in Middle Schools," *American Journal of Preventive Medicine* 24 (2003): 209–17; J. F. Sallis and others, "The Effects of a 2-Year Physical Education Program (SPARK) on Physical Activity and Fitness in Elementary School Students: Sports, Play and Active Recreation for Kids," *American Journal of Public Health* 87, no. 8 (1997): 1328–34.

151. Ashlesha Datar and Roland Sturm, "Physical Education in Elementary School and Body Mass Index: Evidence from the Early Childhood Longitudinal Study," *American Journal of Public Health* 94, no. 9 (2004): 1501–06.

152. French and Story, "Obesity Prevention in Schools" (see note 143).

153. Ibid.

154. Wechsler and others, "Using the School Environment" (see note 43).

155. Martin Luther King Junior Middle School, "The Edible Schoolyard" (www.edibleschoolyard.org [May 20, 2005]).

156. J. L. Morris and S. Zidenberg-Cherr, "Garden-Enhanced Nutrition Curriculum Improves Fourth-Grade School Children's Knowledge of Nutrition and Preferences for Some Vegetables," *Journal of the American Dietetic Association* 102, no. 1 (2002): 91–93.

157. U.S. Environmental Protection Agency, *Travel and Environmental Implications of School Siting*, Report no. EPA 231-R-03-004 (Washington: 2003) (www.epa.gov/smartgrowth/pdf/school_travel.pdf [July 6, 2005)]).

158. Centers for Disease Control and Prevention, "Barriers to Children Walking and Biking to School—United States, 1999," *Morbidity and Mortality Weekly Report* 51, no. 32 (2002): 701–03.

159. Sallis, "Behavioral and Environmental Interventions" (see note 78).

160. C. Tudor-Locke and others, "Objective Physical Activity of Filipino Youth Stratified for Commuting Mode to School," *Medicine & Science in Sports & Exercise* 35, no. 3 (2003): 465–71.

161. Centers for Disease Control and Prevention, "Barriers to Children Walking and Biking to School" (see note 158).

162. U.S. Environmental Protection Agency, *Travel and Environmental Implications of School Siting* (see note 157).

163. Koplan, Liverman, and Kraak, *Preventing Childhood Obesity* (see note 3); U.S. Environmental Protection Agency, *Travel and Environmental Implications of School Siting* (see note 157); Centers for Disease Control and Prevention, "Barriers to Children Walking and Biking to School" (see note 158).

164. "The Walking School Bus Information Website" (www.walkingschoolbus.org/ [June 25, 2005]); Tudor-Locke and others, "Objective Physical Activity of Filipino Youth" (see note 160).

165. Eugene Smolensky and Jennifer Appleton Gootman, *Working Families and Growing Kids: Caring for Children and Adolescents* (Washington: National Academies Press, 2003).

166. Ibid.

167. Robert Wood Johnson Foundation, *Healthy Schools for Healthy Kids* (see note 35).

168. E. Obarzanek and C. A. Pratt, "Girls Health Enrichment Multi-Site Studies (GEMS): New Approaches to Obesity Prevention among Young African-American Girls," *Ethnicity and Disease* 13, no. 1, suppl. 1 (2003): S1–5.

169. Food Research and Action Center, "State of the States, 2005" (see note 24).

170. Fox, Hamilton, and Lin, *Effects of Food Assistance and Nutrition Programs* (see note 17).

171. M. T. Greenberg and others, "Enhancing School-Based Prevention and Youth Development through Coordinated Social, Emotional, and Academic Learning," *American Psychologist* 58, no. 6–7 (2003): 466–74; National Research Council and the Institute of Medicine, Committee on Increasing High School Students' Engagement and Motivation to Learn, Board on Children, Youth, and Families, and Division of Behavioral and Social Sciences and Education, *Engaging Schools: Fostering High School Students' Motivation to Learn* (Washington: National Academies Press, 2004); K. L. Kumpfer and R. Alvarado, "Family-Strengthening Approaches for the Prevention of Youth Problem Behaviors," *American Psychologist* 58, no. 6–7 (2003): 457–65.

172. Ibid.

173. National Research Council and the Institute of Medicine, *Engaging Schools* (see note 171).

174. Centers for Disease Control and Prevention, "Guidelines for School and Community Programs" (see note 75); Centers for Disease Control and Prevention, "Guidelines for School Health Programs to Promote Lifelong Healthy Eating," *Morbidity and Mortality Weekly Report* 45 (1996): 1–37; H. Wechsler and others, "The Role of Schools in Preventing Childhood Obesity," *The State Education Standard* 5, no. 2 (2004): 4–12.

175. Koplan, Liverman, and Kraak, *Preventing Childhood Obesity* (see note 3).

The Role of Child Care Settings in Obesity Prevention

Mary Story, Karen M. Kaphingst, and Simone French

Summary

Mary Story, Karen Kaphingst, and Simone French argue that researchers and policymakers focused on childhood obesity have paid insufficient attention to child care. Although child care settings can be a major force in shaping children's dietary intake, physical activity, and energy balance—and thus in combating the childhood obesity epidemic—researchers know relatively little about either the nutrition or the physical activity environment in the nation's child care facilities. What research exists suggests that the nutritional quality of meals and snacks may be poor and activity levels may be inadequate.

Few uniform standards apply to nutrition or physical activity offerings in the nation's child care centers. With the exception of the federal Head Start program, child care facilities are regulated by states, and state rules vary widely. The authors argue that weak state standards governing physical activity and nutrition represent a missed opportunity to combat obesity. A relatively simple measure, such as specifying how much time children in day care should spend being physically active, could help promote healthful habits among young children.

The authors note that several federal programs provide for the needs of low-income children in child care. The Child and Adult Care Food Program, administered by the Department of Agriculture, provides funds for meals and snacks for almost 3 million children in child care each day. Providers who receive funds must serve meals and snacks that meet certain minimal standards, but the authors argue for toughening those regulations so that meals and snacks meet specific nutrient-based standards. The authors cite Head Start, a federal preschool program serving some 900,000 low-income infants and children up to age five, as a model for other child care programs as it has federal performance standards for nutrition.

Although many child care settings fall short in their nutritional and physical activity offerings, they offer untapped opportunities for developing and evaluating effective obesity-prevention strategies to reach both children and their parents.

www.futureofchildren.org

Mary Story is a professor in the Division of Epidemiology and Community Health, School of Public Health, University of Minnesota, and the director of the Robert Wood Johnson Foundation (RWJF) Healthy Eating Research Program. Karen M. Kaphingst is in the Division of Epidemiology and Community Health, School of Public Health, University of Minnesota, and is the deputy director of the RWJF Healthy Eating Research Program. Simone French is a professor in the Division of Epidemiology and Community Health, School of Public Health, University of Minnesota.

he prevalence of overweight and obesity among American children has been increasing at an alarming rate. Among preschool children aged two to five, overweight has doubled over the past thirty years. Almost one in every four preschoolers is either overweight or at risk of overweight.[1] Prevalence rates are highest among African American, Hispanic, and Native American preschoolers.

Of the nation's 21 million preschool children, 13 million spend a substantial part of their day in child care facilities.[2] Although much has been written on the role of schools in obesity prevention, surprisingly little has been written on how child care settings can help combat childhood obesity. With so many preschool children in attendance, child care settings can be a major force in shaping children's dietary intake, physical activity, and energy balance.

Changing Trends in Maternal Employment

Reliance on child care has grown rapidly in the United States over the past three decades because of changes in demographics, family structure, gender roles, and families' needs for economic security. Traditionally, the number of women in the workforce has driven the demand for child care.[3] From 1970 to 2000, the share of mothers in the labor force (either employed or looking for work) rose from 38 percent to 68 percent; for mothers of children up to age three the rate rose from 24 percent to 57 percent.[4] Today 60 percent of mothers with preschool-aged children are employed, with 70 percent working full-time and 30 percent part-time. Of women with children aged six to seventeen, 75 percent are employed; 78 percent work full-time and 22 percent, part-time.[5] Mandatory work re-

quirements under the 1996 welfare reform law increased the number of low-income parents who work and the number of their children who receive child care.[6]

Child Care Settings

Child care participation in the United States is at an all-time high. Child care, in fact, is now the norm. Parents and child care providers are sharing responsibility for a large and growing number of children during important developmental years, making child care an important setting in which to address the problem of obesity.

Child Care Supply and Participation

According to a study sponsored by the National Child Care Association, Americans paid approximately $38 billion for licensed child care in 2001.[7] Estimates indicate the number of child care facilities in the nation increased more than fourfold in the past thirty years—from 25,000 in 1977, to 40,000 in 1987, and to more than 116,000 in 2004.[8] A precise count of child care settings is not possible for several reasons. First, facilities open and close rapidly. Next, because many family day care homes and some centers and preschools are legally exempt from licensing and registration requirements, they are therefore not on record in state child care licensing offices. Finally, the estimated number of child care facilities does not take into account care provided by nannies, babysitters, and relatives.[9]

Families choose among a variety of day care options: centers (for groups of children in a nonresidential setting, such as a business, church, or school); small family child care homes (typically for six or fewer children in the day care provider's home); large family, or group, child care homes (typically for seven to twelve children cared for by two providers in a provider's home); in-home care (by a nonrelative, such as a nanny or au pair, in the family home); and kith and kin care (by a relative, neighbor, or friend of one family only).[10]

Child Care Patterns for Preschool Children

Preschool children enter care as early as six weeks of age and can be in care for as many as forty hours a week until they reach school age.[11] Forty-one percent of preschool children are in child care for thirty-five or more hours a week. Another 25 percent are in care for fifteen to thirty-four hours a week, while 16 percent are in care for one to fourteen hours. Eighteen percent spend no time in child care.[12]

Nationwide, nearly half of children younger than five with a working mother are cared for in child care centers (32 percent) and family child care homes (16 percent). About 24 percent are cared for by a parent, 23 percent by another relative and 6 percent by a nanny or babysitter. Approximately 80 percent of children aged five and younger with employed mothers are in a child care arrangement for an average of almost forty hours a week.[13]

Child care arrangements vary by race and ethnicity. The 2001 National Household Education Survey collected information about the types of child care arrangements used by families.[14] Some children participate in more than one type of arrangement. Up through age six, Hispanic children are least likely to receive child care in a center-based setting (20 percent) and most likely to be cared for by parents only (53 percent). In addition, 23 percent receive in-home care by a relative, and 12 percent receive in-home care by a nonrelative. African American children are most likely to receive care in a center-based program (41 percent) and least likely to be

cared for in-home by a nonrelative (14 percent); 34 percent are cared for in-home by a relative, and 26 percent receive parental care only. For non-Hispanic white children, similar numbers receive parental care only (38 percent) and attend center-based programs (35 percent), with 20 percent receiving in-home care by a relative and 19 percent being cared for in-home by a nonrelative.

The percentage of children enrolled in formal child care arrangements also varies by state.[15] For example, in Minnesota 55 percent of children under age five are cared for in child care centers or family day care homes, as against 35 percent in California. State differences may be due to demographic and labor patterns, child care subsidies, and costs and supply of child care.[16]

Child Care Patterns for Children Aged Six to Fourteen

A large share of school-aged children also participates in child care. Of the estimated 35 million U.S. children aged six to fourteen, 22 million (63 percent) have an employed mother. According to the U.S. Census Bureau's Survey of Income and Program Participation, the distribution of primary nonschool arrangements for these children was child care centers (5 percent); nonrelative care, including day care homes, babysitters, and nannies (9 percent); organized activities (12 percent); parental care (37 percent); grandparent care (14 percent); care by other relatives (12 percent); and self-care (12 percent). School-aged children spent a significant amount of time in these nonschool arrangements: 63 percent of children aged six to fourteen spent an average of twenty-one hours a week in the care of someone other than a parent before and after school. Children in center-based care average twenty-one hours a week in that setting; those in nonrelative care, such as family child care homes, average nineteen hours a week.[17]

Racial and ethnic differences in child care participation by setting are less pronounced for school-aged children than for preschool children.[18] Most school-aged children rely on parent, grandparent, or other relatives' care outside of school hours (61 percent of white

---

A high-quality diet for young children provides sufficient energy and nutrients to promote normal growth and development, to achieve and maintain a healthy weight, and to attain immediate and long-term health.

---

children, 67 percent of African American children, and 69 percent of Hispanic children).

Nutrition

Obesity prevention involves maintaining energy balance at a healthy weight while achieving overall health and meeting nutritional needs. Technically, energy balance means that energy intake is equivalent to energy expenditure, resulting in no net weight gain or weight loss. But children must be in a slightly positive energy balance to get the energy necessary for normal growth. In children, the goal is to promote growth and development and prevent *excess* weight gain. A primary obesity-prevention approach emphasizes efforts that can help normal-weight children maintain that weight and help overweight children prevent further excess weight gain.[19]

Nutrition Recommendations for Young Children

A high-quality diet for young children provides sufficient energy and nutrients to promote normal growth and development, to achieve and maintain a healthy weight, and to attain immediate and long-term health. The Institute of Medicine Dietary Reference Intakes provide specific daily nutrient needs of children.[20] *The Dietary Guidelines for Americans* provide science-based dietary advice to promote health and reduce the risk for obesity and other chronic diseases through diet and physical activity for Americans older than age two.[21] The 2005 *Dietary Guidelines* make five key recommendations. At least half the grains consumed by children should be whole grains. Children aged two to eight should drink two cups a day of fat-free or low-fat milk or equivalent milk products. Children aged two and older should eat sufficient amounts of fruits and vegetables. Children aged two to three should limit their total fat intake to 30 to 35 percent of calories, and children aged four and older should consume between 25 to 35 percent of calories from fat, with most fats coming from sources of polyunsaturated and monounsaturated fatty acids. Finally, children should get at least sixty minutes of physical activity on most, preferably all, days of the week.

Poor diet is a major contributor, along with physical inactivity, to the obesity epidemic. To reverse the trend toward obesity, children must have access to and consume such healthful foods as fruits and vegetables, consume adequate portion sizes, limit intake of fats and added sugars, and get plenty of physical activity. The diets of most U.S. children do not meet the *Dietary Guidelines*.[22] They tend to be low in fruits and vegetables, calcium-rich foods, and fiber and to be high in total fats, saturated and trans fats, salt, and added sugars. A recent study examined diet quality trends among a nationally representative sample of preschool children aged three to five between 1977 and 1998.[23] Although dietary quality improved slightly over those years, total energy intake increased, as did added sugars and excess juice consumption. Consumption of grains, fruits, and vegetables improved but was still well below recommended levels.

Diets of infants and toddlers are also of concern. In the Feeding Infants and Toddlers Study, a national random sample of 3,022 infants and toddlers from four to twenty-four months old, energy intakes were higher than recommended, according to dietary recall data, suggesting that many caregivers may be overfeeding their children.[24] Up to a third of children aged seven to twenty-four months ate no vegetables or fruits on the day of the dietary recall. For fifteen- to eighteen-month-olds, the vegetable most commonly eaten was french fries. More than 25 percent of nineteen- to twenty-four-month-olds ate french fries or fried potatoes on any day, and 44 percent consumed a sweetened beverage.[25] Although these studies did not distinguish between foods and beverages consumed at home and at child care, they point to troubling aspects of young children's diets.

The overall diets of children must be improved. Early attention to diet would have immediate nutritional benefits, would help prevent obesity, and could reduce chronic disease risk if healthful habits are carried into adulthood. Clearly, establishing healthful dietary and physical activity behaviors needs to begin in childhood. Child care settings can lay the foundations for health and create an environment to ensure that young children are offered healthful foods and regular physical activity.

Table 1. Federal Child and Adult Care Food Program, Fiscal Year 2004

Child care homes	
Average daily participation of children	913,071
Change in child participation in past ten years	−0.6%
Number of participating family child care homes	157,522
Child care centers (includes Head Start)	
Average daily participation of children	1,969,129
Change in child participation in past ten years	62.4%
Number of participating child care centers	44,323
Total federal funding	$1,918,190,945

Sources: Food Research and Action Center, "State of the States, 2005: A Profile of Food and Nutrition Programs across the Nation" (www.frac.org [March 22, 2005]); USDA Food and Nutrition Service (FNS) Nutrition Assistance Programs (available at www.fns.usda.gov/fns/ [May 21, 2005]).

Child Care Meals and Snacks: The Child and Adult Care Food Program

The Child and Adult Care Food Program (CACFP) provides federal funds for meals and snacks served to children in licensed child care homes, child care centers, Head Start programs, after-school care programs, and homeless shelters (see table 1). The program, begun as a pilot program in 1968, became permanent in 1978 and is administered by the Department of Agriculture's Food and Nutrition Service through grants to the states. In most states, the state educational agency administers the program.[26]

Participation and reach. In 2004, CACFP reached almost 2 million children a day in child care centers and Head Start programs and more than 913,000 children in family child care homes. More than 44,000 child care centers and 157,000 family child care homes participated. On an average day, CACFP served meals and snacks to 2.8 million children in these settings.[27]

Eligibility. Programs that may participate in CACFP include eligible public or private nonprofit child care centers, for-profit child care centers serving 25 percent or more low-income children, after-school programs, Head Start programs, and other institutions that are licensed or approved to provide day care services. Because family child care homes tend to be very small businesses, they can participate in CACFP only if they have a recognized sponsor to serve as an intermediary between them and the responsible state agency. Sponsors are responsible for recruiting, for determining that homes meet the

> *In 1996, welfare reform legislation changed the reimbursement structure for child care homes to target benefits more specifically to homes serving low-income children.*

CACFP eligibility criteria, for providing training and other support to family child care providers, for monitoring homes to ensure they comply with federal and state regulations, for verifying the homes' claims for reimbursement, and for distributing the meal reimbursements to the homes.[28]

Funding reimbursement is provided for up to two meals and one snack, or one meal and two snacks, for each child. The Department of Agriculture also makes available donated agricultural commodities or cash in lieu of commodities. Subsidies for food served to children in child care centers are calculated differently than for those paid to family and group day care homes. Under CACFP regulations, meals and snacks served to children in child care centers, Head Start, and outside-

of-school programs are reimbursed at rates based on a child's eligibility for free, reduced-price, or paid meals.[29] Children in Head Start programs categorically receive free meals and snacks, thus qualifying the Head Start center for the highest reimbursement rate.

Reimbursement for meals served in day care homes is based on eligibility for Tier I rates (which targets higher levels of reimbursement to low-income areas, providers, or children) or lower Tier II rates (not located in a low-income area nor operated by a low-income provider).[30] In 1996, welfare reform legislation changed the reimbursement structure for child care homes to target benefits more specifically to homes serving low-income children.[31] As a result, the number of low-income children served in CACFP homes grew by 80 percent between 1995 and 1999, and the number of meal reimbursements for low-income children doubled.[32] A family child care provider serving five low-income children can receive about $4,000 a year in CACFP funds.[33] In fiscal year 2002, the program's total cost, including cash and commodity subsidies, administrative costs, and a payment to states for audits and oversight, was $1.8 billion—$100 million more than the previous year's expenditures.[34]

Meal pattern requirements. To be eligible for federal reimbursement, providers must serve meals and snacks that meet established meal pattern requirements modeled on the food-based menu planning guidelines in the National School Lunch Program and School Breakfast Program. The meal patterns specify foods to be offered at each meal and snack as well as minimum portion sizes, which vary by age.[35] The four food categories are: milk; vegetables, fruit, or 100 percent juice; grains or breads; and meat and meat alternates. Fluid milk must be served at all meals and

Summary of Regulations and Funding for the Child and Adult Care Food Program

Regulations

The U.S. Department of Agriculture's Food and Nutrition Service administers the Child and Adult Care Food Program through grants to the states. Program standards include meal pattern requirements for children in defined age groups: one to two years, three to five years, and six to twelve years. The program also provides a separate meal pattern for infants.

To be eligible for reimbursement, breakfast, lunch, supper, and snacks must contain specified minimum amounts of foods from some or all of the following four components: milk, vegetable or fruit or full-strength (100 percent) juice, bread and grains, and meat and meat alternates. Foods and beverages served to children must be approved, or "creditable," to be reimbursed. The Department of Agriculture, state agencies, and sponsoring organizations make these determinations and issue guidelines and educational materials for providers.

Funding

The CACFP program is an entitlement program. As long as they follow regulations, participating nonresident child care centers and family or group day care homes are guaranteed to receive funds to offer free or reduced-price meals. In addition, outside-of-school programs are entitled to funds for snacks. The program is financed in two ways.

First, child care centers and outside-of-school programs receive a per-meal reimbursement, up to two meals and one snack (or two snacks and one meal), based on the family income of the child receiving the meal. The institution must determine each enrolled participant's eligibility for free and reduced-price meals. Children in families below 130 percent of the poverty line receive free meals. Children in families between 130 and 185 percent of the poverty line receive reduced-price meals. Children in families above 185 percent of the poverty line receive a small per-meal subsidy for full-price ("paid") meals.

The per-meal subsidies are indexed for inflation. In fiscal year 2006, the per-meal reimbursement rates in the forty-eight contiguous U.S. states are: $1.27 for free breakfasts, $2.32 for free lunches and suppers, and $0.63 for free snacks; $0.97 for reduced-price breakfasts, $1.92 for reduced-price lunches and suppers, and $0.31 for reduced-price snacks; and $0.23 for paid breakfasts, $0.22 for paid lunches and suppers, and $0.05 for paid snacks.

Second, family and group day care homes receive reimbursement for up to two meals and one snack (or one meal and two snacks). To participate, family and group child care homes must have a public or private (nonprofit) sponsor. In this instance, the subsidy rate is determined by the area where the child care home is located or by the income level of the provider, with providers in low-income neighborhoods or with low incomes themselves receiving higher subsidies.

For fiscal year 2006 for the forty-eight contiguous U.S. states, Tier I homes, which are located in low-income districts or operated by a provider with a household income that is at or below 185 percent of the poverty line, are reimbursed at the rate of $1.06 for breakfasts, $1.96 for lunches and suppers, and $0.58 for snacks. Tier II homes, which are not located in low-income districts nor operated by a low-income provider, are reimbursed at the rate of $0.39 for breakfasts, $1.18 for lunches and suppers, and $0.16 for snacks. (A Tier II provider can apply for the Tier I rate for low-income children in the family child care home.)

Sources: *Code of Federal Regulations* 226.20; *Federal Register* 70, no. 136, July 18, 2005, pp. 41196–97.

Notes: Rates for both sets of financing are somewhat higher for Alaska and Hawaii. In addition to the rates for lunch and supper, institutions may also receive 17.5 cents in commodities (or cash in lieu of commodities) as additional assistance for each lunch and supper served.

may also be served as part of a snack. No requirements govern whether children older than two should be served whole, 2 percent, 1 percent, or skim milk. Milk and 100 percent fruit or vegetable juices are the only beverages that are reimbursable through the program. CACFP regulations pertain only to foods and beverages for which the provider is seeking federal reimbursement. They do not preclude providers from offering additional low-nutrition, high-calorie foods.

Need for improved nutritional quality in CACFP. CACFP meals and snacks are not required to meet specific nutrient-based standards such as those implemented in the mid-1990s for the school lunch and school breakfast meals.[36] The Healthy Meals for Healthy Americans Act of 1995 required that these school meals be consistent with the *Dietary Guidelines for Americans,* including fat and saturated fat content. Moreover, as noted, the CACFP regulations do not prevent providers from offering additional low-nutrition, high-calorie foods or beverages for which they are not seeking reimbursement. As with schools, comprehensive nutrition policies for the total child care food environment are needed.

Many child care facilities depend on CACFP to defray expenses, and many parents, especially low-income working families, depend on these settings for a substantial portion of their children's nutritional intake.[37] CACFP motivates a family child care home to become licensed, thus coming under applicable health, quality, and safety standards. It interacts regularly with family child care providers, providing monitoring, training, including nutrition education, and other assistance. Further, CACFP is an entitlement program, meaning that all eligible homes and centers must be allowed to partic-

ipate and that all eligible children being cared for in the homes and centers must be served. Immigrant status does not affect eligibility status. CACFP provides a basic nutritional safety net for low-income children. Strengthening the regulations to make CACFP meals, snacks, and beverages comply with the *Dietary Guidelines,* including fat and saturated fat content, could further improve children's nutrition and help prevent child obesity. Increasing the number of licensed family child care homes to enable them to participate in CACFP could extend healthful eating and quality child care to many more at-risk children.[38]

Nutrition Quality of Foods in Child Care Settings

Surprisingly little research has been done to assess the nutritional quality of foods in child care settings. Most studies have focused on CACFP providers. A recent research review identified ten descriptive studies of CACFP in child care settings published between 1982 and 2004, four of which were national studies.[39] Because CACFP does not have nutrient-based standards, almost all of the studies have used the recommendations of the American Dietetic Association (ADA) as evaluation benchmarks. The ADA recommends that food served to children in care for a full day (eight hours or more) meet at least one-half to two-thirds of their daily needs for energy and nutrients and that food served to children in part-time care (four to seven hours) provide at least one-third of their daily needs. These benchmarks are requirements for the Head Start nutrition program.[40] The ADA also recommends that child care meals and snacks be consistent with the *Dietary Guidelines.*

The only comprehensive national study, done in 1995, collected meal and snack data on a nationally representative sample of 1,962 CACFP-participating child care sites (family child care homes and child care centers, including Head Start centers) and food intake data on children aged five and older at 372 centers or homes. Nutrient analysis showed that the most common combinations of meals and snacks offered (breakfast, lunch, and one to two snacks) provided 61 to 71 percent of children's daily energy needs and more than two-thirds of the recommended dietary allowance for key nutrients. Meals and snacks had an average of 13 percent of calories from saturated fat, exceeding the *Dietary Guidelines* of no more than 10 percent. Few providers offered lunches that met the *Dietary Guidelines'* goals for total fat or saturated fat; 50 percent served lunches with more than 35 percent of the calories from fat. Providers that met the dietary fat recommendation were more likely to serve 1 percent or skim milk and fruit, and they were less likely to serve french fries, fried meats, hot dogs, cold cuts, and high-fat condiments. On average 90 percent of the breakfasts and 87 percent of the lunches complied with the meal pattern requirements. The food component most often missing from meals was fruits and vegetables.[41]

A 1999 national study of CACFP meals and snacks conducted in 542 Tier II child care homes (not located in a low-income area nor operated by a low-income provider) found that meals and snacks offered to children aged two and older provided, on average, more than two-thirds of the recommended dietary allowance for calories and key nutrients.[42] Mean saturated fat content exceeded national recommendations. Less than one-third of the morning snacks (31 percent) and afternoon snacks (28 percent) included fresh, canned, or dried fruit. Less than 25 percent of day care homes offered any fresh fruit as

snacks. Only 3 percent of the afternoon snacks included vegetables.

The few smaller-scale studies that have evaluated the menus in child care settings, primarily CACFP sites, show cause for concern.[43] One study collected data on 171 child care centers that participated in CACFP in seven states.[44] It collected copies of menus and menu records for meals and snacks for ten consecutive days. Meal patterns were incon-

---

CACFP meals and snacks are not required to meet specific nutrient-based standards such as those implemented in the mid-1990s for the school lunch and breakfast meals.

---

sistent with the *Dietary Guidelines* regarding fat, sodium, fruits and vegetables, and serving a variety of foods. Menus were high in fat and seldom provided recommended servings of vegetables. Cookies were frequently on the menus. Another study evaluated menus in nine Texas child care centers participating in CACFP and found that only about half the centers included fresh produce; among those that did, the amount was frequently minimal. Food service staff did not always understand the CACFP requirements and had limited nutrition knowledge. One staff member said he never served fresh fruit because he didn't "know how far an apple will go," but he knew exactly how much applesauce to ladle from a can to make the minimum portion required by CACFP. Another staff member thought that bottled orange drink was "full-strength juice" because no water was added.[45]

A recent study compared the dietary intakes of fifty children aged three to nine who attended nine child care centers in Texas with the recommendations of the Food Guide Pyramid for Young Children.[46] Researchers observed children's meals and snacks during child care for three consecutive days and took reports on dietary intakes of the children before and after child care from the parents. During child care, the three-year-olds ate enough fruit, but not enough grains, vegetables, or dairy to meet two-thirds of the Food Guide Pyramid for Young Children recommendations. The four- and five-year-old children consumed adequate dairy only. The vegetables and grains served most often were potatoes and refined flour products. Intakes at home did not compensate. These findings suggest that children attending child care centers are not getting adequate diets at child care centers or at home.

In summary, relatively little is known about the dietary quality and types of foods and beverages offered in child care facilities, especially those that are not licensed or regulated and do not participate in the CACFP program. The nutritional quality of meals and snacks may be poor. Increased attention should thus be paid to the nutritional adequacy of foods served in child care settings. More research is needed on the current food environment in child care, including what foods are served, their nutritional quality, and staff training on nutrition. It has been ten years since any national survey described the nutrient content of meals and snacks in child care centers and day care homes participating in CACFP, and that survey included only children older than five.[47] Given the increased number and use of child care facilities over the past decade, an updated national survey is needed to assess nutrition quality and practices, including types and portion

sizes of foods and beverages offered and consumed by children in child care settings.

Physical Activity

Physical activity is crucial to overall health and to obesity prevention.[48] Reduced physical activity is a likely contributor to increasing obesity rates among children of all ages.[49]

Physical Activity Recommendations for Young Children

The 2005 *Dietary Guidelines* recommend that children and adolescents engage in at least sixty minutes of physical activity on most, preferably all, days of the week.[50] The National Association for Sport and Physical Education's guidelines recommend that toddlers get at least thirty minutes daily of structured physical activity and preschoolers should have at least sixty minutes. It also recommends that toddlers and preschoolers engage in at least sixty minutes a day of unstructured physical activity and not be sedentary for more than sixty minutes at a time except when sleeping. Thus, preschool-aged children should have at least two hours of exercise a day, half in structured physical activity and the remainder in unstructured, free-play settings.[51] Children aged five to twelve should have at least sixty minutes of daily exercise.

To help meet the daily physical activity recommendations for preschoolers, experts recommend incorporating planned physical activity into the daily preschool schedule.[52] Structured activity sessions should be short, about fifteen to twenty minutes, and should emphasize a wide variety of different movements.[53] States vary widely in their physical activity requirements for child care settings, but most address the subject in general, non-quantified terms. The failure to specify how much time children should spend being physically active is an overlooked opportunity to increase physical activity among young children in settings where many spend much of their day.

Physical Activity in Child Care Settings

Surprisingly little is known about the activity levels of children in child care. Russell Pate and several colleagues used accelerometers, or small electronic devices worn around the waist, to record minute-by-minute activity levels of 281 children attending nine preschools (Head Start, church-based, and private) in South Carolina.[54] The children, who wore accelerometers for roughly 4.4 hours a day for an average of 6.6 days, participated in a mean of seven minutes an hour of moderate to vigorous physical activity (MVPA) at the preschools. Activity levels varied widely among schools, averaging from four to ten minutes an hour. The preschool that a child attended was a significant predictor of MVPA. The authors speculated that a child attending preschool for eight hours would engage in about one hour of MVPA and would be unlikely to engage in another hour of MVPA outside the preschool setting, suggesting that many preschool children may not be meeting physical activity recommendations. Another study assessed the physical activity level of 214 children aged three to five enrolled in ten child care centers in South Dakota. Each child wore an accelerometer for two continuous days (forty-eight hours).[55] The child care center was the strongest predictor of physical activity levels, with more than 50 percent of the daily activity counts occurring between 9 a.m. and 5 p.m. These studies suggest that school policies and practices greatly influence the overall physical activity of the nation's young children.[56] The quality and quantity of physical activity in child care settings can vary depending on indoor space, gross motor play equipment, outdoor play area, group size, and the education and training of child care staff.[57]

The only study to evaluate weight-related differences in physical activity during the preschool day compared the physical activity of overweight and normal-weight three- to five-year-old children while attending preschool.[58] The study assessed 245 children, recruited from nine preschools, on multiple days while using both direct observation and accelerometers. It found that overweight boys were significantly less active than normal-weight boys, though it found no weight-related activ-

The 2005 Dietary Guidelines recommend that children and adolescents engage in at least sixty minutes of physical activity on most, preferably all, days of the week.

ity differences in girls. Overweight children may thus be at increased risk for further gains in body fat because of low physical activity levels during the preschool day.

Another study of 266 three- to five-year-old children from nine preschools found that preschool policies and practices influenced children's physical activity.[59] Children in preschools with frequent field trips (four or more a month) and college-educated teachers had significantly higher levels of MVPA. Children in higher-quality preschools, measured by the number of children per classroom, the educational backgrounds of the teachers, and specific features of the facilities, had lower levels of sedentary behavior. Similar levels of physical activity were observed in private, church-based, and Head Start preschool settings. On average, the children failed to meet current recommendations for physical activity.[60] Children in this study were engaged in MVPA about 27 percent of the time, meaning that on average they would have about thirty-two minutes of MVPA in two play periods lasting an hour each. Most notably, the study found higher levels of physical activity in preschools with policies and practices that promoted physical activity.

We could find no studies that assessed children's television and video viewing and computer use in child care centers or day care homes, although it has been reported that children spend more time watching TV in child care homes than in centers.[61] Many studies have found a positive link between children's television viewing and obesity, and the American Academy of Pediatrics recommends limiting children's total television viewing time to no more than one to two hours of quality programming a day.[62] Future studies should examine television policies and practice in child care facilities.

Research has found that many preschool-aged children are not meeting the recommended guidelines of two hours of physical activity a day and that children in child care settings need more physical activity.[63] How active children are in preschools is largely determined by how much time they have to play freely in settings conducive to physical activity, such as outdoor playgrounds, parks, or gyms. One way to ensure that preschoolers get adequate exercise is to provide more time in free-play settings and add structured physical activity to their program.[64] As yet, however, no broad policies govern physical activity for preschool children in child care. Although several national groups have published recommendations, no requirements exist at the federal level. Physical activity policies, where they exist, are set by states and facilities.

Obesity-Prevention Interventions in Preschool Settings

Child care settings offer untapped opportunities for developing and evaluating effective obesity-prevention strategies to reach both children and their parents. But we could locate few published obesity-prevention studies with preschool children.[65] In Hip-Hop to Health Jr., a study of twelve Chicago Head Start preschool programs serving minority children, children in half the preschools participated in a fourteen-week (forty minutes three times a week) program of healthful eating and exercise. Their parents received weekly newsletters with information mirroring the children's curriculum. Children in the other six preschools served as a control group. Children in the program had significantly smaller increases in BMI than did children in the control group at both the one-year and two-year follow-ups.[66] But the study found no significant treatment group differences in food intake or physical activity.

Another study worth noting—and one with implications for obesity-prevention programs—is the "Healthy Start" project. A cardiovascular risk-reduction study involving 1,296 low-income, predominantly minority preschool children in nine Head Start centers in New York, the project modified the food service in some centers and left food service in some centers unchanged as a control.[67] The food service intervention reduced the fat and saturated fat content of preschool meals and reduced children's consumption of saturated fat while at preschool without compromising their intake of energy and essential nutrients, thus demonstrating the feasibility of an intervention to change food service in child care centers.

School-based interventions to reduce television watching in elementary school children, including one conducted by T. N. Robinson, have reported reductions in body fat.[68] One intervention, which involved preschoolers from 2.6 to 5.5 years old, almost all of whom were white, aimed to reduce at-home television viewing.[69] Children in eight child care centers received a seven-session program to reduce television viewing as part of a health-promotion curriculum; children in eight control centers received a safety and injury-prevention program. Parents were given take-home educational materials and participated in parent-child activities. Parents reported that children in the intervention group watched television at home an average of 4.7 hours less a week than children in the control group—a reduction similar to those reported by Robinson.[70] But children in the intervention and in the control group had no significant differences in body fat. Longer and more intensive interventions that target other modifiable obesity risk factors may yield greater results.

Reducing consumption of sweetened beverages, including juice, both in child care settings and at home may be an effective obesity-prevention strategy. Several studies indicate that sweetened beverages may contribute to the increased prevalence of obesity among preschool children. One analysis of National Health and Nutrition Examination Survey data found a positive link between the consumption of carbonated soft drinks and overweight in all age groups, including two- to five-year-olds.[71] Another examined the association between sweet drink consumption and overweight among 10,904 low-income preschool children aged two and three at baseline and then looked at their weight and height one year later.[72] Sweet drinks included juices, fruit drinks, and sodas. Forty-one percent of the children consumed these drinks at least three times a day. Energy intake in-

creased as the consumption of sweet drinks increased. For example, those who consumed less than one drink a day had a mean intake of 1,425 calories a day, as against 2,005 calories a day for those who consumed three or more a day. Preschool children who were at risk for overweight or who were overweight at baseline and who consumed more than

Reducing consumption of sweetened beverages, including juice, both in child care settings and at home may be an effective obesity-prevention strategy.

one drink a day were significantly more likely to become or remain overweight.

A cross-sectional study in 1997 found that two- to five-year-old children who drank twelve or more ounces of fruit juice a day were more likely (32 percent as against 9 percent) to be obese than those who drank less juice.[73] Not all studies have found a link between juice consumption and overweight, but the American Academy of Pediatrics recommends that children aged one to six drink no more than four to six ounces of fruit juice a day.[74] Fruit juice and fruit drinks are easily overconsumed by toddlers and young children because they taste good. They are also conveniently packaged and can be carried around during the day. Because juice is viewed as nutritious, child care providers or parents may not set limits. Like soda, however, it can contribute to obesity. Whole fruit should be encouraged as an alternative because of the fiber benefit and because whole fruit takes longer to eat.

It is not known how much sweetened beverages or juice children consume in child care settings and at home. National data indicate that energy intake, added sugar as a share of total energy, and excess juice consumption (more than six ounces a day) increased significantly among preschoolers between 1977 and 1998.[75] Researchers need to assess sweetened beverage intake among preschoolers in child care facilities and to conduct interventions to remove fruit drinks and soda from child care, to limit juice to six ounces a day, and to examine the effect on weight status.

Head Start

Head Start, a federal preschool program serving infants and children up to age five, includes a varied mix of programs—education, health, nutrition, social services, and parental involvement—that presents a unique opportunity to combat childhood obesity. Created in 1965, Head Start was designed to help break the cycle of poverty by providing preschool children of low-income families with a comprehensive program to meet their educational, emotional, social, health, and nutritional needs.[76] In 2003, 19,200 Head Start sites throughout the country reached more than 900,000 children. The program is racially diverse, and most children are three (34 percent) or four (53 percent) years old.[77] Although Head Start has touched millions of children's lives, it reaches only about 40 percent of those who are eligible.[78]

One objective of Head Start is to ensure that all children are linked to an ongoing source of health care.[79] The emphasis on continuous primary care means that children's height and weight are monitored and that parents receive guidance on nutrition and physical activity. Head Start maintains a Child Health Record for each child and requires a health screening within forty-five days of enrollment.[80] Al-

though each child's height and weight are measured and BMI calculated as part of a routine health examination, it is not clear how these data are used on an individual basis or what information is given to the parents. Nor is it clear whether the BMI data collected are analyzed at a state or national level or used for surveillance or monitoring.

Head Start is also a vital source of nutrition for low-income children. Its federal performance standards require that its meals and snacks provide at least one-third of the daily nutritional needs of children in a part-day center-based setting and one-half to two-third of the needs of children in a full-day program.[81] Head Start sites participate in the CACFP program and must have a registered dietitian review and evaluate their menus. Performance standards also require that parent education activities include "opportunities to assist individual families with food preparation and nutritional skills."[82]

Head Start's federal regulations also require that settings provide opportunities for outdoor and indoor active play, adequate indoor and outdoor space, equipment for active play, and opportunities to develop gross and fine motor skills. The regulations do not specify the amount, frequency, and type of physical activity. No standards or rules govern television use.

Overall, evaluations of Head Start show many benefits for children, families, and communities, though little research has focused on obesity prevention.[83] The only published study to date is Hip-Hop to Health Jr., described above.[84] Because of its multiple components and because it serves low-income, multiethnic children who are at high risk of overweight, Head Start could well be used to strengthen and expand obesity-prevention efforts. The program has national reach and could signifi-

An Innovative State Program

A promising pilot intervention called Nutrition and Physical Activity Self-Assessment for Child Care (NAP SACC) was launched in North Carolina in 2003.[1] Funded by the Centers for Disease Control and the N.C. Department of Health and Human Services, the program's goal is to promote healthful eating and physical activity in young children in child care and preschool settings. The intervention examines the feasibility of using local health professionals to help child care centers assess and improve their nutrition and physical activity environments. The state implemented the pilot in fifteen child care centers, with four control centers. Using an assessment tool with nine nutrition and six physical activity areas, centers self-assessed their policies and practices. Based on the assessments, center staff identified specific areas for improvement. Local health professionals conducted workshops for the center staff and provided ongoing support and technical assistance. The second phase of the project is now under way in 102 child care centers.

1. Nutrition and Physical Activity Self-Assessment for Child Care (NAP SACC) Website (www.napsacc.org [March 25, 2005]).

cantly improve healthful eating and physical activity patterns of young children. Interventions and policy changes could focus on ensuring that meals and snacks adhere to the *Dietary Guidelines*, that physical activity is increased, and that parents are actively involved. BMI screening results could be provided to parents and health providers and could be used for surveillance on state and national levels.

Regulation of Child Care Programs

With the exception of Head Start, the states regulate child care facilities. Each state sets and enforces specific health and safety requirements, which regulated providers must meet to operate legally.[85] All states set minimum health, safety, and nutrition standards for providers. They generally regulate child care homes through licensing, registration, and certification. Most states require family child care providers to be licensed if they care for more than four children. In many states, licensing or registration is voluntary for providers caring for four or fewer children. Almost all child care centers are regulated or licensed in some way.[86]

No uniform quality standards govern all child care and early education programs nation-wide, and many programs are exempt from any regulation or licensing requirements.[87] Although regulations vary across states, they focus mostly on basic safety and health requirements, such as keeping smoke detectors in working order; locking cabinets that contain dangerous materials; specifying the minimum area for indoor or outdoor space, staff-child ratios, the minimum age of caregivers, and preservice training qualifications and inservice requirements for staff; and ensuring that children's immunizations are up to date.[88] Regulations regarding nutrition, physical activity, and media use vary widely across the states and are reviewed below. The American Dietetic Association, American Academy of Pediatrics, American Public Health Association, and National Resource Center for Health and Safety in Child Care have published recommendations, performance standards, and benchmarks for nutrition, food service, and developmentally appropriate activities in child care settings.[89]

Although setting and enforcing child care requirements are primarily state and local responsibilities, the federal government requires states to have basic safety and health regulations in place to receive funds from the

Child Care and Development Block Grant. This federal program subsidizes child care costs for low-income families, helping them afford quality child care and removing a barrier to parental employment.[90] It is a significant public investment. In 2004, the government provided $4.8 billion.[91] To get these funds, states must certify that health and safety requirements are in place and that both regulated and nonregulated providers being paid with block grant funds are in compliance. Washington does not, however, stipulate the contents of the requirements or the means to enforce them, and states vary widely on these points.

Nonregulated Child Care Providers
Most states do not regulate all types of child care providers. Nonregulated providers need not comply with state regulations and are not subject to state enforcement. Some family child care providers caring for small numbers of children are also exempt from regulation, and some states exempt certain types of center-based programs, such as those run by religious groups, school-based preschool, school-based after-school programs, or centers operating part-day or part-year only.[92] Nonregulated providers who receive funds from the federal block grant must, however, meet state and local health and safety requirements.

National advocacy groups have expressed concern about the gaps in child care regulation. The National Health and Safety Performance Standards for Out-of-Home Child Care assert that "every state should have a statute that identifies the regulatory agency and mandates the licensing and regulation of all full-time and part-time out-of-home care of children, regardless of setting, except care provided by parents or legal guardians, grandparents, siblings, aunts, or uncles or when a family engages an individual to care solely for

their children."[93] The National Association for the Education of Young Children states that "any program providing care and education to children from two or more unrelated families should be regulated; there should be no exemptions from this principle."[94]

Regulatory Enforcement
The state child care licensing office enforces its state's child care regulations. With current tight fiscal climates in most states and competing priorities for limited funds, states must make choices about the extent to which they can reasonably carry out this enforcement and the types of providers who will be affected.[95] Regulatory systems in many states are not funded to enforce licensing regulations effectively.[96] Regulatory burdens also affect providers, and costs can be passed along to parents. Providers may choose to leave the market—or choose not to be licensed—if regulatory practices become too cumbersome.

Regulations Governing Food, Physical Activity, and Media Use
The National Resource Center for Health and Safety in Child Care, part of the U.S. Department of Health and Human Services, Health Resources and Services Administration, maintains a website that provides links to the complete child care licensing standards for all fifty states and the District of Columbia.[97] Using this website, we recently conducted an analysis of state child care licensing standards for nutrition, physical activity, and media use. We examined licensing regulations for child care centers, small family child care homes (typically caring for six or fewer children), and large family and group child care homes (usually with seven to twelve children).

We found not only that regulations vary considerably from state to state but that, within a state, regulations may vary for different types of child care settings. Typically child care centers are most heavily regulated, followed by large family and group child care homes, with small family child care homes the least heavily regulated. As noted, many states exempt small family child care homes from licensing requirements and instead rely on voluntary registration. Five states—Delaware, Georgia, Illinois, Mississippi, and Tennessee—have particularly comprehensive policies on nutrition, physical activity, and media use. In the following discussion of licensing regulations in these areas, we describe a state as having a specific regulation if the regulation is mandatory in at least one child care setting.

Nutrition

State nutrition regulations vary widely. Thirty states require the Child and Adult Care Food Program meal patterns or have similar requirements. Fifteen states specify the share of children's daily nutritional requirements to be provided per meal or based on the length of time in care, and twenty-one states specify the number of meals and snacks to be offered to children based on length of time in care. Just two states, Michigan and West Virginia, require that meals and snacks must follow the *Dietary Guidelines for Americans*. Mississippi regulations refer to the *Dietary Guidelines*, noting that they can "provide assistance in planning meals for ages two (2) and older, which will promote health and prevent disease."[98] Ten states limit foods and beverages of low nutritional value. Five states regulate vending machines. Alabama, Georgia, and Louisiana prohibit vending machines in areas used by children. Arkansas permits vending machines in school-age settings provided they are not the only source of snacks and beverages. Mississippi requires food in vending machines to meet the state's nutrition regulations for meals and snacks in child care settings.

Physical Activity

Most states specify that the daily program should promote physical development, including large and small muscle activity; have a balance of active and quiet activities, indoor and outdoor activities, and individual and group activities; include age- and developmentally appropriate activities, equipment, and supplies; and provide enough materials and equipment to avoid excessive competition and long waits. Thirty-three states and the District of Columbia require that the program provide large muscle, or gross motor, activity or development. Nine states require "vigorous" physical activity for children. No states use the term "moderate" to describe the appropriate level of activity. Just two states, Alaska and Massachusetts, specify how long children should engage in physical activity. Alaska mandates "a minimum of 20 minutes of vigorous physical activity for every three hours the facility is open between the hours of 7:00 a.m. and 7:00 p.m." Massachusetts calls for "thirty minutes of physical activity every day." Alaska's regulations pertain to all types of child care settings; the Massachusetts rule affects only child care homes.

Thirty-eight states and the District of Columbia require that children in child care centers and homes have time outdoors each day, health and weather permitting. Eight of these states and the District of Columbia specify how long children should be outdoors; most require at least one hour a day. The District of Columbia and Mississippi require the most daily outdoor time—two hours for a full-day program and at least thirty minutes for a part-day program.

Media Use

Twenty-two states regulate media use, including television, computer, video, video game, radio, and electronic game use. Most simply define appropriate or inappropriate content or define acceptable use of media within the program of activities (for example, media should be used with discretion and not as a substitute for planned activities). Only nine states specify time limits on screen time. Five set a maximum of two hours a day; the others allow less time.

Quality Child Care
Most children in the United States now spend some time in child care during their critical developmental years. A body of evidence has accumulated to show that the quality of care has a lasting impact on a child's well-being and ability to learn.[99] High-quality care and early education help children prepare for school, ready to succeed; improve their skills; and stay safe while their parents work.[100] But quality care arrangements are hard to find, particularly for low-income parents.[101] Much of the care available in the United States is poor to mediocre.[102]

Strong state licensing requirements, expanded to apply to most care settings, can help ensure children's health and well-being. Stricter licensing requirements, such as low staff-to-child ratios and adequate training for providers, can help improve the quality of care. Providers who care for children on a regular basis play an essential role in children's development and experiences.[103] Properly trained and educated teachers enhance children's development. Recruiting and retaining qualified staff pose significant challenges, however, when providers' salaries average $17,610 a year, often without benefits or paid leave.[104] Most states do not require providers to have even a basic knowledge of child development, and they require little or no training before allowing providers to work with children. Several national organizations have called for uniform training

for providers on specific content areas, including nutrition, child growth and development, and health and safety.[105] The American Dietetic Association recommends that child care providers and food service personnel receive appropriate nutrition and food service training.[106] We found no recommendations for training relating specifically to physical activity, though children in preschools with better-educated teachers have been found to have significantly higher levels of MVPA.[107]

Recommendations for Child Care Settings
Largely ignored in the nation's obesity dialogue so far has been the food and physical activity environment in child care settings. But child care represents an untapped rich source of strategies to help children acquire positive healthy habits to prevent obesity. The infrastructure already exists within Head Start and CACFP child care sites to incorporate healthful eating and exercise into these programs, thus reaching many low-income and minority children who are at greatest risk for obesity. But regulations and standards governing physical activity and nutrition need to be strengthened. Child care settings also offer a way to reach parents to make healthful changes at home to reinforce and support healthful eating and regular exercise. The box on the following page lists strategies for creating a healthful environment in child care settings to improve physical activity and eating behaviors to prevent obesity in young children.

Conclusions
The early years spent in child care are crucially important to a child's development. High-quality child care and early education help ensure that a child will develop skills and enter school ready to learn.[108] For a young child, health and education are inseparable. Eating nutritious foods and engaging

Strategies for Achieving a More Healthful Food and Physical Activity Environment in Child Care Settings

Policy Goals

At the federal level, Congress should require all meals and snacks offered by the Child and Adult Care Food Program to meet the *Dietary Guidelines for Americans*. Regulations would apply to all providers in participating child care centers, family child care facilities, and after-school care programs.

States should develop nutrition and physical activity policies for licensed child care facilities that address healthful eating, physical activity, and media use. Policies should also address nutrition and physical activity training for staff and nutrition training for food service staff.

At the local level, licensed preschool and child care facilities should have written nutrition policies that follow the *Dietary Guidelines for Americans* for meals, snacks, and beverages. They should also have written policies to ensure adequate, developmentally appropriate physical activity and to limit screen time.

Research Goals

Researchers should pursue four primary goals. First, they should develop, implement, and evaluate innovative intervention programs focused on promoting healthful eating and physical activity and on preventing obesity in child care facilities, especially facilities serving low-income and minority children who are at highest risk. Second, they should conduct descriptive environmental studies in child care centers, Head Start, and licensed day care homes to assess the food environment (the types and amounts of foods and beverages served for meals and snacks), the physical activity environment (the amount and type of physical activity), and media use. Third, they should conduct a national study of child care programs on the dietary quality of meals and snacks served and how they compare to the *Dietary Guidelines for Americans* and Dietary Reference Intakes. And finally they should evaluate methods to increase parental involvement, to change parental behavior, and to change the home environment through child care–based obesity-prevention interventions.

---

in physical activity on a daily basis are two essential elements for healthy well-being in the early years. Child care settings can and should provide an environment in which young children are offered nutritious foods and regular physical activity through structured and unstructured play so that they learn these healthful lifestyle behaviors at an early age. Child care homes and centers offer many opportunities to form and support healthful eating habits and physical activity patterns in young children. Thus they can play a critical role in laying a foundation for healthy weight. The number of children in the United States aged four and younger is expected to grow by 1.2 million over the next decade, for a 6 percent rise. The number of working parents who depend on child care services is also expected to grow.[109] To help stem the childhood obesity epidemic, the nation must pay more attention to the food and physical activity offered in various child care settings.

Notes

1. U.S. Department of Health and Human Services, *The Surgeon General's Call to Action to Prevent and Decrease Overweight and Obesity* (Rockville, Md.: 2001); A. A. Hedley and others, "Prevalence of Overweight and Obesity among U.S. Children, Adolescents, and Adults, 1999–2002," *Journal of the American Medical Association* 291, no. 23 (2004): 2847–50.

2. National Center for Education Statistics, *Child Care and Early Education Program Participation of Infants, Toddlers, and Preschoolers* (Washington: U.S. Department of Education, 1996).

3. Robert C. Fellmeth, "The Child Care System in the United States," in *Health and Welfare for Families in the 21st Century*, edited by Helen M. Wallace, Gordon Green, and Kenneth J. Jaros (Sudbury, Mass.: Jones & Bartlett Publishers, 2003).

4. Eugene Smolensky and Jennifer Appleton Gootman, eds., Committee on Family and Work Policies, National Research Council (U.S.), *Working Families and Growing Kids: Caring for Children and Adolescents* (Washington: National Academies Press, 2003).

5. U.S. Department of Health and Human Services, *Child Health USA 2002* (Rockville, Md.: 2003).

6. Food Research and Action Center, "State of the States, 2005: A Profile of Food and Nutrition Programs across the Nation" (www.frac.org [March 22, 2005]).

7. M. Cubed, *The National Economic Impacts of the Child Care Sector*, National Child Care Association, fall 2002 (www.nccanet.org/NCCA%20Impact%20Study.pdf [July 29, 2005]).

8. Children's Foundation and National Association for Regulatory Administration, "Family Child Care Licensing Study" (http://128.174.128.220/egi-bin/IMS/Results.asp [March 22, 2005]).

9. Smolensky and Gootman, eds., *Working Families and Growing Kids* (see note 4).

10. National Association for the Education of Young Children, "Licensing and Public Regulation of Early Childhood Programs: A Position Statement of the National Association for the Education of Young Children" (Washington, 1998).

11. Children's Defense Fund, "Child Care Basics" (www.childrensdefense.org/earlychildhood/childcare/child_care_basics_2005.pdf [May 21, 2005]).

12. J. Capizzano and G. Adams, "The Hours That Children under Five Spend in Child Care: Variation across States," no. B-8 (Washington: Urban Institute, 2000).

13. Smolensky and Gootman, eds., *Working Families and Growing Kids* (see note 4).

14. National Center for Education Statistics, *National Household Education Survey 2001* (Washington: U.S. Department of Education, 2002).

15. Cubed, *The National Economic Impacts of the Child Care Sector* (see note 7).

16. Ibid.

17. Smolensky and Gootman, eds., *Working Families and Growing Kids* (see note 4).

18. Ibid.

19. Jeffrey Koplan, Catharyn T. Liverman, and Vivica I. Kraak, *Preventing Childhood Obesity: Health in the Balance* (Washington: National Academies Press, 2005).

20. National Academy of Sciences, Food and Nutrition Information Center, National Research Council, *Dietary Reference Intakes (DRI) and Recommended Dietary Allowances (RDA)* (www.nal.usda.gov/fnic/etext/000105.html [August 15, 2005]).

21. U.S. Department of Health and Human Services and U.S. Department of Agriculture, *Dietary Guidelines for Americans, 2005,* 6th ed. (Government Printing Office, 2005).

22. U.S. Department of Health and Human Services, *Healthy People 2010: Understanding and Improving Health,* 2nd ed. (GPO, 2000).

23. S. Kranz, A. M. Siega-Riz, and A. H. Herring, "Changes in Diet Quality of American Preschoolers between 1977 and 1998," *American Journal of Public Health* 94, no. 9 (2004): 1525–30.

24. B. Devaney and others, "Nutrient Intakes of Infants and Toddlers," *Journal of the American Dietetic Association* 104, no. 1, suppl. 1 (2004): S14–S21.

25. M. K. Fox and others, "Feeding Infants and Toddlers Study: What Foods Are Infants and Toddlers Eating?" *Journal of the American Dietetic Association* 104, no. 1, suppl. 1 (2004): S22–S30.

26. U.S. Department of Agriculture, Food and Nutrition Service, "Child and Adult Care Food Program" (www.fns.usda.gov/cnd/care/cacfp/cacfphome.htm [March 5, 2005]).

27. Food Research and Action Center, "State of the States, 2005" (see note 6).

28. F. Glanz, "Child and Adult Care Food Program, 2004," in *Effects of Food Assistance and Nutrition Programs on Nutrition and Health,* vol. 3: *Literature Review,* edited by M. K. Fox, W. Hamilton, and B. H. Lin. Food Assistance and Nutrition Research Report no. 19-3 (Washington: U.S. Department of Agriculture, Economic Research Service, 2004).

29. For example, for July 2003–04, subsidies for children with family incomes below 130 percent of the poverty line were 60 cents for each snack, $1.20 for each breakfast, and $2.19 for each lunch or supper. For children with family incomes between 130 percent and 185 percent of the poverty line, subsidies were 30 cents for snacks, 90 cents for breakfast, and $1.79 for lunch or supper; for children with family incomes above 185 percent of the poverty line, subsidies were 5 cents for snacks, 22 cents for breakfast, and 21 cents for lunch or supper. These amounts are indexed yearly for inflation. Committee on Ways and Means, U.S. House of Representatives, *2004 Green Book* (GPO, 2004), section 15, pages 15–117.

30. U.S. Department of Agriculture, Food and Nutrition Service, "Child and Adult Care Food Program" (see note 26).

31. Glanz, "Child and Adult Care Food Program, 2004" (see note 28).

32. Ibid.

33. Food Research and Action Center, "State of the States, 2005" (see note 6).

34. Committee on Ways and Means, *2004 Green Book,* pages 15–116 (see note 29).

35. U.S. Department of Agriculture, Food and Nutrition Service, "Child and Adult Care Food Program" (see note 26).

36. Glanz, "Child and Adult Care Food Program, 2004" (see note 28).

37. Lynn Parker, "The Federal Nutrition Programs: A Safety Net for Very Young Children," *Zero to Three* 21, no. 1 (2000): 29–36.

38. Ibid.

39. Glanz, "Child and Adult Care Food Program, 2004" (see note 28).

40. American Dietetic Association, "Position of the American Dietetic Association: Nutrition Standards for Child-Care Programs," *Journal of the American Dietetic Association* 99, no. 8 (1999): 981–88; American Dietetic Association, "Position of the American Dietetic Association: Benchmarks for Nutrition Programs in Child Care Settings," *Journal of the American Dietetic Association* 105, no. 6 (2005): 979–86; U.S. Department of Health and Human Services, Administration for Children and Families, Head Start Bureau, *Head Start Program Performance Standards and Other Regulations* (Washington, 2005).

41. M. K. Fox and others, *Early Childhood and Child Care Study: Nutritional Assessment of the CACFP*, vol. 2: *Final Report* (Washington: U.S. Department of Agriculture, Food and Consumer Service, 1997).

42. Ibid.

43. M. E. Briley, C. Roberts-Gray, and S. Rowe, "What Can Children Learn from the Menu at the Child Care Center?" *Journal of Community Health* 18, no. 6 (1993): 363–77; M. E. Briley, C. Roberts-Gray, and D. Simpson, "Identification of Factors That Influence the Menu at Child Care Centers: A Grounded Theory Approach," *Journal of the American Dietetic Association* 94, no. 3 (1994): 276–81; C. B. Oakley and others, "Evaluation of Menus Planned in Mississippi Child-Care Centers Participating in the Child and Adult Care Food Program," *Journal of the American Dietetic Association* 95, no. 7 (1995): 765–68.

44. Briley, Roberts-Gray, and Rowe, "What Can Children Learn" (see note 43).

45. Briley, Roberts-Gray, and Simpson, "Identification of Factors" (see note 43).

46. A. Padget and M. E. Briley, "Dietary Intakes at Child-Care Centers in Central Texas Fail to Meet Food Guide Pyramid Recommendations," *Journal of the American Dietetic Association* 105, no. 5 (2005): 790–93.

47. Fox and others, *Early Childhood and Child Care Study* (see note 41).

48. Department of Health and Human Services and Department of Agriculture, *Dietary Guidelines for Americans, 2005* (see note 21); Department of Health and Human Services, *Healthy People 2010* (see note 22).

49. Russell R. Pate and others, "Physical Activity among Children Attending Preschools," *Pediatrics* 114, no. 5 (2004): 1258–63.

50. Department of Health and Human Services and Department of Agriculture, *Dietary Guidelines for Americans, 2005* (see note 21).

51. National Association for Sport and Physical Education, *Active Start: A Statement of Physical Activity Guidelines for Children Birth to Five Years* (Reston, Va.: National Association for Sport and Physical Education, 2002).

52. M. Dowda and others, "Influences of Preschool Policies and Practices on Children's Physical Activity," *Journal of Community Health* 29, no. 3 (2004): 183–96.

53. National Association for Sport and Physical Education, *Active Start* (see note 51); American Academy of Pediatrics, Committee on Sports Medicine and Fitness and Committee on School Health, "Organized Sports for Children and Preadolescents," *Pediatrics* 107 (2001): 1459–62.

54. Pate and others, "Physical Activity among Children" (see note 49).

55. K. Finn, N. Johannsen, and B. Specker, "Factors Associated with Physical Activity in Preschool Children," *Journal of Pediatrics* 140, no. 1 (2002): 81–85.

56. Pate and others, "Physical Activity among Children" (see note 49).

57. Dowda and others, "Influences of Preschool Policies" (see note 52); Finn, Johannsen, and Specker, "Factors Associated with Physical Activity" (see note 55).

58. S. G. Trost and others, "Physical Activity in Overweight and Nonoverweight Preschool Children," *International Journal of Obesity & Related Metabolic Disorders* 27, no. 7 (2003): 834–39.

59. Dowda and others, "Influences of Preschool Policies" (see note 52).

60. National Association for Sport and Physical Education, *Active Start* (see note 51).

61. Smolensky and Gootman, eds., *Working Families and Growing Kids* (see note 4).

62. American Academy of Pediatrics, "Children, Adolescents, and Television," *Pediatrics* 107, no. 2 (2001): 423–26.

63. Dowda and others, "Influences of Preschool Policies" (see note 52); Pate and others, "Physical Activity among Children" (see note 49); Finn, Johannsen, and Specker, "Factors Associated with Physical Activity" (see note 55).

64. Dowda and others, "Influences of Preschool Policies" (see note 52); Pate and others, "Physical Activity among Children" (see note 49).

65. M. L. Fitzgibbon and others, "Two-Year Follow-up Results for Hip-Hop to Health Jr.: A Randomized Controlled Trial for Overweight Prevention in Preschool Minority Children," *Journal of Pediatrics* 146, no. 5 (2005): 618–25; M. L. Fitzgibbon and others, "A Community-Based Obesity Prevention Program for Minority Children: Rationale and Study Design for Hip-Hop to Health Jr.," *Preventive Medicine* 34, no. 2 (2002): 289–97.

66. Fitzgibbon and others, "Two-Year Follow-up Results" (see note 65). The difference at the one-year follow-up was 0.06 vs. 0.59 kg/m^2 ; the difference at the two-year follow-up was 0.54 vs. 1.08 kg/m^2.

67. Christine L. Williams and others, "Cardiovascular Risk Reduction in Preschool Children: The 'Healthy Start' Project," *Journal of the American College of Nutrition* 23, no. 2 (2004): 117–23; C. L. Williams and others, "'Healthy-Start': Outcome of an Intervention to Promote a Heart Healthy Diet in Preschool Children," *Journal of the American College of Nutrition* 21, no. 1 (2002): 62–71.

68. T. N. Robinson, "Reducing Children's Television Viewing to Prevent Obesity: A Randomized Controlled Trial," *Journal of the American Medical Association* 282, no. 16 (1999): 1561–67; S. L. Gortmaker and others, "Reducing Obesity via a School-Based Interdisciplinary Intervention among Youth: Planet Health," *Archives of Pediatrics and Adolescent Medicine* 153, no. 4 (1999): 409–18.

69. B. A. Dennison and others, "An Intervention to Reduce Television Viewing by Preschool Children," *Archives of Pediatrics & Adolescent Medicine* 158, no. 2 (2004): 170–76.

70. Robinson, "Reducing Children's Television Viewing" (see note 68).

71. R. P. Troiano and others, "Energy and Fat Intakes of Children and Adolescents in the United States: Data from the National Health and Nutrition Examination Surveys," *American Journal of Clinical Nutrition* 72, no. 5, suppl. (2000): S1343–S53.

72. J. A. Welsh and others, "Overweight among Low-Income Preschool Children Associated with the Consumption of Sweet Drinks: Missouri, 1999–2002," *Pediatrics* 115, no. 2 (2005): e223–29.

73. B. A. Dennison, H. L. Rockwell, and S. L. Baker, "Excess Fruit Juice Consumption by Preschool-Aged Children Is Associated with Short Stature and Obesity," *Pediatrics* 99, no. 1 (1997): 15–22. Erratum appears in *Pediatrics* 100, no. 4 (1997): 733.

74. American Academy of Pediatrics, Committee on Nutrition, "The Use and Misuse of Fruit Juice in Pediatrics," *Pediatrics* 107, no. 5 (2001): 1210–13.

75. Kranz, Siega-Riz, and Herring, "Changes in Diet Quality" (see note 23).

76. U.S. Department of Health and Human Services, Administration for Children and Families, Head Start Bureau, "About Head Start" (www.acf.hhs.gov/programs/hsb/about [March 22, 2005]).

77. U.S. Department of Health and Human Services, Administration for Children and Families, Head Start Bureau, "Head Start Fact Sheets" (www.acf.hhs.gov/programs/hsb/research/factsheets.htm [March 22, 2005]).

78. Smolensky and Gootman, eds., *Working Families and Growing Kids* (see note 4).

79. U.S. Department of Health and Human Services, Administration for Children and Families, Head Start Bureau, *Head Start Program Performance Standards and Other Regulations* (Washington, 2005).

80. Ibid.

81. Ibid.

82. Ibid.

83. Wallace, Green, and Jaros, eds., *Health and Welfare for Families in the 21st Century* (see note 3).

84. Fitzgibbon and others, "Two-Year Follow-up Results" (see note 65).

85. U.S. General Accounting Office, *Child Care: State Efforts to Enforce Safety and Health Requirements,* GAO/HEHS-00-28 (Washington, January 2000).

86. Sandra L. Hofferth, "Child Care in the United States Today," *Future of Children* 6, no. 2 (1996): 41–61.

87. H. Blank, "Challenges of Child Care," in *About Children: An Authoritative Resource on the State of Childhood Today*, edited by A. G. Cosby and others (Elk Grove Village, Ill.: American Academy of Pediatrics, 2005).

88. U.S. General Accounting Office, *Child Care* (see note 85); Hofferth, "Child Care in the United States Today" (see note 86).

89. American Dietetic Association, "Position of the American Dietetic Association: Nutrition Standards" (see note 40); American Dietetic Association, "Position of the American Dietetic Association: Benchmarks for Nutrition Programs" (see note 40); American Academy of Pediatrics, American Public Health Association, and National Resource Center for Health and Safety in Child Care, *Caring for Our Children: National Health and Safety Performance Standards—Guidelines for Out-of-Home Child Care*, 2nd ed. (Elk Grove Village, Ill.: 2002).

90. U.S. General Accounting Office, *Child Care* (see note 85).

91. Children's Defense Fund, "Child Care Basics" (see note 11).

92. U.S. General Accounting Office, *Child Care* (see note 85); American Academy of Pediatrics, American Public Health Association, and National Resource Center for Health and Safety in Child Care, *Caring for Our Children* (see note 89).

93. American Academy of Pediatrics, American Public Health Association, and National Resource Center for Health and Safety in Child Care, *Caring for Our Children* (see note 89), p. 383.

94. National Association for the Education of Young Children, "Licensing and Public Regulation" (see note 10), p. 4.

95. U.S. General Accounting Office, *Child Care* (see note 85).

96. National Association for the Education of Young Children, "Licensing and Public Regulation" (see note 10).

97. National Resource Center for Health and Safety in Child Care, U.S. Department of Health and Human Services, Health Resources and Services Administration, "Individual States' Child Care Licensure Regulations" (http://nrc.uchs.edu/STATES/states.htm [March 22, 2005]).

98. Ibid.

99. Carnegie Corporation of New York, *Starting Points: Meeting the Needs of Our Youngest Children* (New York, August 1994).

100. Blank, "Challenges of Child Care" (see note 87).

101. Children's Defense Fund, "Child Care Basics" (see note 11).

102. Ibid.; Blank, "Challenges of Child Care" (see note 87).

103. Blank, "Challenges of Child Care (see note 87).

104. U.S. Department of Labor, Bureau of Labor Statistics, *November 2003 National Occupational Employment and Wage Estimates* (Washington, 2003) (www.bls.gov/news.release/ocwage.t01.htm [August 2, 2005]); C. Howes, M. Whitebook, and D. Phillips, *Worthy Work, Unlivable Wages: The National Child Care Staffing Study, 1988–1997* (Washington: Center for the Child Care Workforce, 1998); S. Helburn and others, *Cost, Quality, and Child Outcomes Study* (Denver, Colo.: University of Colorado, 1995).

105. American Academy of Pediatrics, American Public Health Association, and National Resource Center for Health and Safety in Child Care, *Caring for Our Children* (see note 89); National Association for the Education of Young Children, Division of Early Childhood Council for Exceptional Children, National Board for Professional Teaching Standards, *Guidelines for Preparation of Early Childhood Professionals* (Washington, 1996).

106. American Dietetic Association, "Position of the American Dietetic Association: Nutrition Standards" (see note 40); American Dietetic Association, "Position of the American Dietetic Association: Benchmarks for Nutrition Programs" (see note 40).

107. Dowda and others, "Influences of Preschool Policies" (see note 52).

108. Blank, "Challenges of Child Care" (see note 87).

109. Cubed, *The National Economic Impacts* (see note 7).

The Role of Parents in Preventing Childhood Obesity

*Ana C. Lindsay, Katarina M. Sussner, Juhee Kim,
and Steven Gortmaker*

Summary

As researchers continue to analyze the role of parenting both in the development of childhood overweight and in obesity prevention, studies of child nutrition and growth are detailing the ways in which parents affect their children's development of food- and activity-related behaviors. Ana Lindsay, Katarina Sussner, Juhee Kim, and Steven Gortmaker argue that interventions aimed at preventing childhood overweight and obesity should involve parents as important forces for change in their children's behaviors.

The authors begin by reviewing evidence on how parents can help their children develop and maintain healthful eating and physical activity habits, thereby ultimately helping prevent childhood overweight and obesity. They show how important it is for parents to understand how their roles in preventing obesity change as their children move through critical developmental periods, from before birth and through adolescence. They point out that researchers, policymakers, and practitioners should also make use of such information to develop more effective interventions and educational programs that address childhood obesity right where it starts—at home.

The authors review research evaluating school-based obesity-prevention interventions that include components targeted at parents. Although much research has been done on how parents shape their children's eating and physical activity habits, surprisingly few high-quality data exist on the effectiveness of such programs. The authors call for more programs and cost-effectiveness studies aimed at improving parents' ability to shape healthful eating and physical activity behaviors in their children.

The authors conclude that preventing and controlling childhood obesity will require multifaceted and community-wide programs and policies, with parents having a critical role to play. Successful intervention efforts, they argue, must involve and work directly with parents from the earliest stages of child development to support healthful practices both in and outside of the home.

www.futureofchildren.org

Ana C. Lindsay is a research scientist in the Department of Nutrition at the Harvard School of Public Health. Katarina M. Sussner is a doctoral candidate in the Department of Biological Anthropology at the Harvard Graduate School of Arts and Sciences. Juhee Kim is a research fellow in the Department of Nutrition at the Harvard School of Public Health. Steven Gortmaker is a professor of the practice of health sociology in the Department of Society, Human Development, and Health at the Harvard School of Public Health.

Parents are key to developing a home environment that fosters healthful eating and physical activity among children and adolescents. Parents shape their children's dietary practices, physical activity, sedentary behaviors, and ultimately their weight status in many ways. Parents' knowledge of nutrition; their influence over food selection, meal structure, and home eating patterns; their modeling of healthful eating practices; their levels of physical activity; and their modeling of sedentary habits including television viewing are all influential in their children's development of lifelong habits that contribute to normal weight or to overweight and obesity.[1]

Because the parents' roles at home in promoting healthful eating practices and levels of physical activity—and thus in preventing obesity—are so critical, they should also be central to collective efforts to combat the nation's childhood obesity epidemic. L. Epstein offers three reasons for involving parents in obesity-prevention interventions. First, obesity runs in families, and it may be unrealistic to intervene with one member of a family while other family members are modeling and supporting behaviors that run counter to the intervention's goals. Second, parents serve as models and reinforce and support the acquisition and maintenance of eating and exercise behaviors. Finally, to produce maximal behavior change in children, it may be necessary to teach parents to use specific behavior-change strategies such as positive reinforcement.[2] Several successful school-based health-promotion interventions, such as Planet Health and Eat Well and Keep Moving, already include a component targeted at improving parenting behaviors, as does the well-established Special Supplemental Nutrition Program for Women, Infants, and Children (WIC) public health and educational program.[3] Because research shows how the parents' roles in influencing the development of overweight and obesity differ at different stages of their children's development, these parenting components will be most effective if they are targeted at children in particular age groups.

Parental Roles during a Child's Development

Parenting influences the development of overweight and obesity in various ways at different stages of a child's development. The following discussion is structured around three time periods in children's lives: gestation and early infancy; early childhood, when children are toddlers or preschoolers; and middle childhood and adolescence, when children are attending school.[4]

Gestation and Infancy

Before an infant is even born, aspects of his mother's pregnancy can put him at risk of overweight in childhood and later in life.[5] An unfavorable intrauterine environment, for example, can increase a fetus's future risk of developing adult metabolic abnormalities, including obesity, hypertension, and non-insulin-dependent diabetes mellitus.[6] The children of mothers who suffer from diabetes mellitus, gestational diabetes, and undernutrition and overnutrition during pregnancy are at particular risk for obesity, with the greatest risk factor being gestational diabetes.[7] A key strategy for obesity prevention at this stage of a child's development, therefore, is to focus on screening for and preventing diabetes during pregnancy.

Parents also have an important role to play during infancy, when a child is establishing the foundation for dietary habits and nutritional adequacy over a lifetime.[8] Although debate over whether breast-feeding can help prevent obesity later in life continues, many researchers believe that breast-feeding infants does have a protective effect against obesity. Several studies, for example, have documented lower rates of overweight among children who were breast-fed for longer durations.[9] Their findings, however, were limited to non-Hispanic whites and did not apply to other racial or ethnic groups.[10] One explanation for the protective effect of breast-feeding is that it helps infants better regulate their food intake than does bottle-feeding. Encouraging an infant to empty a bottle and using formulas more concentrated in energy and nutrients than breast milk may make it more difficult for the baby to attend to his or her own normal feelings of satiety. If such experiences occur early in infancy and continue, an infant may not develop reliable control over food intake. None of the recent studies of breast-feeding, however, rules out the possibility that the protective effect of breast-feeding on obesity later in life may be due to confounding factors such as parental weight status or social and economic status.[11]

Toddlers and Preschool Children

As toddlers and preschoolers develop habits related to eating and physical activity, parents can shape their early environments in ways that encourage them to be more healthful.[12]

Parents and Healthful Food Behaviors

Children come equipped with a biological set of taste predispositions: they like sweet and salty tastes and energy-dense foods, and they dislike bitter and sour tastes.[13] But they develop most of their food habits through exposure and repeated experience. Research suggests that individual differences in the physiologic regulation of energy intake appear as early as the preschool years and that parents have enormous influence on these

differences.[14] Current data, although limited, suggest that the way parents feed their children contributes to individual differences in how well children can regulate their food intake and perhaps to the origins of energy imbalance.[15] Especially in the early years of a child's life, parents have a direct role in providing experiences that encourage the child's control of food intake. Around preschool age, when children particularly dislike new foods, it is important for parents to model healthful eating habits and to offer a variety of healthful foods to their children. When parents provide early exposure to nutritious foods, even fruits and vegetables, children like and eat more of such foods.[16] But parents should observe a clearly defined role in offering the foods to their children. As described by W. Dietz and L. Stern, parents "are responsible for offering a healthful variety of foods," while children themselves "are responsible for deciding what and how much they want to eat from what they are offered."[17]

Although children are predisposed to respond to the energy content of foods in controlling their intake, they are also responsive to their parents' control attempts. Research has shown that these attempts can refocus the child away from responsiveness to internal cues of hunger and satiety and toward such external factors as the presence of palatable foods.[18] Parents who control or restrict what their young children eat may believe they are doing what is best for their child, but recent research challenges this assumption. Imposing stringent controls can increase preferences for high-fat, energy-dense foods, perhaps causing children's normal internal cues to self-regulate hunger and satiety to become unbalanced.[19]

Parents should also be aware of the social contexts in which foods are consumed. Studies have found that children develop preferences for foods offered in positive contexts and, conversely, are more likely to dislike foods offered in negative contexts.[20] Offering healthful foods in positive contexts will encourage youngsters to enjoy and eat such foods.

Another important influence on the types of food young children consume is a household's food choices. At an early age children will eat

Parents who control or restrict what their young children eat may believe they are doing what is best for their child, but recent research challenges this assumption.

what their parents, especially their mothers, eat.[21] And if parents overeat, their children may too. Thus the parents' own eating behaviors may contribute to the development of overweight in their children.[22] The types of food available and accessible in the home are also linked with the weight status of preschool children. Research suggests, for example, that increased consumption of sugar-sweetened drinks, like fruit juice, might raise the risk of overweight among preschool children.[23] One study found that children aged two to five years who drank more than twelve ounces of fruit juice a day were more likely to be overweight than those who drank less.[24] More recently, a study of two- to three-year-old children found that for those who are at risk for overweight, consuming sweet drinks as infrequently as once or twice daily in-

creased their odds of becoming overweight.[25] These findings are consistent with those of long-term studies and interventions focused on sugar-sweetened beverages among school-aged children, although some smaller long-term studies in children found no significant link between fruit juice intake and overweight.[26]

Parents and Physical Activity during Early Childhood

Physical activity is a key component of energy balance, and keeping small children active is an essential part of preventing child overweight.[27] Research has found that physical activity is associated with lower risks of accelerated weight gain and excess adiposity among preschool-aged children.[28] An eight-year study of three- to five-year-old children found that the most active children had significantly lower body mass index (BMI) than their less active counterparts.[29] A study of three- to five-year-old children attending preschool found that overweight boys were significantly less active than normal-weight boys during the preschool day.[30]

Few studies have examined the relationship between the activity levels of parents and their young children. The Framingham Children's Study, however, monitored physical activity with a mechanical device—the Caltrac accelerometer—in four- to seven-year-old children and their parents and found that the children of active mothers were twice as likely to be active as children of inactive mothers. When both parents were active, these children were 5.8 times more likely to be active than the children of two sedentary parents.[31]

A few studies of preschool children have found that the more time children spend outdoors, the higher their activity levels.[32] These findings suggest that parents can and should encourage outdoor play. Questions of safety and accessibility, however, may make it more difficult for some parents and children to spend time outdoors. Minority and lower-income parents, for example, are more likely to live in communities with fewer parks, sports facilities, bike paths, and other places for children to be active and safe.[33]

Although most research on television viewing's influence on child obesity has been conducted among older children and adolescents, some studies have focused on preschool-aged children. A study of five- and six-year-old His-panic (predominantly Mexican American) children in Chicago found a link between TV viewing and overweight.[34] R. H. DuRant and several colleagues directly observed three- and four-year-old children in their homes and found that children who watched TV more hours a day and children who watched for longer periods of time at one sitting were less likely to engage in physical activity.[35] Another study of 2,761 adults with children aged one to five years from forty-nine New York State WIC agencies found that viewing TV and videos and having a TV in the bedroom were both linked with the prevalence of child over-weight.[36] These studies indicate that parents should limit preschoolers' TV and video viewing and keep televisions out of their bedrooms.

School-Aged Children and Youth

National data indicate that 16 percent of children aged six to nineteen years are over-weight.[37] As children grow older and as they focus less on family and more on school, peers, and different media, parental influence wanes. As adolescents, children spend increasingly more time away from home, become more exposed to environments that encourage obesity, and have greater choices in their own diet and physical activities. When children make critical decisions about nutrition and physical activity on their own, parents' roles become even more challenging. Nevertheless, parents and family members can still provide a healthful home nutrition and physical activity environment.

Parents and Healthful Eating in School-Aged Children

Parents can encourage healthful eating habits at home by increasing the number of family meals eaten together, making healthful foods available, and reducing the availability of sugar-sweetened beverages and sodas.

Studies show that eating dinner together as a family promotes healthful eating among children and adolescents by increasing their consumption of fruits, vegetables, and whole grains and reducing their consumption of fats and soft drinks.[38] These same studies, however, show that families eat dinner together less often as children grow older. One study found that nine-year-olds ate dinner with their family roughly half the time, while four-teen-year-olds ate dinner with their families only a third of the time.[39] It is crucial, there-fore, that parents maintain family eating practices throughout adolescence.

As with preschool-aged children, the availability of foods at home is a major influence on older children's diets. Studies have found that making fruits and vegetables available at home increases children's consumption of these foods.[40] And parents must not only provide healthful foods at home, but also eat these foods themselves.

Between 1965 and 1996, adolescents' soft drink consumption increased 150 percent while their consumption of fruit drinks increased 89 percent. As with young children, several studies indicate that sugar-sweetened beverages may play an important role in the childhood obesity epidemic.[41] A long-term study of children that began when they were eleven and twelve years old found that their odds of becoming overweight increased 60 percent for each additional serving of sugar-sweetened drinks consumed daily.[42] A second long-term study, this one beginning when children were nine to fourteen years old, linked consumption of sugar-added beverages with increased weight gains.[43] In a randomized controlled trial in England, reducing consumption of carbonated beverages lowered the prevalence of overweight among seven- to eleven-year-olds.[44] Such findings show how important it is for parents to limit their children's consumption of these beverages at home. Now that many schools are making a commitment to soda-free hallways and cafeterias, parents can follow their lead and keep their homes free of sugar-sweetened beverages as well.

Parents and Older Children's Activity Levels

Children and adolescents spend more time watching television than they do in almost any other activity. By the time they reach school-age, about half of U.S. children watch television more than two hours a day, and 17 percent of African American children watch more than five hours a day.[45] Many studies link TV viewing with overweight.[46] Randomized controlled trials indicate that watching fewer hours of TV can reduce children's body mass index and obesity risk.[47] TV viewing, therefore, may be one important cause of childhood obesity that parents can modify at home.

TV viewing may increase overweight both by reducing children's physical activity and by encouraging poor eating habits in children by exposing them to commercials for unhealthful foods.[48] Experimental results suggest both factors are at work.[49] According to a recent nationally representative survey, children from third through twelfth grade spend an estimated eight hours a day of media time —using computers, listening to music, watching movies, playing computer and video games, and watching TV. About 26 percent of children are "media multitaskers" who go online while they watch TV, resulting in more exposure to the media environment simultaneously.[50]

Studies of the contents of television advertisements document that children are exposed to a vast number of TV ads for sodas, cereal, candy, and fast food.[51] And other research suggests that exposure to food commercials influences children's preferences and food requests and can contribute to confusion among children about the relative health benefits of foods.

Recent data indicate that 68 percent of children have a TV in their bedroom, and half have a video game player and a VCR or DVD player as well. Increasing numbers of children also have cable or satellite TV, computer, and Internet access in their bedrooms. Despite such widespread access, more than half of children report that they have no parental rules on TV watching hours. Among those reporting such rules, only 20 percent said parents enforce them "most" of the time.[52] Limiting physical access to TV may help children reduce their TV viewing.[53] Children with a TV in their room spend an estimated 1.5 hours more a day watching TV than do those without a set in their room.[54]

Parents can also help by limiting their own TV watching and sedentary behavior. Studies show that when parents are sedentary, their

A Word of Caution to Parents about Encouraging Child Dieting

Even though childhood obesity experts discourage dieting, parents who feel the need to control a child's weight commonly encourage dieting. Studies on dieting behaviors consistently report that their parents' inducement to diet is the most significant factor in causing children to begin dieting. Their parents' direct verbal encouragement is more influential than the parents' own dieting behaviors.

Many adolescents whose parents urged them to diet report engaging in unhealthful dieting behaviors. Focusing on dieting for weight control may overemphasize the thinness ideal and over time may even lead to an increased risk for obesity. It is important for parents of overweight children to learn about the dangers of dieting and to talk with their child's doctor or health care provider about ways to promote healthful habits.

Sources: L. L. Birch and J. O. Fisher, "Development of Eating Behaviors among Children and Adolescents," *Pediatrics* 101, no. 3, pt. 2 (1998): 539–49; K. G. Strong and G. F. Huon, "An Evaluation of a Structural Model for Studies of the Initiation of Dieting among Adolescent Girls," *Journal of Psychosomatic Research* 44, no. 3–4 (1998): 315–26; R. Dixon, V. Adair, and S. O'Connor, "Parental Influences on the Dieting Beliefs and Behaviors of Adolescent Females in New Zealand," *Journal of Adolescent Health* 19, no. 4 (1996): 303–07; G. B. Schreiber and others, "Weight Modification Efforts Reported by Black and White Preadolescent Girls: National Heart, Lung, and Blood Institute Growth and Health Study," *Pediatrics* 98, no. 1 (1996): 63–70; S. Saarilehto and others, "Connections between Parental Eating Attitudes and Children's Meagre Eating: Questionnaire Findings," *Acta Paediatrica* 90 (2001): 333–38; L. Smolak, M. P. Levine, and F. Schermer, "Parental Input and Weight Concerns among Elementary School Children," *International Journal of Eating Disorders* 25, no. 3 (1999): 263–71; J. A. Fulkerson and others, "Weight-Related Attitudes and Behaviors of Adolescent Boys and Girls Who Are Encouraged to Diet by Their Mothers," *International Journal of Obesity and Related Metabolic Disorders* 26, no. 12 (2002): 1579–87.

children are more likely to be sedentary as well.[55] Adolescents whose parents watch TV more than two hours a day are more than twice as likely to be physically inactive as those children whose parents watch less.[56]

During the transition from childhood to adolescence, children's physical activity drops off dramatically.[57] Although current guidelines recommend at least sixty minutes of physical activity for older children on most, preferably all, days of the week, only 63 percent of adolescents reported meeting those guidelines in 1999.[58] Parents can encourage older children to be more active. Studies suggest that participating in sports teams or exercise programs can help adolescents reduce their body mass index.[59]

Some studies have found that children are more likely to be active if their parents are active, while others do not find this relationship and rather emphasize the importance of parental support.[60] Many studies show that parents can promote children's physical activity by providing support and encouragement.[61] Further, those parents who realize the importance of physical activity may offer even greater support.[62] That support can take many forms: arranging access to after-school or community sports and activity programs, watching children's activities, or simply playing with their children.[63] Parents' views about their children's competence and task orientation may also affect their physical activity.[64] Concerns about traffic, drug dealers, crime, and violence may cause parents to limit places where their child can play, thereby reducing their opportunities for activity.[65]

Family-Based Obesity-Prevention Programs

Although a great deal of research has been done on how parents shape their children's eating and physical activity habits, surprisingly few high-quality data exist on the effectiveness of obesity-prevention programs for children that center on parental involvement. One reason for the paucity of data is that, despite some studies that indicate promising results, few programs are solely parent-based. Most efforts to involve parents are components of more comprehensive interventions. For example, many school-based programs aimed at preventing childhood obesity are targeted at children within school settings but include parental components that help parents set lim-

---

Creating more programs to improve parenting behaviors relevant to childhood overweight is a highly promising strategy.

---

its on TV viewing and provide electronic "lock-out" devices.[66] Likewise, health care–based interventions may add a parenting focus. Meanwhile, a WIC-sponsored nutrition intervention will take place within the context of WIC, but it might add a parental component aimed at reducing TV time.[67]

As yet little to no information is available on the cost-effectiveness of obesity-prevention interventions that have a parenting component. One middle-school program called Planet Health was found to be highly cost-effective—in fact, more cost-effective even than commonly accepted preventive interventions such as screening and treatment for hypertension.[68] Precisely what influence the program's parental component specifically generated, however, is unclear. Nevertheless, creating more programs to improve parenting behaviors relevant to childhood overweight is a highly promising strategy. Such

programs would be most effective if they were targeted at children of various ages based on research that shows how parents can best help children at different developmental stages. Researchers should carefully evaluate the programs' effectiveness.

Solely Parent-Based Interventions
One solely parent-based intervention consisted of twenty-eight families of seven- to twelve-year-old African American children who received primary care at an urban community clinic serving a low-income population. Families were randomly selected to receive counseling alone or counseling plus a behavioral intervention that included an electronic television time manager. Both groups reported similar decreases in their children's use of television, videotapes, and video games. The behavioral intervention group reported significantly greater increases in organized physical activity and somewhat greater increases in playing outside. Changes in overall household television use and in meals eaten while watching television also appeared to favor the behavioral intervention, with small to medium effect sizes, but these differences were not statistically significant.[69]

Another recent solely family-based intervention tested two versions of a culturally relevant program to prevent excess weight gain in pre-adolescent African American girls. The girls, aged eight to ten years, were divided into two groups, both of which participated in highly interactive weekly group sessions. In one group, the sessions targeted the girls; in the other, the sessions were geared toward their parents or caregivers. Girls in both groups demonstrated a trend toward reduced body mass index and waist circumference. In addition, girls in both groups reduced their consumption of sugar-sweetened beverages, increased their level of moderate to vigorous activity, and increased their daily serving of water.[70]

Comprehensive Interventions with a Parenting Component

Most interventions aimed at preventing over-weight and obesity have been school-based, and all have improved health knowledge and health-related behaviors to some extent.[71] Some of the most successful school-based in-terventions, however, have included a parent-ing component. These interventions have re-sulted in dramatic changes in health behaviors associated with child obesity and overweight as well as in changes in body mass index or obesity.

School-based interventions at the preschool level are scarce, but one study's findings pro-vide strong support for establishing such pro-grams. The Hip-Hop to Health Jr. program targeted three- to five-year-old minority chil-dren enrolled in Head Start programs in Chicago, with the aim of reducing the ten-dency toward overweight and obesity in African American and Latino preschool chil-dren. The intervention presented a develop-mentally, culturally, and linguistically appro-priate dietary and physical activity curriculum for preschoolers, and a parent component addressed the families' dietary and physical activity patterns. Each week of the intervention covered a particular topic, such as the importance of "Go and Grow" foods, eating fruit, and reducing TV viewing. Parents received weekly newsletters with in-formation that mirrored the children's cur-riculum on healthful eating and exercise as well as a five- to fifteen-minute homework assignment that reinforced concepts pre-sented in the weekly newsletters. During the fourteen-week intervention, children in a control group attended a twenty-minute class once a week in which they learned about var-ious general health concepts, such as dental health, immunization, seat belt safety, and 911 procedures. Their parents' weekly newsletters mirrored these sessions. A recent two-year follow-up study found that the in-tervention group's children had significantly smaller increases in body mass index than did those in the control group.[72]

Another recent study assessed the impact of the school-based Child and Adolescent Trial for Cardiovascular Health (CATCH) inter-vention among primarily Hispanic, low-income elementary school children. The in-tervention tested the effectiveness of changes in school food service, physical education, classroom curricula, and family activities. The family component consisted primarily of skill-building activity packets that students took home to complete with their parents. Third and fourth graders and their families were also invited to participate in Family Fun Nights at the school. The family component supplemented the classroom curriculum, which focused on improving the children's di-etary and physical activity knowledge, atti-tudes, and self-reported behaviors, and rein-forced the concepts, activities, and skills of the curriculum. Among both boys and girls, the intervention reduced overweight or the risk of overweight.[73]

Another successful elementary school–based health behavior intervention on diet and physical activity was the Eat Well and Keep Moving program. Classroom teachers in math, science, language arts, and social stud-ies classes taught the quasi-experimental, two-year field trial among children in grades four and five, with six intervention and eight matched control schools. The intervention provided links to school food services and families and provided training and wellness programs for teachers and other staff members. Its aim was to decrease the consumption of foods high in total and saturated fat, to increase fruit and vegetable intake, to reduce television viewing, and to increase physical activity. Compared with students in the control schools, students in the intervention schools reduced their share of total energy from fat and saturated fat. They also increased their fruit and vegetable intake, vita-

---

A systematic review of research on family involvement in weight control recently found that relatively few intervention studies exist, but those few suggest that parental involvement helps children lose weight.

---

min C intake, and fiber consumption. They reduced their television viewing marginally.[74]

Recently, a pilot study divided children in four elementary schools into an intervention group and a control group and evaluated how a school-based health report card affected family awareness of and concerns about child weight status, plans for weight control, and preventive behaviors. Parents of overweight children (including those at risk of overweight) in the intervention group had greater awareness of their children's weight status and initiated more activities to control weight than did the parents of children in the control group.[75]

Planet Health was a two-year, school-based health behavior intervention targeting mid-

dle school–aged boys and girls in sixth through eighth grades. Students participated in a school-based interdisciplinary program that used existing classroom teachers and took place in four major subjects and physical education classes. Sessions focused on decreasing both television viewing and the consumption of high-fat foods and on increasing both fruit and vegetable intake and physical activity, with no explicit discussion of obesity. Compared with girls in the control group, girls in the intervention group reduced their prevalence of obesity; no differences were found among boys. The intervention reduced television hours among both girls and boys, increased fruit and vegetable consumption among both girls and boys, and reduced total energy intake among girls in the intervention group compared with girls in the control group. Among girls, obesity prevalence was reduced for each hour that television viewing was reduced. Although not primarily a parent-focused program, Planet Health had several family components, including an activity called "Power Down," where the household together engaged in a TV charting exercise to reduce TV time.[76] Further analysis of Planet Health found a reduced risk of disordered, or unhealthy, weight control behaviors in girls. An economic analysis found the program substantially cost-effective.[77]

Obesity-related interventions have also focused on limiting television viewing.[78] A recent randomized control trial called "Switch-Play" aimed to replace TV viewing time with more physical activities. More than half the children reported reducing their TV viewing while less than half increased physical activity. Most of the children enjoyed alternative activity programs, and only 7 to 17 percent had difficulty turning off their favorite TV shows.[79]

An after-school intervention known as the GEMS pilot study tested the feasibility, acceptability, and potential efficacy of after-school dance classes and a family-based intervention to reduce television viewing and weight gain among African American girls in Stanford, California. At the follow-up, girls in the intervention group exhibited trends toward lower body mass index and waist circumference, increased after-school physical activity, and reduced television, videotape, and video game use, as compared with the control group. The treatment group also reported significantly reduced household television viewing and fewer dinners eaten while watching TV.[80]

Although intervention studies show the benefit of cutting TV hours, such practical barriers as long hours of parental work and inadequate child care options make it difficult for families to implement these changes. For many families, particularly in low-income, urban areas without safe places to play outdoors, TV is a substitute babysitter. Mothers are often more concerned with the types of TV programs their children watch than with how much time their children spend watching TV. These mothers raise the issue of affordable and accessible recreation facilities and programs and say the lack of such options contributes to their children's watching more TV at home.[81]

A systematic review of research on family involvement in weight control recently found that relatively few intervention studies exist, but those few suggest that parental involvement helps children lose weight.[82] The studies also indicate that results, in terms of weight loss and behavioral changes, are better when children are treated together with their parents.[83] Involving at least one parent in a weight-loss process improves overall short- and long-term weight regulation, as does overall support from family and friends.[84] For families with several members battling overweight, family treatment can substantially reduce the per-person costs of obesity treatment, and children and their parents can achieve similar percentages of overweight change.[85]

Conclusion

Parents play a critical role at home in preventing childhood obesity, with their role changing at different stages of their child's development. By better understanding their own role in influencing their child's dietary practices, physical activity, sedentary behaviors, and ultimately weight status, parents can learn how to create a healthful nutrition environment in their home, provide opportunities for physical activity, discourage sedentary behaviors such as TV viewing, and serve as role models themselves. Obesity-related intervention programs can use parental involvement as one key to success in developing an environment that fosters healthy eating and physical activity among children and adolescents.

Although few interventions solely target parents, current evidence suggests that parenting interventions may work best as a component of comprehensive interventions within a variety of settings, including schools, health services, or such programs as WIC. Recent research highlights the success of school-based programs, such as Planet Health, CATCH, Eat Well and Keep Moving, and the GEMS pilot study, that incorporate parenting and at-home components into their curricula.[86] Another potential avenue is to incorporate parenting education modules into well-established public health and educational programs, such as WIC, Head Start, and birthing classes, following the model of such programs as Hip-Hop to Health Jr.[87]

As more of these interventions are created, researchers should carefully evaluate their cost-effectiveness. New interventions should replace those that are based either in school alone or in a health center alone with strategies that affect multiple settings at the same time.[88] Community, statewide, and national obesity-prevention programs should emphasize an educational collaboration among schools, health centers, and parents.

Achieving the goal of preventing and controlling the childhood obesity epidemic requires multifaceted and community-wide programs and policies. But even in such broad and comprehensive programs, parents have a critical and influential role to play. Interventions should involve and work directly with parents from the very earliest stages of child development and growth both to make healthful changes at home and to reinforce and support healthful eating and regular physical activity.

Notes

1. J. P. Kaplan, C. T. Liverman, and V. I. Kraak, eds., *Preventing Childhood Obesity: Health in the Balance* (Washington: National Academies Press, 2004).

2. L. Epstein, "Family-Based Behavioural Intervention for Obese Children," *International Journal of Obesity and Related Metabolic Disorders* 20, suppl. 1 (1996): S14–21.

3. S. L. Gortmaker and others, "Reducing Obesity via a School-Based Interdisciplinary Intervention among Youth: Planet Health," *Archives of Pediatric and Adolescent Medicine* 153, no. 9 (1999): 1–10; S. L. Gortmaker and others, "Impact of a School-Based Interdisciplinary Intervention on Diet and Physical Activity among Urban Primary School Children: Eat Well and Keep Moving," *Archives of Pediatric and Adolescent Medicine* 153, no. 9 (1999): 975–83.

4. W. H. Dietz, "Critical Periods in Childhood for the Development of Obesity," *American Journal of Clinical Nutrition* 59, no. 5 (1994): 955–59; M. M. Abrantes, J. A. Lamounier, and E. A. Colosimo, "Overweight and Obesity Prevalence among Children and Adolescents from Northeast and Southeast Regions of Brazil," *Journal of Pediatrics (Rio J)* 78, no. 4 (2002): 335–40; D. J. Barker and C. H. Fall, "Fetal and Infant Origins of Cardiovascular Disease," *Archives of Disease in Childhood* 68, no. 6 (1993): 797–99; K. Krishnaswamy and others, "Fetal Malnutrition and Adult Chronic Disease," *Nutrition Review* 60, no. 5, pt. 2 (2002): S35–39.

5. Barker and Fall, "Fetal and Infant Origins" (see note 4); C. Power and T. Parsons, "Nutritional and Other Influences in Childhood as Predictors of Adult Obesity," *Proceedings of the Nutrition Society* 59, no. 2 (2000): 267–72; C. Maffeis and L. Tatò, "Long-Term Effects of Childhood Obesity on Morbidity and Mortality," *Hormone Research* 55, suppl. 1 (2001): 42–45.

6. Power and Parsons, "Nutritional and Other Influences" (see note 5); Maffeis and Tatò, "Long-Term Effects" (see note 5).

7. R. C. Whitaker and W. H. Dietz, "Role of the Prenatal Environment in the Development of Obesity," *Journal of Pediatrics* 132, no. 5 (1998): 768–76.

8. J. Westenhoefer, "Establishing Dietary Habits during Childhood for Long-Term Weight Control," *Annals of Nutrition and Metabolism* 46 (2002): 18–23.

9. M. L. P. Hediger and others, "Association between Infant Breastfeeding and Overweight in Young Children," *Journal of the American Medical Association* 285, no. 19 (2001): 2453–60; K. K. L. Ong and others, "Size at Birth and Early Childhood Growth in Relation to Maternal Smoking, Parity, and Infant Breast-Feeding: Longitudinal Birth Cohort Study and Analysis," *Pediatric Research* 52, no. 6 (2002): 863–67; M. W. Gillman and others, "Risk of Overweight among Adolescents Who Were Breastfed as Infants," *Journal of the American Medical Association* 285, no. 19 (2001): 2461–67; R. von Kries and others, "Breast Feeding and Obesity: Cross Sectional Study," *British Medical Journal* 319, no. 7203 (1999): 147–50; L. M. Grummer-Strawn and A. Mei, "Does Breastfeeding Protect against Pediatric Overweight? Analysis of Longitudinal Data from the Centers for Disease Control and Prevention Pediatric Nutrition Surveillance System," *Pediatrics* 113, no. 2 (2004): e81–86.

10. Grummer-Strawn and Mei, "Does Breastfeeding Protect?" (see note 9).

11. Hediger and others, "Association between Infant Breastfeeding" (see note 9); Ong and others, "Size at Birth" (see note 9); Gillman and others, "Risk of Overweight among Adolescents" (see note 9); von Kries and others, "Breast Feeding and Obesity" (see note 9).

12. L. L. Birch and J. O. Fisher, "Development of Eating Behaviors among Children and Adolescents," *Pediatrics* 101, no. 3, pt. 2 (1998): 539–49; L. L. Birch and J. O. Fisher, "Mothers' Child-Feeding Practices Influence Daughters' Eating and Weight," *American Journal of Clinical Nutrition* 71, no. 5 (2000): 1054–61; J. Wardle and others, "Parental Feeding Style and the Inter-Generational Transmission of Obesity Risk," *Obesity Research* 10, no. 6 (2002): 453–62; T. N. Robinson, "Television Viewing and Childhood Obesity," *Pediatric Clinics of North America* 48, no. 4 (2001): 1017–25; D. Spruijt-Metz and others, "Relation between Mothers' Child-Feeding Practices and Children's Adiposity," *American Journal of Clinical Nutrition* 75, no. 3 (2002): 581–86; W. C. Heird, "Parental Feeding Behavior and Children's Fat Mass," *American Journal of Clinical Nutrition* 75, no. 3 (2002): 451–52; V. Burke, L. J. Beilin, and D. Dunbar, "Family Lifestyle and Parental Body Mass Index as Predictors of Body Mass Index in Australian Children: A Longitudinal Study," *International Journal of Obesity and Related Metabolic Disorders* 25, no. 2 (2001): 147–57; K. Dettwyler, "Styles of Infant Feeding: Parental/Caretaker Control of Food Consumption in Young Children," *American Anthropology* 91 (1989): 696–703; R. C. Klesges and others, "Parental Influence on Food Selection in Young Children and Its Relationships to Childhood Obesity," *American Journal of Clinical Nutrition* 53, no. 4 (1991): 859–64.

13. A. J. Hill, "Developmental Issues in Attitudes to Food and Diet," *Proceedings of the Nutrition Society* 61, no. 2 (2002): 259–66.

14. L. S. Birch, "Development of Food Acceptance Patterns in the First Years of Life," *Proceedings of the Nutrition Society* 57, no. 4 (1998): 617–24.

15. Ibid.

16. Hill, "Developmental Issues" (see note 13).

17. W. Dietz and L. Stern, *Guide to Your Child's Nutrition* (New York: Villard, American Academy of Pediatrics, 1999).

18. Birch and Fisher, "Development of Eating Behaviors" (see note 12).

19. Ibid.; Birch, "Development of Food Acceptance" (see note 14).

20. U. K. Koivisto Hursti, "Factors Influencing Children's Food Choice," *Annals of Medicine* 31, suppl. 1 (1999): 26–32.

21. S. A. Oliveria and others, "Parent-Child Relationships in Nutrient Intake: The Framingham Children's Study," *American Journal of Clinical Nutrition* 56, no. 3 (1992): 593–98.

22. M. Y. Hood and others, "Parental Eating Attitudes and the Development of Obesity in Children: The Framingham Children's Study," *International Journal of Obesity* 24, no. 10 (2000): 1319.

23. B. S. Dennison, H. L. Rockwell, and S. L. Baker, "Excess Fruit Juice Consumption by Preschool-Aged Children Is Associated with Short Stature and Obesity," *Pediatrics* 99, no. 1 (1997): 15–22; U. Alexy and others, "Fruit Juice Consumption and the Prevalence of Obesity and Short Stature in German Preschool Children: Results of the DONALD Study—Dortmund Nutritional and Anthropometrical Longitudinally Designed," *Journal of Pediatric Gastroenterology and Nutrition* 29, no. 3 (1999): 343–49; J. D. Skinner and others, "Fruit Juice Intake Is Not Related to Children's Growth," *Pediatrics* 103, no. 1 (1999): 58–64; J. A. Welsh and others, "Overweight among Low-Income Preschool Children Associated with the Consumption of Sweet Drinks: Missouri, 1999–2002," *Pediatrics* 115, no. 2 (2005): e223–29.

24. Dennison, Rockwell, and Baker, "Excess Fruit Juice" (see note 23).

25. Welsh and others, "Overweight among Low-Income Preschool Children" (see note 23).

26. Alexy and others, "Fruit Juice Consumption" (see note 23); Skinner and others, "Fruit Juice Intake" (see note 23); J. D. Skinner and B. R. Carruth, "A Longitudinal Study of Children's Juice Intake and Growth: The Juice Controversy Revisited," *Journal of the American Dietetic Association* 101, no. 4 (2001): 432–37.

27. H. W. Kohl III and K. E. Hobbs, "Development of Physical Activity Behaviors among Children and Adolescents," *Pediatrics* 101, no. 3 (1998): 549–54.

28. R. C. K. Klesges and M. Lisa, "A Longitudinal Analysis of Accelerated Weight Gain in Preschool Children," *Pediatrics* 95, no. 1 (1995): 126; L. L. Moore and others, "Preschool Physical Activity Level and Change in Body Fatness in Young Children: The Framingham Children's Study," *American Journal of Epidemiology* 142, no. 9 (1995): 982–88.

29. Moore and others, "Preschool Physical Activity" (see note 28).

30. S. G. Trost and others, "Evaluating a Model of Parental Influence on Youth Physical Activity," *American Journal of Preventive Medicine* 25, no. 4 (2003): 277–82.

31. Hood and others, "Parental Eating Attitudes" (see note 22).

32. T. Baranowski and others, "Observations on Physical Activity in Physical Locations: Age, Gender, Ethnicity, and Month Effects," *Research Quarterly for Exercise and Sport* 64, no. 2 (1993): 127–33; J. F. Sallis and others, "Correlates of Physical Activity at Home in Mexican-American and Anglo-American Preschool Children," *Health Psychology* 12, no. 5 (1993): 390–98.

33. K. E. Powell, L. M. Martin, and P. P. Chowdhury, "Places to Walk: Convenience and Regular Physical Activity," *American Journal of Public Health* 93, no. 9 (2003): 1519–21.

34. A. J. Ariza and others, "Risk Factors for Overweight in Five- to Six-Year-Old Hispanic-American Children: A Pilot Study," *Journal of Urban Health* 81, no. 1 (2004): 150–61.

35. R. H. DuRant and others, "The Relationship among Television Watching, Physical Activity, and Body Composition of Young Children," *Pediatrics* 94, no. 4, pt. 1(1994): 449–55.

36. B. A. Dennison, T. A. Erb, and P. L. Jenkins, "Television Viewing and Television in Bedroom Associated with Overweight Risk among Low-Income Preschool Children," *Pediatrics* 109, no. 6 (2002): 1028–35.

37. A. A. Hedley and others, "Prevalence of Overweight and Obesity among U.S. Children, Adolescents, and Adults, 1999–2002," *Journal of the American Medical Association* 291, no. 23 (2004): 2847–50.

38. M. W. Gillman and others, "Family Dinner and Diet Quality among Older Children and Adolescents," *Archives of Family Medicine* 9, no. 3 (2000): 235–40; D. Neumark-Sztainer and others, "Family Meal Patterns: Associations with Sociodemographic Characteristics and Improved Dietary Intake among Adolescents," *Journal of the American Dietetic Association* 103, no. 3 (2003): 317–22.

39. Gillman and others, "Family Dinner" (see note 38).

40. K. W. Cullen and others, "Availability, Accessibility, and Preferences for Fruit, 100% Fruit Juice, and Vegetables Influence Children's Dietary Behavior," *Health Education Behavior* 30, no. 5 (2003): 615–26; Neumark-Sztainer and others, "Family Meal Patterns" (see note 38).

41. J. Putman and J. Allshouse, *Food Consumption, Price, and Expenditures, 1970–97* (U.S. Department of Agriculture, 1999); C. Cavadini, A. M. Siega-Riz, and B. M. Popkin, "U.S. Adolescent Food Intake Trends

from 1965 to 1996," *Archives of Disease in Childhood* 83, no. 1 (2000): 18–24 (erratum in *Archives of Disease in Childhood* 87, no. 1 [2002]: 85).

42. D. S. Ludwig, K. E. Peterson, and S. L. Gortmaker, "Relation between Consumption of Sugar-Sweetened Drinks and Childhood Obesity: A Prospective, Observational Analysis," *Lancet* 357, no. 9255 (2001): 505–08.

43. C. S. Berkey and others, "Sugar-Added Beverages and Adolescent Weight Change," *Obesity Research* 12, no. 5 (2004): 778–88.

44. J. James and others, "Preventing Childhood Obesity by Reducing Consumption of Carbonated Drinks: Cluster Randomised Controlled Trial," *British Medical Journal* 328, no. 7450 (2004): 1237.

45. C. J. Crespo and others, "Television Watching, Energy Intake, and Obesity in U.S. Children: Results from the Third National Health and Nutrition Examination Survey, 1988–1994," *Archives of Pediatric and Adolescent Medicine* 155, no. 3 (2001): 360–65.

46. W. H. J. Dietz and S. L. Gortmaker, "Do We Fatten Our Children at the Television Set? Obesity and Television Viewing in Children and Adolescents," *Pediatrics* 75, no. 5 (1985): 807–12; S. L. Gortmaker and others, "Television Viewing as a Cause of Increasing Obesity among Children in the United States, 1986–1990," *Archives of Pediatric and Adolescent Medicine* 150, no. 4 (1996): 356–62; R. Pate and J. Ross, "The National Children and Youth Fitness Study II: Factors Associated with Health-Related Fitness," *Journal of Physical Education, Recreation, and Dance* 58 (1987): 93–95; L. A. Tucker, "The Relationship of Television Viewing to Physical Fitness and Obesity," *Adolescence* 21, no. 84 (1986): 797–806; C. S. Berkey and others, "One-Year Changes in Activity and in Inactivity among 10- to 15-Year-Old Boys and Girls: Relationship to Change in Body Mass Index," *Pediatrics* 111, no. 4 (2003): 836–43; R. J. Hancox, B. J. Milne, and R. Poulton, "Association between Child and Adolescent Television Viewing and Adult Health: A Longitudinal Birth Cohort Study," *Lancet* 364, no. 9430 (2004): 257–62.

47. T. N. Robinson, "Reducing Children's Television Viewing to Prevent Obesity: A Randomized Controlled Trial," *Journal of the American Medical Association* 282, no. 16 (1999): 1561–67; S. L. Gortmaker and others, "Reducing Obesity" (see note 3).

48. D. S. Ludwig and S. L. Gortmaker, "Programming Obesity in Childhood," *Lancet* 364, no. 9430 (2004): 226–27.

49. L. H. Epstein and others, "Effects of Manipulating Sedentary Behavior on Physical Activity and Food Intake," *Journal of Pediatrics* 140, no. 3 (2002): 334–39.

50. D. F. Roberts, U. G. Foehr, and U. Rideout, *Generation M: Media in the Lives of 8–18 Year-Olds* (Menlo Park, Calif.: Henry J. Kaiser Family Foundation, 2005).

51. S. A. Bowman and others, "Effects of Fast-Food Consumption on Energy Intake and Diet Quality among Children in a National Household Survey," *Pediatrics* 113, no. 1 (2004): 112–18; J. M. McGinnis, J. A. Gootman, and V. I. Kraak, eds., *Food Marketing to Youth: Threat or Opportunity?* (Washington: National Academies Press, 2005).

52. Roberts, Foehr, and Rideout, *Generation M* (see note 50).

53. Ibid.; J. L. Wiecha and others, "Household Television Access: Associations with Screen Time, Reading, and Homework among Youth," *Ambulatory Pediatrics* 1, no. 5 (2001): 244–51.

54. Roberts, Foehr, and Rideout, *Generation M* (see note 50).

55. M. Fogelholm and others, "Parent-Child Relationship of Physical Activity Patterns and Obesity," *International Journal of Obesity* 23 (1999): 1262; M. T. McGuire and others, "Parental Correlates of Physical Activity in a Racially/Ethnically Diverse Adolescent Sample," *Journal of Adolescent Health* 30, no. 4 (2002): 253–61.

56. A. Wagner and others, "Parent-Child Physical Activity Relationships in 12-Year-Old French Students Do Not Depend on Family Socioeconomic Status," *Diabetes & Metabolism* 30, no. 4 (2004): 359–66.

57. S. Y. Kimm and others, "Longitudinal Changes in Physical Activity in a Biracial Cohort during Adolescence," *Medicine & Science in Sports & Exercise* 32, no. 8 (2000): 1445–54; J. F. Sallis, J. J. Prochaska, and W. C. Taylor, "A Review of Correlates of Physical Activity of Children and Adolescents," *Medicine & Science in Sports & Exercise* 32, no. 5 (2000): 963–75.

58. U.S. Department of Health and Human Services, "*Healthy People 2010*" (U.S. Government Printing Office, 2000); National Association for Sports and Physical Education, *Physical Activity for Children: A Statement of Guidelines for Children 5–12* (Reston, Va., 2004); L. Kann and others, "Youth Risk Behavior Surveillance–United States, 1999," *MMWR CDC Surveillance Summaries* 49, no. 5 (2000): 1–32.

59. R. A. Forshee, P. A. Anderson, and M. L. Story, "The Role of Beverage Consumption, Physical Activity, Sedentary Behavior, and Demographics on Body Mass Index of Adolescents," *International Journal of Food Science and Nutrition* 55, no. 6 (2004): 463–78.

60. L. L. Moore and others, "Influence of Parents' Physical Activity Levels on Activity Levels of Young Children," *Journal of Pediatrics* 118, no. 2 (1991): 215–19; Trost and others, "Evaluating a Model" (see note 30).

61. McGuire and others, "Parental Correlates" (see note 55); Sallis, Prochaska, and Taylor, "A Review of Correlates" (see note 57); J. F. Sallis and others, "Parental Behavior in Relation to Physical Activity and Fitness in 9-Year-Old Children," *American Journal of Diseases of Children* 146, no. 11 (1992): 1383–88.

62. Trost and others, "Evaluating a Model" (see note 30).

63. Ibid.; Sallis and others, "Parental Behavior" (see note 61).

64. J. C. Kimiecik and T. S. Horn, "Parental Beliefs and Children's Moderate-to-Vigorous Physical Activity," *Research Quarterly for Exercise and Sport* 69, no. 2 (1998): 163–75.

65. A. C. Gielen and others, "Child Pedestrians: The Role of Parental Beliefs and Practices in Promoting Safe Walking in Urban Neighborhoods," *Journal of Urban Health* 81, no. 4 (2004): 545–55.

66. T. N. Robinson and others, "Dance and Reducing Television Viewing to Prevent Weight Gain in African-American Girls: The Stanford GEMS Pilot Study," *Ethnicity and Disease* 13, no. 1, suppl. 1 (2003): S65–77.

67. D. B. Johnson and others, "Statewide Intervention to Reduce Television Viewing in WIC Clients and Staff," *American Journal of Health Promotion* 19, no. 6 (2005): 418–21.

68. L. Y. Wang and others, "Economic Analysis of a School-Based Obesity Prevention Program," *Obesity Research* 11, no. 11 (2003): 1313–24.

69. B. S. Ford and others, "Primary Care Interventions to Reduce Television Viewing in African-American Children," *American Journal of Preventive Medicine* 22, no. 2 (2002): 106–09.

70. B. M. Beech and others, "Child- and Parent-Targeted Interventions: The Memphis GEMS Pilot Study," *Ethnicity and Disease* 13, no. 1, suppl. 1 (2003): S40–53.

71. M. J. Muller, S. Danielzik, and S. Pust, "School- and Family-Based Interventions to Prevent Overweight in Children," *Proceedings of the Nutrition Society* 64, no. 2 (2005): 249–54.

72. M. L. Fitzgibbon and others, "Two-Year Follow-up Results for Hip-Hop to Health Jr.: A Randomized Controlled Trial for Overweight Prevention in Preschool Minority Children," *Journal of Pediatrics* 146, no. 5 (2005): 618–25.

73. K. T. Coleman and others, "Prevention of the Epidemic Increase in Child Risk of Overweight in Low-Income Schools: The El Paso Coordinated Approach to Child Health," *Archives of Pediatric and Adolescent Medicine* 159, no. 3 (2005): 217–24.

74. Gortmaker and others, "Impact of a School-Based Interdisciplinary Intervention" (see note 3).

75. V. R. Chomitz and others, "Promoting Healthy Weight among Elementary School Children via a Health Report Card Approach," *Archives of Pediatric and Adolescent Medicine* 157, no. 8 (2003): 765–72.

76. Gortmaker, "Reducing Obesity" (see note 3).

77. Wang, "Economic Analysis of a School-Based Obesity Prevention Program" (see note 68); S. B. Austin and others, "The Impact of a School-Based Obesity Prevention Trial on Disordered Weight-Control Behaviors in Early Adolescent Girls," *Archives of Pediatric and Adolescent Medicine* 159, no. 3 (2005): 225–30.

78. U.S. Department of Health and Human Services, "*Healthy People 2010*" (see note 58); Gortmaker and others, "Impact of a School-Based Interdisciplinary Intervention" (see note 3); Robinson and others, "Dance and Reducing Television Viewing" (see note 66).

79. J. Salmon and others, "Reducing Sedentary Behaviour and Increasing Physical Activity among 10-Year-Old Children: Overview and Process Evaluation of the 'Switch-Play' Intervention," *Health Promotion International* 20, no. 1 (2005): 7–17.

80. Robinson and others, "Dance and Reducing Television Viewing" (see note 66).

81. P. Gordon-Larsen and others, "Barriers to Physical Activity: Qualitative Data on Caregiver-Daughter Perceptions and Practices," *American Journal of Preventive Medicine* 27, no. 3 (2004): 218–23.

82. N. McLean and others, "Family Involvement in Weight Control, Weight Maintenance, and Weight-Loss Interventions: A Systematic Review of Randomized Trials," *International Journal of Obesity and Related Metabolic Disorders* 27, no. 9 (2003): 987–1005.

83. Muller, Danielzik, and Pust, "School- and Family-Based Interventions" (see note 71); M. Golan and others, "Parents as the Exclusive Agents of Change in the Treatment of Childhood Obesity," *American Journal of Clinical Nutrition* 67, no. 6 (1998): 1130–35.

84. Epstein, "Family-Based Behavioural Intervention" (see note 2).

85. G. S. Goldfield and others, "Cost-Effectiveness of Group and Mixed Family-Based Treatment for Childhood Obesity," *International Journal of Obesity and Related Metabolic Disorders* 25, no. 12 (2001): 1843–49.

86. Gortmaker and others, "Impact of a School-Based Interdisciplinary Intervention" (see note 3); Coleman and others, "Prevention of the Epidemic Increase" (see note 73); Robinson and others, "Dance and Reducing Television Viewing" (see note 66).

87. Fitzgibbon and others, "Two-Year Follow-up Results" (see note 72).

88. Muller, Danielzik, and Pust, "School- and Family-Based Interventions" (see note 71).

Targeting Interventions for Ethnic Minority and Low-Income Populations

Shiriki Kumanyika and Sonya Grier

Summary

Although rates of childhood obesity among the general population are alarmingly high, they are higher still in ethnic minority and low-income communities. The disparities pose a major challenge for policymakers and practitioners planning strategies for obesity prevention. In this article Shiriki Kumanyika and Sonya Grier summarize differences in childhood obesity prevalence by race and ethnicity and by socioeconomic status. They show how various environmental factors can have larger effects on disadvantaged and minority children than on their advantaged white peers—and thus contribute to disparities in obesity rates.

The authors show, for example, that low-income and minority children watch more television than white, non-poor children and are potentially exposed to more commercials advertising high-calorie, low-nutrient food during an average hour of TV programming. They note that neighborhoods where low-income and minority children live typically have more fast-food restaurants and fewer vendors of healthful foods than do wealthier or predominantly white neighborhoods. They cite such obstacles to physical activity as unsafe streets, dilapidated parks, and lack of facilities. In the schools that low-income and minority children attend, however, they see opportunities to lead the way to effective obesity prevention. Finally, the authors examine several aspects of the home environment—breast-feeding, television viewing, and parental behaviors—that may contribute to childhood obesity but be amenable to change through targeted intervention.

Kumanyika and Grier point out that policymakers aiming to prevent obesity can use many existing policy levers to reach ethnic minority and low-income children and families: Medicaid, the State Child Health Insurance Program, and federal nutrition "safety net" programs. Ultimately, winning the fight against childhood obesity in minority and low-income communities will depend on the nation's will to change the social and physical environments in which these communities exist.

www.futureofchildren.org

Shiriki Kumanyika is a professor of biostatistics and epidemiology and pediatrics (nutrition) at the University of Pennsylvania School of Medicine. Sonya Grier is a Robert Wood Johnson Foundation Health and Society Scholar at the University of Pennsylvania.

Rates of childhood obesity, now far too high among all U.S. children, are even higher among the nation's ethnic minority and low-income children.[1] These ethnic and socioeconomic disparities in childhood obesity rates present yet another challenge for researchers, policymakers, and practitioners who are focusing on obesity prevention.

In this article, we present and summarize data from multiple sources on racial, ethnic, and related socioeconomic correlates of obesity. We document differences in child obesity across race and ethnic groups and between low- and high-income children. We then consider which obesity-promoting factors might be more prevalent or more intensified among low-income and ethnic minority children than among the general population, with an eye toward identifying modifications that would do the most to prevent obesity. We try to highlight issues for diverse minority populations, but because far more information is available about African Americans and Hispanic Americans than about other groups, the discussion focuses mostly on these two populations.[2]

Obesity Prevalence among Minority and Low-Income Children

No single data source provides information on trends in child obesity for all the major racial and ethnic groups in the United States. The National Health and Nutrition Examination Survey (NHANES), a nationally representative survey that has been conducted periodically since the early 1970s, has large enough samples of white, African American, and (since 1982) Mexican American children to estimate obesity rates within racial and ethnic groups at different points in time.

Table 1, which is based on NHANES data, shows rates of obesity for white, African American, and Mexican American boys and girls in two age groups, ages six to eleven and twelve to nineteen, for three time periods since the mid-1970s. Although obesity rates have increased for boys and girls within each ethnic and racial group, they have increased more for African American and Mexican American children. By 1999–2002, obesity rates were higher for both of these two groups than for white children within each age and gender group. In some cases, obesity rates for ethnic minority children exceeded rates for white children by 10 to 12 percentage points. For boys of both age groups, the obesity rate among Mexican Americans exceeded that among African Americans. For example, nearly a quarter of Mexican American adolescent boys were obese in 1999–2002, as against 19 percent of African Americans and 15 percent of whites. This pattern differs for girls, with the highest obesity rates found among African American girls. For example, among adolescent girls, 24 percent of African Americans, 20 percent of Mexican Americans, and 13 percent of whites were obese.

Several other ethnic minority groups have high rates of child obesity. Measures of obesity for preschool children participating in Hawaii's Supplemental Nutrition Program for Women, Infants, and Children (WIC) indicate that more than a quarter of Samoan children are obese, a rate more than double that for any other ethnic subgroup represented in the sample.[3] Note, however, that the WIC sample is not representative—families must be low-income and nutritionally "at risk" to qualify. Obesity rates are also high among American Indian children. A large Indian Health Service study estimated obesity prevalence at 22 percent for boys and 18 percent for girls based on data for more than 12,000 five- to seventeen-

Table 1. Percentage of U.S. Children and Adolescents Who Are Obese (BMI ≥ 95th Percentile), by Sex, Age, Race, and Hispanic Origin, 1976–2002

Sex	Race and Hispanic origin[a]	1976–80[b]	1988–94	1999–2002
	6–11 years of age			
Boys	White	6.1	10.7	14.0
	African American	6.8	12.3	17.0
	Mexican American	13.3	17.5	26.5
Girls	White	5.2	9.8[c]	13.1
	African American	11.2	17.0	22.8
	Mexican American	9.8	15.3	17.1
	12–19 years of age			
Boys	White	3.8	11.6	14.6
	African American	6.1	10.7	18.7
	Mexican American	7.7	14.1	24.7
Girls	White	4.6	8.9	12.7
	African American	10.7	16.3	23.6
	Mexican American	8.8	13.4[c]	19.6

Source: National Center for Health Statistics, *Health, United States, 2004, with Chartbook on Trends in the Health of Americans* (Hyattsville, Md., 2004), table 70.

a. Data for whites and African Americans are specifically for those without Hispanic or Latino origin; Mexican Americans may be of any race.

b. Data for Mexican Americans are for 1982–84.

c. Estimates are considered unreliable (standard error: 20 to 30 percent).

year-old American Indian children in North and South Dakota, Iowa, and Nebraska.[4] A study of seven American Indian communities in Arizona, New Mexico, and South Dakota reported obesity prevalence of 26.8 percent for boys and 30.5 percent for girls based on data for 1,704 elementary school children with an average age of 7.6 years.[5] As with U.S. children generally, trend data for Navajo six- to twelve-year-olds showed an increase in obesity rates over time.[6]

Asian American children are an exception to the general pattern of higher obesity rates among ethnic minority groups. A 2003 study of New York City elementary school children found obesity rates of 31 percent for Hispanics, 23 percent for African Americans, 16 percent for whites, and 14 percent for Asian Americans.[7] Another study compared overweight (with an 85th percentile BMI cutoff)

for white, African American, Hispanic, and Asian American adolescents in 1996, using data from the National Longitudinal Study of Adolescent Health.[8] This survey of more than 14,000 students in seventh through twelfth grade indicates that Asian American adolescents have relatively low rates of overweight. The share of boys that were overweight was 23 percent among Asian Americans, 26 percent among African Americans, 27 percent among whites, and 28 percent among Hispanics. Among girls, only 10 percent of Asian Americans were overweight, as against 22 percent of whites, 30 percent of Hispanics, and 38 percent of African Americans. However, in adults, a BMI below the usual cutoff for obesity is associated with higher health risks in people of Asian origin when compared to other populations.[9] If this case is also true in children, the lower prevalence of obesity in Asian American children does not necessarily reflect an equivalent lower level of health risk.

Low-income children are at excess risk of obesity regardless of ethnicity, although ethnic differences in pediatric obesity appear at lower-income levels.[10] Several authors have analyzed NHANES data on the links between socioeconomic status and obesity among children and youth overall and in specific age groups.[11] One analysis of two- to nineteen-

---

Low-income children are at excess risk of obesity regardless of ethnicity, although ethnic differences in pediatric obesity appear at lower-income levels.

---

year-old children in NHANES surveys between 1971–74 and 1999–2002 finds higher rates of obesity among low-income children than among all children after 1976–80.[12] Similarly, the National Longitudinal Survey of Youth for four- to twelve-year-olds indicates that low-income children have higher obesity rates than do wealthier children.[13]

The association between socioeconomic status and obesity in school-aged children and adolescents varies by ethnicity and gender and appears to be quite complex.[14] In general, among white children, obesity typically declines as income and parental education increase. Different patterns have been found for children from ethnic minority groups. For example, among twelve- to seventeen-year-old non-Hispanic white children in the 1988–94 NHANES survey, rates of obesity decline for both boys and girls as family in-

come increases. By contrast, among African Americans and Mexican Americans, girls' obesity rates increase with income; boys' rates show no consistent pattern.[15] Another study found that although rates of obesity for white girls decrease as family income rises, rates for African American girls are higher in the lowest and highest income ranges than in the in-between bracket.[16] For both groups, however, obesity rates decline with higher parental education. An analysis of the National Heart, Lung, and Blood Institute Growth and Health Study also noted ethnic differences in the relationship between socioeconomic status and obesity.[17] It found the expected inverse link between obesity and both parental income and education—with obesity decreasing as income or education increased—in white girls but not in African American girls. Overall, these studies indicate that differences in obesity rates across race and ethnic groups do not simply reflect differences in the average socioeconomic status across groups.

In summary, obesity rates are higher for African American and Hispanic children and adolescents than for their white peers. Among African Americans rates are particularly high among girls, although the disparity varies by age and socioeconomic status. Hispanic boys seem to be at particularly high risk for obesity. Obesity rates for American Indian children appear to be comparable to or in some cases higher than those for African American children. Samoan children are also at high risk. Asian American children, by contrast, are less likely than those from other ethnic groups to be obese by standard definitions although the applicability of the standard definitions to Asian Americans is unclear. Although poorer children are more likely to be obese when all children are considered, this link varies across ethnic and racial groups.

Health Effects of Childhood Obesity on Minority and Low-Income Populations

Early observers tracking the increase in childhood obesity were concerned that obese children would become obese adults and suffer obesity-related health complications.[18] Their concerns, however, are now more immediate: obese children are already suffering from these complications. Stephen Daniels, in an article in this volume, documents the many health problems that accompany childhood obesity. Obesity-related diseases seen in children include precursors of cardiovascular disease, type 2 diabetes, and sleep-disordered breathing.[19]

Ethnic minority and low-income children appear more likely to experience some of the obesity-related health problems. Type 2 diabetes provides a useful example. Among adults, type 2 diabetes is more common among African Americans and Hispanics than among whites. Although many of the data on type 2 diabetes in children come from clinic records or case studies rather than from population samples, the data strongly suggest that the patterns of diabetes risk for children and adolescents parallel those for adults.[20] Similarly, symptoms of metabolic syndrome—an important risk factor for diabetes and cardiovascular disease among adults—are more prevalent in some although not all minority youth populations.[21] In the 1988–94 NHANES, the metabolic syndrome was more prevalent in Mexican American adolescents than in whites (girls only) but less prevalent in blacks than in whites (both sexes).[22] Left ventricular hypertrophy, or thickening of the heart's main pumping chamber, and sleep apnea are two other health consequences of pediatric obesity that are also more prevalent in some ethnic minority groups. For example, one study of a sample of children (with an average age of 13.6 years) being evaluated for high blood pressure found left ventricular hypertrophy in 70 percent of Hispanics, 39 percent of African Americans, and 33 percent of whites.[23] In an overnight sleep-monitoring study of children aged two to eighteen years, African Americans had higher odds than whites of having sleep apnea.[24]

The higher rates of obesity among ethnic minority and low-income children, when combined with the adverse health effects of child obesity, are likely to produce continued racial and economic differences in health outcomes. Preventing obesity for all children may be a way to reduce socioeconomic and ethnic health disparities.

Understanding and Closing the Gap

Effectively addressing ethnic and socioeconomic disparities in childhood obesity requires understanding which causes of obesity might be especially prevalent or intensified in ethnic minority and low-income populations; understanding how aspects of the social, cultural, and economic environments of minority and low-income children might magnify the effects of factors that cause obesity; and determining which changes in those environments would help most to reduce obesity. In what follows, we discuss these issues in relation to media and marketing influences, community food access, built environments, schools, and home environments, noting in each case how factors that may promote obesity are particularly likely to affect low-income and minority youth.

Media and Marketing

Research suggests that low-income and ethnic minority youth are disproportionately exposed to marketing activities.[25] A Kaiser

Foundation report found that among children eight to eighteen years old, ethnic minorities use entertainment media more heavily than majority youth do. African Americans and Hispanics spend significantly more time watching TV and movies and playing video games than do white youth.[26] African American youth also watch on-screen media (TV, DVDs, videos, movies) more than Hispanics and whites do, and Hispanics watch such media significantly more than whites do. Television is especially prevalent in African American and low-income households. Media use differs, as well, by socioeconomic status. Low-income children watch TV for more hours and have significantly higher levels of total media exposure than higher-income children.[27] Consumers in low-income households, who are heavy viewers of daytime television, are more likely to view television advertising as authoritative and as helpful in selecting products, and they may prefer it to print media.[28]

Because of their heavy media use, ethnic minority and low-income youth are exposed to a great deal of food advertising at home. Research has found that such advertising can affect children's food preferences after even brief exposure.[29] A study of media use among Latino preschoolers confirmed just how influential such commercials can be. Sixty-three percent of mothers said that in the past week their preschooler had asked for a toy advertised on television, 55 percent reported that their preschooler had asked for an advertised food or drink, and 67 percent noted that their preschooler had asked to go to an advertised store or restaurant.[30] Older elementary school children exposed to television commercials for sweets and other snacks were more likely to choose candy and sugary drinks and less likely to choose fruit and orange juice when offered a snack.[31]

Most research on food advertising, however, does not focus on ethnic minority or low-income youth. A systematic review of the effects of food promotion on children examined more than 100 articles, fewer than six of which dealt explicitly with ethnic minority or low-income children.[32] Experimental evidence, however, indicates that ethnic minorities seem especially responsive to targeted ads.[33] African American adolescents, for example, identify with black characters in advertisements, and they rate advertisements featuring these characters more favorably.[34] Such responses may lead them to buy and consume less nutritious food products when advertised by these characters.

Ethnic minority and low-income children may also be exposed to a different mix of information than are other children. Content analyses of television advertising have found that shows featuring African Americans have more food commercials than do general prime-time shows and that these commercials feature more energy-dense foods.[35] Advertisements for such products appear to be particularly effective in increasing children's total caloric consumption.[36] Advertisements in African American adult magazines are also dominated by low-cost, low-nutrition, energy-dense foods, and the magazines are less likely to contain health-oriented messages.[37] Similarly, a content analysis of the products advertised to low-income consumers found that most featured food and drinks, largely items such as cookies and other snacks.[38] Such an imbalanced information environment makes it harder for parents to know about and to provide more healthful options.

Food and food-related images, such as body size, are also pervasive in various media. A content analysis of movies—and ethnic minorities watch movies more often than whites do—found stereotypical food-related behaviors with respect to body shape, gender, and ethnic background.[39] More healthful, low-fat foods often appeared in scenes involving well-educated and affluent characters. Overweight characters were underrepresented, but when they did appear, they ate more high-fat, high-calorie foods than did their thinner counterparts. There is no evidence, however, on whether the movies' representation of food and food-related images affects how children perceive themselves or alters the foods they consume.

More research on the specific marketing environments of ethnic minority and low-income consumers is urgently needed. Policymakers and practitioners should consider policy interventions, including strengthening marketing and advertising guidelines in ways that reduce the overexposure of all children to marketing for high-calorie, high-fat foods.[40] Because ethnic minority and low-income children are exposed to more media than other children, policies that improve marketing and advertising may be most beneficial for these groups of children. Researchers have also suggested that schools can reduce the negative effects of advertising on minority and low-income children by teaching media literacy courses that make children aware of the many messages they receive daily from the media and how those messages can affect their attitudes and behavior.[41]

Food Access and Availability
The characteristics of communities in which ethnic minority and low-income children live may affect the foods that are available for their consumption. Compared with more affluent communities, minority and low-income communities have fewer than average supermarkets and convenience stores that stock fresh, good-quality, affordable foods such as whole grains or low-fat dairy products and meats.[42] A 1995 study estimated that supermarket flight from the inner cities left the typical low-income neighborhood with 30 percent fewer supermarkets than higher-income areas. At least one study

---

Content analyses of television advertising have found that shows featuring African Americans have more food commercials than do general prime-time shows and that these commercials feature more energy-dense foods.

---

that included a large cohort of African Americans has linked supermarket availability directly to fruit and vegetable intake.[43]

With fewer supermarkets available, low-income minority families may be more likely to shop in small corner stores or bodegas. These stores tend to offer markedly less healthful foods in lower-income neighborhoods, as demonstrated in a New York study comparing in-store food availability in low-income, minority East Harlem and the adjacent, affluent Upper East Side.[44] Prices of more healthful foods may also be higher in bodegas and corner stores than in supermarkets. One study reported that although low-fat milk was available in more than two-thirds of the bodegas in areas where residents were less educated, had lower incomes, and were Latino, some such stores charged more for low-fat milk than for regular milk.[45] Evidence shows that higher prices for more healthful foods have an effect on children's weight. A recent study based on a nationally representative sample of elementary school children concludes that children living in areas with lower prices of fruits and vegetables had significantly lower gains in BMI between kindergarten and third grade. Further, these effects were larger for children in poverty, children who were obese or overweight in kindergarten, and Asian and Hispanic children.[46] This evidence is consistent with that from a study of low-income women in Baltimore that

---

A study in New Orleans found that black neighborhoods had more fast-food restaurants per square mile than did white neighborhoods.

---

found the cost of fresh produce kept them from eating more fruits and vegetables.[47]

African American and low-income neighborhoods also have many fast-food restaurants. A recent study found that African American adults ate more fast foods than did whites, perhaps because of their greater availability.[48] A study in New Orleans found that black neighborhoods had more fast-food restaurants per square mile than did white neighborhoods.[49] Another study found that areas of South Los Angeles with fewer African American residents (8 percent on average) were twice as likely as areas with more African Americans (36 percent on average) to have full-service rather than limited-service, fast-food restaurants.[50]

Studies of parents' attitudes toward fast-food restaurants highlight the problems that may

be produced by having fast-food outlets nearby as well as the reasons why fast-food outlets are popular among low-income families. Hispanic women in a low-income community reported that the overabundance of fast-food restaurants and their intensive marketing interfered with their ability to exercise control over their children's eating habits. They also reported that acculturation to fast food caused their children to reject more healthful, traditional Hispanic foods.[51] But Latino women in a California study preferred fast-food restaurants and especially valued their family- and child-friendly aspects.[52]

On the important question of whether living near fast-food restaurants increases the chance that children become obese, the evidence is inconclusive. Research has found that foods served in fast-food outlets are much more energy-dense and have a higher fat content than meals consumed at home.[53] Furthermore, there is a correlation between fast-food consumption and body weight, at least among adults. In a survey of women aged twenty to seventy years in North Carolina, those who reported eating at fast-food restaurants "usually" or "often" had higher energy and fat intakes and higher body mass indexes than those who reported eating at them "rarely" or "never."[54] In the Coronary Artery Risk Development in Young Adults (CARDIA) Study, which followed for fifteen years a group of young adults aged eighteen to thirty at the time of enrollment, those who ate at fast-food restaurants more than twice a week weighed an average of 4.5 kilograms more than those who ate in them less than once a week.[55]

This evidence suggests that if children who live close to fast-food outlets consume more fast food, they may be more likely to become obese. But the few studies that specifically examine how the proximity of fast-food outlets affects children's fast-food consumption and their weight status do not find a connection. Living close to fast-food restaurants was not linked with being overweight among three- to five-year-old children in Cincinnati or to the self-reported frequency of fast-food restaurant use among seventh- to twelfth-grade students in Minnesota.[56] Researchers require more evidence, based on children from more geographical regions and age groups, before they can draw a definitive conclusion on this issue.

Built Environments

Where and how often children and adolescents engage in physical activity depends on the physical design and quality of their neighborhoods.[57] In low-income urban communities, the built environment affects children's physical activity much more than it affects that of adults. Because many adults do not own cars and must depend on public transportation, they often have to be physically active just to get to and from work or shopping.[58] By contrast, for safety reasons, parents may restrict their children's outdoor activities by using a combination of TV and easy access to snack foods to get children to go straight home from school and stay there. Children's limited access to parks and recreational facilities may also curtail their physical activity.[59] Neighborhood or community constraints on children's physical activity are likely to vary regionally and across ethnic groups. In low-income communities, family work schedules, discretionary time, money, and car ownership may make it hard for parents and caregivers to transport children to sports and other recreational activities, suggesting the need to develop nearby after-school or community-based, supervised programs.

Despite the logic that inadequate opportunities for physical activity should adversely af-

fect children's weight, the evidence on this issue is limited. Several observational studies have failed to link children's weight status to the availability of neighborhood parks or to parental perceptions about safety.[60] A better approach would be to study direct links between specific neighborhood-based physical activity options and the types and amounts of physical activity in which children engage, taking into account how their family or home life, as well as the neighborhood's social organization, affects their access to these options. Additional research on this topic that focuses on low-income and minority children is needed.

School Settings

Schools offer opportunities for improving children's nutrition, increasing their physical activity, and preventing obesity. But schools in inner-city or low-income communities may be unable to take advantage of these opportunities, as most obesity-prevention initiatives proposed to date require significant funding and some depend on a school's physical facilities and neighborhood characteristics.[61] In addition, school officials, teachers, and parents have many competing priorities, such as new academic accountability standards and efforts to prevent drug abuse and violence.

Research on whether schools in low-income areas are less able to provide students with healthful foods or physical activity options is inconclusive. Several reports have compared environmental quality, resources, and per-student spending in schools with differing community income or differing shares of minority students. A report by the U.S. General Accounting Office (GAO) focused on such school problems as inadequate or unsatisfactory buildings, building features, or environmental conditions as well as expenses above the national average. Schools reporting the most problems in all areas were large schools, central-city schools, schools in the western United States, schools with populations of at least 50.5 percent minority students, and schools with 70 percent or more poor students.[62] The differences, however, were often not striking, and the greatest variations were often by state.

A Centers for Disease Control and Prevention analysis addressed general health and safety issues as well as conditions and policies with more direct implications for physical activity and nutrition. It included athletic facilities and playground equipment, kitchen facilities and equipment, the presence of a cafeteria, soft drink vending contracts, and junk food promotion.[63] Contrary to expectation, schools in urban areas, schools with a high share of minority children, and schools with a low share of college-bound students were not worse off than other schools. Schools with the best health-protective environments turned out to be elementary schools, public schools, and larger schools.

Poorer children benefit from the National School Lunch and National School Breakfast Programs. These food programs, which provide free or reduced-price meals to low-income children, disproportionately enroll minority children. In 2004, in fourth grade, for example, nearly 70 percent of African American students, as against 23 percent of whites, were eligible for free or reduced-price lunches. Nearly half of African American students, as against only 5 percent of whites, attended schools where most children are eligible for subsidized meals.[64] Because these meals must meet federally set nutritional standards, these programs offer an opportunity to improve the nutrition of low-income minority children.

Although poorer children are eligible for free or reduced-price lunches in school, many schools offer a wide variety of "competitive" foods that do not meet nutritional standards. Schools that participate in the school lunch program face some federal restrictions on what foods they can serve during lunch periods in the school cafeteria, and many states and school districts are imposing additional standards.[65] But children can often purchase sodas and high-fat, high-sugar foods at school. As noted by the Government Accountability Office, these unregulated competitive foods undermine the school breakfast and school lunch programs, with negative nutrition implications for the children, but they may generate substantial revenue for the schools.[66] The GAO report does not indicate whether schools with limited resources depend more on revenue from competitive food sales than do wealthier schools. If they do, limitations on competitive food sales may impose a relatively larger burden on low-income schools. More research on this topic is needed. If in fact low-income schools will be disproportionately harmed by restrictions on competitive foods, then new regulations on competitive food sales might be coupled with compensatory financing for the schools most harmed.

In addition to restricting the sales of less healthful foods, many schools are considering interventions to promote the consumption of more nutritious foods. Some of these initiatives may be more effective in schools serving low-income children than in schools with more resources. For example, an intervention that lowered the prices of fruits and vegetables had a greater impact in inner-city schools than in suburban schools and suggests that making nutritious foods more accessible in these schools can increase demand.[67] In-school free fruit and vegetable distribution should be of particular benefit to low-income children, who have less access to fruits and vegetables than their more affluent counterparts. Such approaches as salad bars with links to local farmers' markets or even student gardening programs could also be useful.[68] But before any such programs can begin on a large scale, comparative analysis of the availability of the community resources required for feasibility is essential.

Home and Family Settings

Another important question for researchers analyzing ethnic and socioeconomic disparities in childhood obesity is whether differences in home environments contribute to differences in child obesity rates. There are various underlying reasons why parenting practices may differ across ethnic and socioeconomic groups. Minority and low-income households have a higher share of female-headed families, lower parental education, and higher rates of teen parenting, all of which may profoundly affect the home environment.[69] Economic insecurity can influence food choices directly, by encouraging the purchase of cheaper, energy-dense foods, and indirectly, by producing psychosocial stress that affects parenting.[70] The higher prevalence of obesity among adults in minority and low-income populations may also affect children's weight status.[71] Maternal obesity and diabetes, both relatively more common among minority women, may predispose children to obesity.[72] In addition, obesity among parents may affect both the weight norms their children develop and the modeling of eating behaviors and physical activity they observe.

In what follows, we focus on three aspects of the home environment—breast-feeding, television viewing, and parental attitudes and behaviors. Each may be of particular importance for the development of obesity in ethnic minority and low-income children and may be amenable to change through targeted interventions.

Breast-feeding. Although breast-feeding rates for all groups have increased notably in recent years, disadvantaged minority groups still have lower rates than others.[73] As of 2001, the rates of breast-feeding for African American infants were 53 percent in-hospital and 22 percent at age six months. For Hispanics, the

---

Schools with the best health-protective environments turned out to be elementary schools, public schools, and larger schools.

---

rates were 73 percent in-hospital and 33 percent at six months, whereas for whites, the rates were 72 percent in-hospital and 34 percent at six months.[74] High rates of teen pregnancy may contribute to lower breast-feeding rates, early introduction of solid foods, and early feeding of high-sugar foods for African American infants.[75] In another article in this volume Ana Lindsay and several colleagues note that the evidence on whether children who are breast-fed longer are less likely to become obese is inconclusive. Instead, mothers who choose to breast-feed may be more likely to adopt other behaviors that reduce the chance of obesity. Nonetheless, the link between longer breast-feeding and a lower risk of obesity, combined with the other well-documented benefits of breast-feeding, argues for efforts to increase breast-feeding among ethnic minority families.

Television viewing. TV watching may contribute to obesity by increasing sedentary behavior, increasing snacking while watching TV, and exposing children to advertisements for unhealthful foods and beverages.[76] The Institute of Medicine has recommended that parents restrict their children's television watching to fewer than two hours a day.[77]

Television's pervasive role in the lives of minority and low-income children, however,

---

High rates of teen pregnancy may contribute to lower breast-feeding rates, early introduction of solid foods, and early feeding of high-sugar foods for African American infants.

---

may make it hard for parents to turn off the TV. As noted, ethnic minority and low-income children have, as a group, high average levels of television viewing. African American households that can afford them are more likely than others to have premium channels and to have three or more TV sets.[78] Interestingly, the lower their parents' education, the higher the likelihood that a child will have a VCR or DVD in the bedroom. African American children are also more likely than whites to report having televisions in their bedrooms, along with DVDs, cable and satellite connections, premium channels, and video game consoles. Youth from the lowest income group are the most likely to have their own television sets. Watching television during meals is also more common in families with lower parental education, or lower income, as well as among Hispanics and African Americans. The National Heart,

Lung, and Blood Institute Growth and Health Study found that eating while watching TV was more common among African American girls. This practice is also linked with reported higher caloric intake.[79]

Developing interventions, possibly school- or child care center–based, to help low-income and minority parents reduce their children's TV time is important. Such interventions could also teach parents to help their children learn to evaluate critically the advertisements and programs they see at home.

Parental attitudes and behaviors. Efforts to get parents to pay closer attention to their children's weight and BMI can be controversial, because some parents can become overly restrictive about their children's food intake. Addressing childhood obesity issues with parents in minority and lower-income communities requires particular sensitivity to differences in attitudes about weight that may be the products of culture or economic insecurity.

Societal attitudes about weight may be changing as more and more adults become overweight and obese. But in communities where most women or adults are obese, as in many ethnic minority and low-income communities, attitudes, norms, behaviors, and cultural influences may be in equilibrium with a high level of obesity. There may be a mixture of positive and negative attitudes about being overweight, especially where people who are thin are thought to be sick, addicted to drugs, too poor to have enough to eat, or to risk "wasting away" in the case of food shortage or of serious illness.[80] In such environments, parents and other family members may consider being overweight as normal, perhaps determined by heredity. Shapeliness, robustness, and nurturing qualities may be standards of female attractiveness that encourage the overall acceptance of people who—by BMI standards—are otherwise considered overweight or obese. One study found that African American girls were more likely than white girls to try to gain weight, largely because their parents told them they were too thin.[81]

Several child feeding attitudes or practices that are theoretically associated with obesity development are common among low-income mothers. Among them are heightened concerns about a child being hungry; greater difficulty withholding food from a child, even one who has just eaten; and concern about underweight even if a child is above normal weight.[82] Focus groups have found that low-income parents may see their overweight or obese children as "thick or solid." And other family members might challenge parents if they try to control their child's diet.[83] The view that "a fat child is a healthy child" or that children's weight follows a natural trajectory where heavy children will "grow out of it" may be more common among families that are food insecure or where hunger concerns are part of a group's identity.

In spite of such cultural differences, programs to motivate and educate low-income parents and caregivers in diverse ethnic minority populations about how to promote healthful eating and physical activity in their children, combined with programs for the children themselves, have yielded promising results.[84] Childhood obesity-prevention programs should also work with parents on their own weight issues. By promoting an understanding of the core principles of energy balance and by helping parents model the targeted nutrition and physical activity behaviors for their children, such programs

could lead to favorable changes at home. Given the challenges of parenting in low-income communities, these programs should lessen rather than increase the stresses on parents by helping them and their children in ways that go beyond eating and physical activity. For example, after-school programs could include tutoring and time to do homework in addition to providing healthful snacks, dance, and active play.[85] Working with girls and their mothers together—counseling mothers about weight control and having them interact with their daughters—may be particularly effective for African American preadolescent or adolescent girls.[86] The ideal program simultaneously addresses many issues, including empowerment strategies, in the community, school, and home.

Conclusions and Implications

Any strategy to address childhood obesity in the overall population must include targeted interventions for children in the nation's minority and low-income families. Preventing child obesity in ethnic minority and low-income populations requires thinking through all the issues that apply to the population at large and then considering how these issues might differ in a population with different socio-cultural characteristics and usually less favorable health profiles, environmental circumstances, and life chances.

To date, the research on childhood obesity that is specifically focused on ethnic minority and low-income populations is limited. But the available evidence clearly shows that the higher rates of obesity in minority and low-income communities are associated with a plethora of unfavorable influences—economic stresses, reduced access to affordable healthful foods and opportunities for physical activity, overexposure to targeted advertising and marketing of energy-dense foods, and factors related to family ecologies. Simply counseling parents and children about weight control will be almost pointless in environments that work against carrying out recommendations for healthful eating and physical activity. To identify environmental changes that will most likely reduce childhood obesity in minority and low-income communities requires more investigation. Researchers also should focus on how culturally influenced attitudes and practices interact with environmental variables.

Although reducing obesity prevalence among minority and low-income children will not be possible without also improving their social and economic environments, clearly tremendous opportunities exist for targeted policies and interventions. In particular, policymakers can reinforce current programs that foster nutritional equity—food stamps, school and child care center feeding programs, and the supplemental WIC program—by adding a specific component on childhood obesity. They may also strengthen both routine and specialized health care services for obesity treatment and prevention for low-income and minority children through improvements in Medicaid, the State Children's Health Insurance Program, and services delivered in federally qualified and locally supported community health centers.[87] Such reforms, however, will almost certainly require a significant financial commitment.

Policies must also improve access to healthful foods and physical activity in low-income and minority communities. Families need more protection from the "invisible hand of the free market" as the primary determinant of affordable, accessible, and healthful food options. Food availability, access, and the closely related media and marketing issues should be top policy priorities in schools, families, and communities alike. The built environment must offer children more options for physical activity. Researchers and policymakers must face head-on the safety issues, such as violence and drug trafficking, that compromise socially disadvantaged inner-city neighborhoods. Because attention to these issues is highly specific for any locality and influenced by local policies, a feasible overall obesity-prevention strategy might address food-related and media-related initiatives at the national or regional level and built environment issues at the local level.

Underlying all these conclusions is one main message. Making serious progress in the fight against childhood obesity in minority and low-income communities will depend on our national will to radically alter the negative effects of the social and physical environments in which these communities exist.

Notes

1. In this article, "obesity" refers to children up to age eighteen whose body mass index (BMI, calculated as weight in kilograms divided by the square of height in meters) is at or above the 95th percentile of the appropriate age- and gender-specific BMI reference curve. Children with BMI values at or above the 85th percentile are classified as being "overweight." Note that this terminology differs from that used by the Centers for Disease Control and Prevention, which refers to children with BMI values at or above the 95th percentile as "overweight" and those with BMI values at or above the 85th percentile as "at risk for overweight."

2. Minority status is assigned to a set of diverse populations and subpopulations that fit the "non-white" U.S. Census Bureau's racial and ethnic classifications. The major minority group categories are African American, Hispanic or Latino, American Indian and Alaska Native, Native Hawaiian, Asian American, and Pacific Islander. These broad groupings mask substantial heterogeneity within groups. For example, the group "Hispanic or Latino" may include individuals of any race and includes U.S.-born and immigrant populations from Mexico, Puerto Rico, Cuba, Central and South America, and Spain. American Indians and Alaska Natives include hundreds of different federally recognized groups. Asian Americans come from all parts of Asia and are often classified together with Pacific Islanders, which can be misleading. Obesity rates may vary substantially across these subgroups.

3. G. Baruffi and others, "Ethnic Differences in the Prevalence of Overweight among Young Children in Hawaii," *Journal of the American Dietetic Association* 104, no. 11 (2004): 1701–07.

4. E. Zephier, J. H. Himes, and M. Story, "Prevalence of Overweight and Obesity in American Indian School Children and Adolescents in the Aberdeen Area: A Population Study," *International Journal of Obesity and Related Metabolic Disorders* 23, suppl. 2 (1999): S28–30.

5. B. Caballero and others, "Pathways: A School-Based, Randomized Controlled Trial for the Prevention of Obesity in American Indian Schoolchildren," *American Journal of Clinical Nutrition* 78, no. 5 (2003): 1030–38.

6. J. C. Eisenmann and others, "Growth and Overweight of Navajo Youth: Secular Changes from 1955 to 1997," *International Journal of Obesity and Related Metabolic Disorders* 24, no. 2 (2000): 211–18.

7. L. E. Thorpe and others, "Childhood Obesity in New York City Elementary School Students," *American Journal of Public Health* 94, no. 9 (2004): 1496–1500.

8. P. Gordon-Larsen, L. S. Adair, and B. M. Popkin, "The Relationship of Ethnicity, Socioeconomic Factors, and Overweight in U.S. Adolescents," *Obesity Research* 11, no. 1 (2003): 121–29 (erratum in *Obesity Research* 11, no. 4 [2003]: 597).

9. World Health Organization Expert Consultation, "Appropriate Body-Mass Index for Asian Populations and Its Implications for Policy and Intervention Strategies," *Lancet* 363, no. 9403 (2004): 157–63 (erratum in *Lancet* 363, no. 9412 [2004]: 902); M. J. McNeely and E. J. Boyko, "Type 2 Diabetes Prevalence in Asian Americans: Results of a National Health Survey," *Diabetes Care* 27, no. 1 (2004): 66–69.

10. B. Sherry and others, "Trends in State-Specific Prevalence of Overweight and Underweight in 2- through 4-Year-Old Children from Low-Income Families from 1989 through 2000," *Archives of Pediatric and Adolescent Medicine* 158, no. 12 (2004): 1116–24; Baruffi and others, "Ethnic Differences in the Prevalence of

Overweight among Young Children in Hawaii" (see note 3); N. Stettler and others, "High Prevalence of Overweight among Pediatric Users of Community Health Centers," *Pediatrics* 116, no 3 (2005): e381–88.

11. R. P. Troiano and others, "Overweight Prevalence and Trends for Children and Adolescents: The National Health and Nutrition Examination Surveys, 1963 to 1991," *Archives of Pediatric and Adolescent Medicine* 149, no. 10 (1995): 1085–91; and Bing-Hwan Lin, "Nutrition and Health Characteristics of Low-Income Populations: Body Weight Status," U.S. Department of Agriculture, Economic Research Service, Agriculture Information Bulletin 796-3, February 2005. See also Patricia Anderson and Kristin Butcher's article in this volume.

12. See Patricia Anderson and Kristin Butcher's article in this volume.

13. R. S. Strauss and H. A. Pollack, "Epidemic Increase in Childhood Overweight, 1986–1998," *Journal of the American Medical Association* 286, no. 22 (2001): 2845–88.

14. R. P. Troiano and K. M. Flegal, "Overweight Children and Adolescents: Description, Epidemiology, and Demographics," *Pediatrics* 101, no. 3, pt. 2 (1998): 497–504; Gordon-Larsen, Adair, and Popkin, "The Relationship of Ethnicity, Socioeconomic Factors, and Overweight" (see note 8); S. Y. Kimm, and others, "Race, Socioeconomic Status, and Obesity in 9- to 10-Year-Old Girls: The NHLBI Growth and Health Study," *Annals of Epidemiology* 6, no. 4 (1996): 266–75.

15. Troiano and Flegal, "Overweight Children and Adolescents" (note 14).

16. Gordon-Larsen, Adair, and Popkin, "The Relationship of Ethnicity, Socioeconomic Factors, and Overweight" (see note 8).

17. S. Y. Kimm and others, "Race" (see note 14).

18. R. C. Whitaker and others, "Predicting Obesity in Young Adulthood from Childhood and Parental Obesity," *New England Journal of Medicine* 337 (1997): 869–73.

19. See Stephen Daniels's article in this volume.

20. A. Fagot-Campagna, "Emergence of Type 2 Diabetes Mellitus in Children: Epidemiological Evidence," *Journal of Pediatric Endocrinology and Metabolism* 3, suppl. 6 (2000): 1395–402; J. E. Oeltmann and others, "Prevalence of Diagnosed Diabetes among African-American and Non-Hispanic White Youth, 1999," *Diabetes Care* 26, no. 9 (2003): 2531–35.

21. Although there is as yet no accepted definition of metabolic syndrome in adolescents, its prevalence among U.S. twelve- to nineteen-year-olds, when defined by a combination of abdominal obesity and elevated cardiovascular risk factors, adapted from the definition in adults, is strongly associated with weight status. Prevalence jumps from 0.1 in youths below the 85th BMI percentile to 6.8 percent in youths between the 85th and 95th BMI percentiles and to 28.7 percent in those above the 95th percentile. See S. Cook and others, "Prevalence of a Metabolic Syndrome Phenotype in Adolescents: Findings from the Third National Health and Nutrition Examination Survey, 1988–1994," *Archives of Pediatric and Adolescent Medicine* 157, no. 8 (2003): 821–27.

22. Cook and others, "Prevalence of a Metabolic Syndrome Phenotype" (see note 21).

23. C. Hanevold and others, "The Effects of Obesity, Gender, and Ethnic Group on Left Ventricular Hypertrophy and Geometry in Hypertensive Children: A Collaborative Study of the International Pediatric Hypertension Association," *Pediatrics* 113, no. 2 (2004): 328–33 (erratum in *Pediatrics* 115, no. 4 [2005]: 1118).

24. S. Redline and others, "Risk Factors for Sleep-Disordered Breathing in Children: Associations with Obesity, Race, and Respiratory Problems," *American Journal of Respiratory and Critical Care Medicine* 159, no. 5, pt. 1 (1999): 1527–32.

25. D. F. Roberts, U. G. Foehr, and V. J. Rideout, *Kids and Media at the New Millennium* (Menlo Park, Calif.: Kaiser Family Foundation, 1999); E. H. Woodard IV and N. Gridina, *Media in the Home, 2000: The Fifth Annual Survey of Parents and Children* (Philadelphia, Pa.: Annenberg Public Policy Center of the University of Pennsylvania, 2000); D. F. Roberts and others, *Kids and Media in America* (New York: Cambridge University Press, 2004).

26. Roberts and others, *Kids and Media in America* (see note 25).

27. Roberts and others, *Kids and Media at the New Millennium* (see note 25).

28. L. F. Alwitt and T. D. Donley, *The Low-Income Consumer: Adjusting the Balance of Exchange* (Thousand Oaks, Calif.: Sage Publications, 1996).

29. D. L. G. Borzekowski and T. N. Robinson, "The 30-Second Effect: An Experiment Revealing the Impact of Television Commercials on Food Preferences of Preschoolers," *Journal of the American Dietetic Association* 101 (2001): 42–46.

30. D. L. G. Borzekowski and A. F. Poussaint, *Latino American Preschoolers and the Media* (Washington: Annenberg Public Policy Center, 1998).

31. G. Gorn and M. E. Goldberg, "Behavioral Evidence on the Effects of Televised Food Messages on Children," *Journal of Consumer Research: An Interdisciplinary Quarterly* 9, no. 2 (1982): 200–05.

32. G. Hastings and others, *Review of Research on the Effects of Food Promotion to Children* Final Report Prepared for the Food Standards Agency, Centre for Social Marketing, University of Strathclyde, September 22, 2003.

33. S. A. Grier and A. M. Brumbaugh, "Noticing Cultural Differences: Ad Meanings Created by Target and Non-Target Markets," *Journal of Advertising* (Spring 1999): 79–93; J. L. Aaker, A. M. Brumbaugh, and S. A. Grier, "Nontarget Markets and Viewer Distinctiveness: The Impact of Target Marketing on Advertising," *Journal of Consumer Psychology* 9 (2000): 127–40; S. A. Grier and A. M. Brumbaugh, "Consumer Distinctiveness and Advertising Persuasion," in *Diversity in Advertising*, edited by Jerome D. Williams, Wei-Na Lee, and Curtis P. Haugtvedt (Hillsdale, N.J.: Lawrence Erlbaum Associates, Inc., 2004).

34. O. Appiah, "Black, White, Hispanic, and Asian American Adolescents' Responses to Culturally Embedded Ads," *Howard Journal of Communications* 12, no. 1 (2001): 29–48; O. Appiah, "Ethnic Identification on Adolescents' Evaluations of Advertisements," *Journal of Advertising Research*, September–October (2001): 7–22; O. Appiah, "It Must Be the Cues: Racial Differences in Adolescents' Responses to Culturally Embedded Ads," in *Diversity in Advertising*, edited by Williams, Lee, and Haugtvedt (see note 33).

35. M. A. Tirodkar and A. Jain, "Food Messages on African American Television Shows," *American Journal of Public Health* 93, no. 3 (2003): 439–41; V. R. Henderson and B. Kelly, "Food Advertising in the Age of Obesity: Content Analysis of Food Advertising on General Market and African American Television," *Journal of Nutrition Education and Behavior* 37, no. 4 (2005): 191–96.

36. D. B. Jeffrey, R. W. McLellarn, and D. T. Fox, "The Development of Children's Eating Habits: The Role of Television Commercials," *Health Education Quarterly* 9, no. 2–3 (1982): 174–89.

37. C. A. Pratt and C. B. Pratt, "Comparative Content Analysis of Food and Nutrition Advertisements in *Ebony, Essence,* and *Ladies' Home Journal,*" *Journal of Nutrition Education* 27, no. 1 (1995): 11–18; C. A. Pratt and C. B. Pratt, "Nutrition Advertisements in Consumer Magazines: Health Implications for African Americans," *Journal of Black Studies* 26, no. 4 (1996): 504–23; S. C. Duerksen and others, "Health Disparities and Advertising Content of Women's Magazines: A Cross-Sectional Study," *BMC Public Health* 5 (2005): 85.

38. Alwitt and Donley, *The Low-Income Consumer* (see note 28).

39. G. P. Sylvester and others, "Food and Nutrition Messages in Film," *Annals of the New York Academy of Sciences* 699 (1993): 294–95; Roberts, Foehr, and Rideout, *Kids and Media at the New Millennium* (see note 25).

40. J. Michael McGinnis, Jennifer A. Grootman, and Vivica I. Kraak, *Food Marketing to Children and Youth: Threat or Opportunity?* (Washington: National Academies Press, 2006).

41. A. Silverblatt, *Media Literacy: Keys to Interpreting Media Messages* (Westport, Conn.: Praeger, 1995).

42. K. Morland and others, "Neighborhood Characteristics Associated with the Location of Food Stores and Food Service Places," *American Journal of Preventive Medicine* 22, no. 1 (2002): 23–29; Philadelphia Food Trust, "Food for Every Child: The Need for More Supermarkets in Philadelphia," 2005 (www.thefoodtrust.org/pdf/supermar.pdf) [November 28, 2005]); C. R. Horowitz and others, "Barriers to Buying Healthy Foods for People with Diabetes: Evidence of Environmental Disparities," *American Journal of Public Health* 94, no. 9 (2004): 1549–54; S. N. Zenk and others, "Fruit and Vegetable Intake in African-Americans: Income and Store Characteristics," *American Journal of Preventive Medicine* 29, no. 1 (2005): 1–9; D. D. Sloane and others, REACH Coalition of the African American Building a Legacy of Health Project, "Improving the Nutritional Resource Environment for Healthy Living through Community-Based Participatory Research," *Journal of General Internal Medicine* 18, no. 7 (2003): 568–75; Rodolpho M. Nayga Jr. and Zy Weinberg, "Supermarket Access in the Inner Cities," *Journal of Retailing and Consumer Services* 6 (1999): 141–45.

43. K. Morland, S. Wing, and A. Diez-Roux, "The Contextual Effect of the Local Food Environment on Residents' Diets: The Atherosclerosis Risk in Communities Study," *American Journal of Public Health* 92, no. 11 (2002): 1761–67.

44. Horowitz and others, "Barriers to Buying Healthy Foods for People with Diabetes" (see note 42).

45. H. Wechsler and others, "The Availability of Low-Fat Milk in an Inner-City Latino Community: Implications for Nutrition Education," *American Journal of Public Health* 85, no. 12 (1995): 1690–92.

46. R. Sturm and A. Datar, "Body Mass Index in Elementary School Children, Metropolitan Area Food Prices and Food Outlet Density," *Public Health* 119, no. 12 (2005): 1059–68.

47. S. Shankar and A. Klassen, "Influences on Fruit and Vegetable Procurement and Consumption among Urban African-American Public Housing Residents, and Potential Strategies for Intervention," *Family Economics and Nutrition Review* 13, no. 2 (2001): 34–46.

48. M. A. Pereira and others, "Fast-Food Habits, Weight Gain, and Insulin Resistance (The CARDIA Study): 15-Year Prospective Analysis," *Lancet* 365, no. 9453 (2005): 36–42.

49. J. P. Block and others, "Fast Food, Race/Ethnicity and Income," *American Journal of Preventive Medicine* 27, no. 3 (2004): 211–17.

50. L. B. Lewis and others, "African Americans' Access to Healthy Food Options in South Los Angeles Restaurants," *American Journal of Public Health* 95, no. 4 (2005): 668–73.

51. S. J. Jones, "The Measurement of Food Security at the Community Level: Geographic Information Systems and Participatory Ethnographic Methods." Ph.D. dissertation, University of North Carolina at Chapel Hill, 2002.

52. G. X. Ayala and others, "Restaurant and Food Shopping Selections among Latino Women in Southern California," *Journal of the American Dietetic Association* 105, no. 1 (2005): 38–45.

53. A. M. Prentice and S. A. Jebb, "Fast Foods, Energy Density, and Obesity: A Possible Mechanistic Link," *Obesity Review* 4, no. 4 (2003): 187–94; B. H. Lin, J. Guthrie, and E. Frazao, "Quality of Children's Diets at and Away from Home, 1994–96," *Food Review* 22, no. 1 (1999): 2–10.

54. J. A. Satia, J. A. Galanko, and A. M. Siega-Riz, "Eating at Fast-Food Restaurants Is Associated with Dietary Intake, Demographic, Psychosocial, and Behavioral Factors among African Americans in North Carolina," *Public Health and Nutrition* 7, no. 3 (2004): 369–80.

55. Pereira and others, "Fast-Food Habits, Weight Gain, and Insulin Resistance" (see note 47).

56. H. L. Burdette and R. C. Whitaker, "Neighborhood Playgrounds, Fast-Food Restaurants, and Crime: Relationships to Overweight in Low-Income Preschool Children," *Preventive Medicine* 38, no. 1 (2004): 57–63; S. A. French and others, "Fast-Food Restaurant Use among Adolescents: Associations with Nutrient Intake, Food Choices, and Behavioral and Psychosocial Variables," *International Journal of Obesity and Related Metabolic Disorders* 25, no. 12 (2001): 1823–33.

57. See the article by James Sallis and Karen Glanz in this volume.

58. C. M. Hoehner and others, "Perceived and Objective Environmental Measures and Physical Activity among Urban Adults," *American Journal of Preventive Medicine* 28, 2 suppl. 2 (2005): 105–16.

59. L. M. Powell, S. Slater, and F. J. Chaloupka, "The Relationship between Community Physical Activity Settings and Race, Ethnicity, and Socioeconomic Status," *Evidence-Based Preventive Medicine* 1, no. 2 (2004): 135–44.

60. Burdette and Whitaker, "Neighborhood Playgrounds, Fast-Food Restaurants, and Crime" (see note 55); H. L. Burdette and R. C. Whitaker, "A National Study of Neighborhood Safety, Outdoor Play, Television Viewing, and Obesity in Preschool Children," *Pediatrics* 116, no. 3 (2005): 657–62; A. J. Romero and others, "Are Perceived Neighborhood Hazards a Barrier to Physical Activity in Children?" *Archives of Pediatric and Adolescent Medicine* 155, no. 10 (2001): 1143–48.

61. J. Koplan, C. Liverman, and V. Kraak, eds., *Preventing Childhood Obesity: Health in the Balance* (Washington: National Academies Press, 2005).

62. General Accounting Office, Health, Education, and Human Services Division, "School Facilities: America's Schools Report Differing Conditions," GAO/HEHS-96-103 (Washington, June 14, 1996).

63. S. E. Jones, N. D. Brener, and T. McManus, "Prevalence of School Policies, Programs, and Facilities That Promote a Healthy Physical School Environment," *American Journal of Public Health* 93, no. 9 (2003): 1570–75.

64. J. Wirt and others, *The Condition of Education 2004 (NCES 2004-077). Indicator 5: Concentration of Enrollment by Race/Ethnicity and Poverty* (Washington: U.S. Department of Education, National Center for Education Statistics, 2004) (www.nces.ed.gov/programs/coe/list/index.asp [accessed Dec. 27, 2005]).

65. See Mary Story, Karen M. Kaphingst, and Simone French's article entitled "The Role of Schools in Obesity Prevention" in this volume.

66. U.S. Government Accountability Office, "School Meal Programs: Competitive Foods Are Widely Available and Generate Substantial Revenues for Schools," Report no. GAO-05-563 (August 2005).

67. S. A. French and others, "Pricing Strategy to Promote Fruit and Vegetable Purchase in High School Cafeterias," *Journal of the American Dietetic Association* 97, no. 9 (1997): 1008–10.

68. S. A. French and H. Wechsler, "School-Based Research and Initiatives: Fruit and Vegetable Environment, Policy, and Pricing Workshop," *Preventive Medicine* 39, suppl. 2 (2004): S101–07.

69. Dennis P. Andrulis, "Moving beyond the Status Quo in Reducing Racial and Ethnic Disparities in Children's Health," *Public Health Reports* 120 (2005): 370–77.

70. M. S. Townsend and others, "Food Insecurity Is Positively Related to Overweight in Women," *Journal of Nutrition* 131 (2001): 1738–45; A. Drewnowski and N. Darmon, "The Economics of Obesity: Dietary Energy Density and Energy Cost," *American Journal of Clinical Nutrition* 82, 1 suppl. (2005): S265–73; V. C. McLoyd, "The Impact of Economic Hardship on Black Families and Children: Psychological Distress, Parenting, and Socioemotional Development," *Child Development* 61, no. 2 (1990): 311–46.

71. A. A. Hedley and others, "Prevalence of Overweight and Obesity among U.S. Children, Adolescents, and Adults, 1999–2002," *Journal of the American Medical Association* 291, no. 23 (2004): 2847–50; J. W. Lucas, J. S. Schiller, and V. Benson, "Summary Health Statistics for U.S. Adults: National Health Interview Survey, 2001," *Vital Health Statistics* 10, no. 218 (2004): 1–134.

72. T. J. Rosenberg and others, "Pre-Pregnancy Weight and Adverse Perinatal Outcomes in an Ethnically Diverse Population," *Obstetrics and Gynecology* 102, no. 5, pt. 1 (2003): 1022–27; T. J. Rosenberg and others, "Maternal Obesity and Diabetes as Risk Factors for Adverse Pregnancy Outcomes: Differences among Four Racial/Ethnic Groups," *American Journal of Public Health* 95, no. 9 (2005): 1545–51.

73. National Center for Health Statistics, *Health, United States, 2004, with Chartbook on Trends in the Health of Americans* (Hyattsville, Md., 2004), table 18.

74. A. S. Ryan, Z. Wenjun, and A. Acosta, "Breastfeeding Continues to Increase into the New Millennium," *Pediatrics* 110, no. 6 (2002): 1103–09.

75. M. Bentley and others, "Infant Feeding Practices of Low-Income, African-American, Adolescent Mothers: An Ecological, Multigenerational Perspective," *Social Science and Medicine* 49, no. 8 (1999): 1085–100.

76. See article by Ana Lindsay and her colleagues in this volume.

77. Koplan, Livermore, and Kraak, *Preventing Childhood Obesity* (see note 61).

78. D. F. Roberts, U. G. Foehr, and V. Rideout, *Generation M: Media in the Lives of 8–18 Year Olds* (Menlo Park, Calif.: Kaiser Family Foundation, 2005); Roberts, Foehr, and Rideout, *Kids and Media at the New Millennium* (see note 25).

79. S. W. McNutt and others, "A Longitudinal Study of the Dietary Practices of Black and White Girls 9 and 10 Years Old at Enrollment: The NHLBI Growth and Health Study," *Journal of Adolescent Health* 20, no. 1 (1997): 27–37.

80. A. Jain and others, "Why Don't Low-Income Mothers Worry about Their Preschoolers Being Overweight?" *Pediatrics* 107, no. 5 (2001): 1138–46.

81. G. B. Schreiber and others, "Weight Modification Efforts Reported by Black and White Preadolescent Girls: National Heart, Lung, and Blood Institute Growth and Health Study," *Pediatrics* 98, no. 1 (1996): 63–70.

82. A. E. Baughcum and others, "Maternal Feeding Practices and Beliefs and Their Relationships to Overweight in Early Childhood," *Journal of Developmental and Behavioral Pediatrics* 22, no. 6 (2001): 391–408.

83. Jain and others, "Why Don't Low-Income Mothers Worry?" (see note 80).

84. T. A. Wadden and others, "Obesity in Black Adolescent Girls: A Controlled Clinical Trial of Treatment by Diet, Behavior Modification, and Parental Support," *Pediatrics* 85, no. 3 (1990): 345–52; B. M. Beech and others, "Child- and Parent-Targeted Interventions: The Memphis GEMS Pilot Study," *Ethnicity and Disease* 13, no. 1, suppl. 1 (2003): S40–53; T. N. Robinson and others, "Dance and Reducing Television Viewing to Prevent Weight Gain in African-American Girls: The Stanford GEMS Pilot Study," *Ethnicity and Disease* 13, no. 1, suppl. 1 (2003): S65–77; M. L. Fitzgibbon and others, "Two-Year Follow-Up Results for Hip-Hop to Health Jr.: A Randomized Controlled Trial for Overweight Prevention in Preschool Minority Children," *Journal of Pediatrics* 146, no. 5 (2005): 618–25.

85. Robinson and others, "Dance and Reducing Television Viewing" (see note 84).

86. Wadden and others, "Obesity in Black Adolescent Girls" (see note 84); Beech and others, "Child- and Parent-Targeted Interventions" (see note 84).

87. Stettler and others, "High Prevalence of Overweight among Pediatric Users" (see note 10).

Treating Child Obesity and Associated Medical Conditions

Sonia Caprio

Summary

With American children on course to grow into the most obese generation of adults in history, Sonia Caprio argues that it is critical to develop more effective strategies for preventing childhood obesity and treating serious obesity-related health complications. She notes that although pediatricians are concerned about the obesity problem, most are ineffective in addressing it.

Treatment should begin, Caprio explains, with a thorough medical exam, an assessment of nutrition and physical activity, an appraisal of the degree of obesity and associated health complications, a family history, and full information about current medications. Caprio also summarizes the current use of medications and surgery in treating child obesity and argues that for severe forms of obesity, the future lies in developing new and more effective drugs.

Caprio explains that today's most effective obesity treatment programs have been carried out in academic centers through an approach that combines a dietary component, behavioral modification, physical activity, and parental involvement. Such programs, however, have yet to be translated to primary pediatric care centers. Successfully treating obesity, she argues, will require a major shift in pediatric care that builds on the findings of these academic centers regarding structured intervention programs.

To ensure that pediatricians are well trained in implementing such programs, the American Medical Association is working with federal agencies, medical specialty societies, and public health organizations to teach doctors how to prevent and manage obesity in both children and adults. Such training should be a part of undergraduate and graduate medical education and of continuing medical education programs.

Caprio also addresses the problem of reimbursement for obesity treatment. Despite the health risks of obesity, patients get little support from health insurers, thus putting long-term weight-management programs beyond the reach of most. Caprio argues that obesity should be recognized as a disease and receive coverage for its treatment just as other diseases do.

www.futureofchildren.org

Sonia Caprio, M.D., is a professor of pediatric endocrinology at the Yale University School of Medicine.

Sonia Caprio

Since the mid-1980s prevalence rates of childhood and adolescent obesity in the United States have more than doubled.[1] American children are on course to grow into the most obese generation of adults in history. The worsening obesity epidemic makes it critical to continue examining and developing new and more effective treatment strategies. And because many obese youngsters suffer obesity-associated metabolic, orthopedic, and other health complications that tend to increase with the severity of obesity, it is essential not only to identify the obese child but to recognize, treat, and monitor the associated obesity-related diseases.[2]

Although pediatricians are concerned about the problem of obesity, most feel unprepared, ill equipped, and ineffective in addressing it. Many studies, as well as a survey of pediatricians, dietitians, and pediatric nurse practitioners, confirm that pediatricians do indeed face many challenges in treating childhood obesity.[3] Most pediatric primary care providers are not trained to provide the extensive counseling on nutrition, exercise, and lifestyle changes that is required to treat obesity, and most are pessimistic that treatment can be successful. Most also have insufficient time and attention to dedicate to the obese child, a problem compounded by the lack of reimbursement by third-party payers. Pediatricians also lack support services, especially access to mental health professionals, nutritionists, or exercise physiologists. And they are frustrated by insufficient patient motivation and a lack of parental concern.[4] In a study of obese African American children, many parents neither perceived their children as very overweight nor felt that weight was a health problem for their child.[5] Although comparable data are not available for white children, this

study suggests that many African American parents do not perceive obesity as a pediatric health concern.

Given the magnitude of the childhood obesity problem, however, pediatricians and other health care providers are going to have to step up and take a major role in the care and health of the obese child. Successfully treating obesity will require a major shift in pediatric care.

The Role Pediatricians Should Take in Treating Obesity

In 1998 the Maternal and Child Health Bureau, an agency of the U.S. Department of Health and Human Services, convened a committee of pediatric experts to develop recommendations to guide physicians, nurse practitioners, and nutritionists in evaluating and treating overweight children and adolescents.[6] A group of pediatricians, nurse practitioners, and nutritionists reviewed the recommendations and approved their appropriateness for practitioners. Although the document is not entirely evidence-based, it represents the consensus from experts in pediatric obesity and is the gold standard of care for all practitioners evaluating and treating the obese child.

Evaluating the obese child should begin with a detailed medical examination, together with an assessment of nutrition, physical activity, and behaviors that are linked to obesity, followed by an appraisal of the degree of obesity and its associated metabolic complications. The goals of the medical exam are to identify and treat diseases associated with childhood obesity, to rule out possible underlying causes of obesity, and to assess the child's readiness for change. The focus should be on the child's entire family and any other caregivers or role models living at home.[7] The examination should include a family history of parental obesity, gestational diabetes, dyslipidemia (abnormal levels of fat in the blood), and cardiovascular disease, as well as type 2 diabetes.[8] It should also gather information about any medication the child uses, because so many common medicines, such as glucocorticoids and antipsychotic medications, influence weight.[9] A nutritional history should include the quality and portion size of the meals, when and where the child eats, and levels of satiety and fullness following a meal. It should also record the amount and quality of snacks and daily consumption of juice and soft drinks, which often replace milk in children's and adolescents' diets and are a major contributing factor to high calorie intake.[10] Finally, it should inquire how often the child eats "fast food," because children who frequently eat at fast-food restaurants consume more total energy, more energy per gram of food, more total fat and carbohydrates, more added sugars, less fiber, and fewer fruits and vegetables than children who do not.[11]

The child's activity level should also be assessed. Studies that use motion sensors show that children who spend less time in moderate activity are at a higher risk than their more active counterparts of becoming obese during childhood and adolescence.[12] Television watching and video games contribute to more sedentary leisure activities as well as to increased snacking and inappropriate food choices prompted by television advertising. Many hours of television viewing are positively correlated with overweight, especially in older children and adolescents.[13]

Overweight in both children and adolescents can profoundly affect quality of life, self-esteem, and social competence.[14] Among severely obese adolescents, 48 percent have moderate to severe depressive symptoms.

Overweight adolescents often engage in significantly more unhealthy behaviors and experience more psychosocial distress than their normal weight peers.[15] Because psychological disorders may cause or be related to obesity, it is important for a pediatrician to recognize them and to be able to refer a child to a therapist as needed.

Assessment of Obesity: The Body Mass Index

The initial assessment should begin with an accurate measure of height and weight, which is used to calculate, record, and plot the child's age- and gender-specific body mass index (BMI) on the Centers for Disease Control and Prevention 2000 BMI charts.[16] BMI in children provides a consistent measure of obesity across age groups, correlating with measures of body fatness in children and adolescents. Although some controversy attends the use of BMI to assess obesity in children, as detailed in the article in this volume by Patricia Anderson and Kristen Butcher, the International Task Force on Obesity finds BMI a reasonable index of adiposity.[17]

Early recognition of excessive weight gain relative to normal growth is an essential component of the physical examination and should be part of any visit in primary health care. In 2003, the American Academy of Pediatrics recommended that pediatricians calculate and plot BMI in all children and adolescents.[18] Most health care providers, however, fail to address it in the pediatric population. A 2002 study of pediatricians, pediatric nurse practitioners, and dietitians showed that fewer than 20 percent of pediatricians assessed body mass index.[19] And two recent studies indicate that screening practices for overweight using BMI during routine visits have not been adopted.[20] Many pediatricians, it seems clear, are overlooking

Racial Disparities in the Care of Childhood Obesity

African American and Hispanic children and adolescents have higher prevalence rates of obesity than do white children and adolescents, but they receive less care.[1] The disparity is particularly disconcerting because black and Hispanic children are at greater risk for obesity-associated complications, such as type 2 diabetes, than are white children.[2]

In a national survey of ambulatory pediatric visits, Stephen Cook and several colleagues report disturbing racial and health-related disparities. Blood pressure screening differed by race and insurance status, with 47.7 percent of visits of white children including such screening as against 29 percent of visits of black children. Diet and exercise counseling also varied by age, insurance type, and clinician type. Exercise counseling occurred half as often in visits by black children.[3] A recent report by Karen Dorsey and several colleagues on the diagnosis, evaluation, and treatment of childhood obesity in pediatric practice also found large disparities in treatment.[4] In their study of four pediatric clinics (two community health centers and two hospital-based clinics) in New Haven that are serving an urban population with many racial and ethnic minorities insured by Medicaid, they report that providers may be under-diagnosing girls, children who are Hispanic, those insured through Medicaid, and those living apart from their biological parents. The authors also document a lack of testing for diabetes or lipid disorders among this at-risk population of children. Efforts should be invested to understand and correct these racial disparities.

Health professionals of different ethnic backgrounds should develop and implement ethnicity-based management programs for children and adolescents with diverse ethnic, racial, and cultural backgrounds. The United States has few black and Hispanic obesity specialists, nutritionists, and exercise physiologists, and the enormous racial and ethnic gap in providers must be filled. Pediatricians must also address these health disparities in the community through other means, such as working with the local news media. The state of Illinois has recently proposed three pieces of childhood obesity legislation that are likely to be enacted soon. The first urges the U.S. Department of Agriculture to update nutritional labels for foods distributed through the Supplemental Nutrition Program for Women and Children (WIC). The second requires each school board in the state to establish a school district office of nutrition to help prevent childhood obesity. The third urges the state board of education to develop guidelines showing how schools can meet standards for saturated fat in school meals and provide healthy alternatives. Many other states are also working in the same direction, and more legislation to prevent and treat childhood obesity is likely.

1. C. L. Ogden and K. M. Flegal, "Prevalence and Trends in Overweight among U.S. Children and Adolescents, 1999–2000," *Journal of the American Medical Association* 288 (2002): 1728–32.

2. A. L. Rosenbloom and others, "Emerging Epidemic of Type 2 Diabetes in Youth," *Diabetes Care* 22, no. 2 (1999): 345–54.

3. Stephen Cook and others, "Screening and Counseling Associated with Obesity Diagnosis in a National Survey of Ambulatory Pediatric Visits," *Pediatrics* 116 (2005): 112–16.

4. Karen B. Dorsey and others, "Evaluation and Treatment of Childhood Obesity in Pediatric Practice," *Archives of Pediatric and Adolescent Medicine* 159 (2005): 632–38.

obesity during well child visits. Why such screening practices have not been adopted is unclear. In a recent report from the U.S. Preventive Task Force in the journal *Pediatrics,* Evelyn Whitlock and several colleagues concluded that the existing evidence is insuffi-cient to recommend for or against routine screening using the BMI for overweight in children and adolescents in primary care settings.[21] But the report should be interpreted carefully: according to an article by Nancy Krebs in the same journal, the report should not lead to complacency but rather serve as a call for action.[22] Despite the uncertainties and controversy surrounding BMI's use in pediatrics, assessing children's BMI and BMI percentiles beginning at age two can prompt health care providers to address weight-to-height ratios during well child visits and should be part of the routine physical exam.

Assessment of Obesity-Related Diseases

To identify the obesity-related diseases that are being seen increasingly in children, laboratory tests should include a fasting lipid profile, which measures cholesterol and triglyceride levels, a liver function test, and fasting glucose and insulin levels.[23] A consensus panel of the American Diabetes Association recommends that overweight children with two additional risk factors, such as a family history of type 2 diabetes, race or ethnicity (American Indian, African American, Hispanic, or Asian Pacific), signs of insulin insensitivity, or hypertension, be considered for further testing.[24] Another consensus report finds that patients with obesity-related diseases, such as type 2 diabetes, hypertension, polycystic ovarian syndrome, dyslipidemia, nonalcoholic steatohepatitis, and sleep apnea, will require the expertise of the pediatric endocrinologist, cardiologist, gastroenterologist, and pulmonologist.[25] These conditions are described in detail in the article by Stephen Daniels in this volume. Children with these conditions should be cared for within specialized obesity clinics.

Current Specialized Treatment Programs and Interventions

Surprisingly little evidence-based, high-quality research exists on interventions to treat childhood obesity. A summary of the research behind obesity interventions for both adults and children was published in April 2004 in the *British Medical Journal*.[26]

Most of the effective treatment programs have been carried out in academic centers through an interdisciplinary approach that combines a dietary component, behavioral modification, physical activity, and parental involvement.[27] L. H. Epstein and his team at the State University of New York at Buffalo have been in the forefront of developing programs that reduce adiposity in childhood through this multidisciplinary approach. The most important finding of these interventions may be that relatively modest but sustainable changes in lifestyles may have more long-term impact on obesity than radical regimens that enable patients to lose weight rapidly but not to maintain their new, lower weight afterward. In perhaps the only successful long-term intervention, Epstein used such behavioral strategies as contracting, self-monitoring, and social reinforcement with obese children and their parents to limit consumption of fatty foods and to increase exercise.[28] Although research has demonstrated that intensive group programs can be successful, such programs have yet to be translated to primary care centers. In the absence of well-established, office-based evaluation and treatment programs, the Maternal and Child Health Bureau and the National Center for Education in Maternal and Child Health have issued recommendations for the obese child's evaluation and treatment that are strongly based on comprehensive interventions like those Epstein developed.

Dietary Components of Treatment

Most lifestyle intervention programs in children use a diet that mildly restricts calories. The classic example is the Traffic Light Diet, which color-codes foods as green, yellow, and red to signal whether they are safe to eat in any quantity (green), require moderation and caution (yellow), or should generally be avoided (red). Combining comprehensive obesity-treatment programs with the Traffic Light Diet can significantly change eating patterns.[29] Indeed, one study found that the diet continued to affect the eating habits of children five to ten years after treatment began.[30] Diets more restricted in calories, including high-protein diets, are used rarely and only in more severe forms of obesity. Given their potential danger, they should be implemented under strict medical control, possibly in a clinical setting.

Thus emerging data would suggest that eliminating carbonated drinks or other sugary drinks from the diet can significantly reduce caloric intake and obesity.

Interest is also growing in whether low-carbohydrate diets can help reduce adiposity in adults.[31] A recent study showed that obese men and women lost more weight and had more significant reductions in plasma triglyceride concentrations on a low-carbohydrate diet than on conventional low-fat diets.[32] And limited evidence suggests that the nature or quality of ingested carbohydrates may modulate weight gain in childhood. Although the relationship between carbohydrates and weight gain is still highly controversial, studies by D. Ludwig and several colleagues strongly link consumption of sugar-sweetened drinks with obesity.[33] Thus emerging data would suggest that eliminating carbonated drinks or other sugary drinks from the diet can significantly reduce caloric intake and obesity.[34] But low-carbohydrate diets should not be used for children and adoles-

cents until more information is available regarding their effects on insulin resistance and their long-term effects on weight and metabolic health.

Role of Physical Exercise

Physical activity is a critical component of obesity treatment in both adults and children. Increasing the caloric expenditure of obese children may not only accelerate their weight loss, but also make it easier to maintain weight changes. Exercise in the absence of dietary intervention, however, has not been found to affect weight significantly. And for the obese child, exercising can be difficult. Few studies have explored the effects of aerobic exercise on children's body weight and cardiovascular fitness. Nor is much information available regarding the effects of resistance exercise on children's metabolism and body weight. But because the capacity for voluntary exercise declines with the increasing severity of obesity, resistance exercise may prove more effective than more strenuous aerobic exercise. As yet there are no evidence-based guidelines by which to design exercise programs for obese children. Epstein and his team have suggested reducing sedentary behaviors as an alternative to increasing physical activity, an interesting approach that may be helpful both in treating and in preventing obesity. Inactivity can be decreased in many ways, usually most successfully when a parent is involved. The best example is reducing the time that the child spends watching television.[35]

Pharmacologic Approaches in Pediatrics

Many experts in pediatric obesity argue that behavioral treatment alone is ineffective, particularly in the case of severe obesity. Few if any guidelines exist for using medications in treating child obesity. In general, however, experts suggest that children and adolescents with a BMI greater than the 95th percentile for age and sex and with obesity-related medical complications that may be corrected or improved through weight reduction should be considered for intensive regimens, including medication.[36] Most medications approved for weight loss in the United States either suppress appetite or reduce nutrient absorption. A third emerging therapy is not aimed directly at controlling weight but rather targets insulin resistance to reduce the metabolic complications associated with obesity.

The Food and Drug Administration (FDA) approved sibutramine (Meridia), an appetite suppressant, for weight loss and maintenance in conjunction with reduced caloric intake in adults and adolescents older than age sixteen.[37] R. I. Berkowitz and several colleagues provided the first randomized, placebo-controlled trial of sibutramine in treating obese adolescents.[38] The double-blind study followed eighty-two adolescents with a BMI of 32 to 44 for six months, and then all patients received the drug without being blind to the treatment for another six months. Including sibutramine as part of a comprehensive behavioral program resulted in greater weight loss in obese adolescents than the traditional behavioral treatment alone, but the weight loss plateaued after six months of therapy. Serious side effects, such as hypertension and tachycardia (rapid heart rate), were reported in nineteen out of forty-three youngsters; in five, the drug dose had to be reduced or discontinued. The study found no major improvement in insulin resistance and dyslipidemia. A. Matos-Godoy and several colleagues also evaluated the efficacy and safety of sibutramine in a six-month double-blind, placebo-controlled trial in sixty obese adolescents.[39] Unlike the Berkowitz study, it found no clinically significant changes in blood pressure.[40] Both studies concluded

that sibutramine should be used for weight loss in adolescents and children only on an experimental basis until more extensive safety and efficacy data are available.

In future tests of sibutramine in children and adolescents with severe obesity, researchers could experiment with different strategies. For example, introducing the drug after a period of weight reduction with traditional approaches may reduce the potential for such side effects as hypertension.

Orlistat (Xenical), a drug that decreases nutrient absorption, cuts intestinal fat absorption by up to 30 percent. The FDA approved its use in children older than age twelve. A multicenter, one-year randomized, placebo-controlled trial in 539 obese adolescents found that those who used orlistat lost weight and had significantly greater reductions in BMI and body fat than those given the placebo.[41] But the two groups saw no significant differences with respect to changes in lipid or glucose levels. The explanation for the failure of lipid and glucose levels to improve may be that the body weight loss was small (5 percent). Although researchers do not yet know how much BMI must be reduced to provide short- and long-term health benefits in children and adolescents, the above study would suggest that small changes in weight do not affect the metabolic risk factors.

The third class of drugs used in treating obesity are those that target insulin resistance, which, along with the associated high insulin levels, are often present in obese children and adolescents and which vary with the degree and severity of overweight. Both disorders may not only contribute to the metabolic complications of obesity but also accentuate weight gain in children and adolescents by promoting lipid storage. Thus targeting insulin resistance may have a dual effect—preventing further weight gain and improving the associated metabolic complications. Metformin, for example, is used in treating type 2 diabetes.[42] It is approved for adolescents. Only two small studies have used metformin in a randomized trial in obese adolescents.[43] Both found small but statistically significant effects on BMI and significant effects on fasting blood sugar, insulin, and lipids. The studies are encouraging and should be repeated in a larger sample and for a longer duration.

When possible, it is always best to treat obesity without using drugs. Unfortunately, however, once both adult and child patients have lost weight, their efforts to maintain their new weight often fail. That so many people regain weight after stopping medication clearly suggests that obesity is a chronic condition that requires continuous treatment. And even though environmental factors have played an important role in childhood obesity's dramatic rise over the past two decades, clearly there is a genetic component to body weight. Indeed, recent data suggest that 5 percent of cases of severe obesity in children younger than ten are due to genetic mutations.[44] These children and adolescents need multiple strategies, including drugs, used in combination in a carefully designed treatment program.

Research over the past decade has dramatically advanced knowledge about the molecular mechanisms regulating body fat and the central regulation of energy intake. Ultimately, for the severe forms of obesity, the future lies in developing new and more effective medications. Researchers should continue to investigate the causes of childhood obesity and to refine obesity's classifications and diagnoses based on health risks.

Surgical Approaches

Surgery is used to treat obesity in adults only when patients are severely obese (or their BMI greater than 40) or when they have a BMI greater than 35 together with severe obesity-related health complications. In the Swedish Obese Subjects (SOS) Study, a large study evaluating surgery's efficacy, patients were equally divided among surgical and non-surgical groups.[45] After two years, the surgical patients had lost 28 kilograms (62 pounds); those in the control group, 0.5 kilograms. After eight years, the average weight loss was 20 kilograms in surgical patients and 0.7 kilograms in controls. Thus overall, surgery promoted substantial, prolonged weight loss in patients with severe obesity.[46] Results in the relatively few published surgical trials in obese children and adolescents seem to parallel those of adult trials.[47] Nevertheless, evidence-based guidelines should be developed for surgery as a treatment of childhood obesity.

Primary and Specialized Care

Chronically obese children are increasingly being referred to pediatric endocrinology centers, often years after the onset of obesity. A study by T. Quattrin and several colleagues found that most of the children who were referred to specialists had developed obesity in their preschool years, when preventive measures are likely to be most effective, if implemented. Two years after the first visit to the specialist, only 38 percent of the children were less overweight than they were on their first visit.[48] The study concluded that such referrals are ineffective, and efforts should go, instead, to developing and making available to pediatricians early family-based, behavioral lifestyle intervention programs. The study's primary point, however, was not to address where the child should receive care but to emphasize that effectively treating obesity in children and adolescents requires a well-designed, multifaceted intervention program. Given the chronic nature of obesity, frequent visits for treatment are indispensable. The traditional, sporadic, every-six-months visit that a normal primary care practice provides is not adequate. Because many obese children and adolescents also suffer from one or more metabolic complications, the role of the pediatric endocrinologist is critical in the multidisciplinary approach to the problem. Both pediatricians and patients must realize that the goal of treatment is not the initial weight loss alone but also weight management to achieve the best possible weight for improved health. The growing prevalence of childhood obesity indicates an urgent need to develop effective strategies for prevention and treatment.

How Well Equipped Are Pediatricians to Handle "Adult" Diseases?

The typical medical complications of obesity, once confined to adulthood, are now emerging in childhood.[49] During the past decade, pediatricians were confronted with unusual diseases like type 2 diabetes, nonalcoholic fatty liver disease, and polycystic ovary disorder.[50] To slow or reverse the increase in childhood obesity and its associated health risks, it is necessary to treat childhood obesity as soon as it is detected. Given the limits to treating long-standing obesity, early pediatric interventions to limit excessive weight gain in preschool and preadolescent children appear to be the best way to tackle the problem. The most effective way to prevent complications of obesity in teenagers and adults is to introduce, model, and reinforce healthful behaviors and lifestyles early in childhood.

Because so many children suffer from overweight and obesity, such interventions are most appropriately based in the primary pediatric care setting, preferably with the support of registered dietitians and structured intervention programs. Especially when caring for the younger child, managing excessive weight gain should be the province of the primary care pediatrician. Although, as noted, few overweight children are now actively treated in the primary care setting and many are referred to specialists, the epidemic of childhood obesity and the paucity of pediatric obesity subspecialists have overwhelmed specialized treatment programs' capacities to handle the demand for their services.

The most effective way to prevent complications of obesity in teenagers and adults is to introduce, model, and reinforce healthful behaviors and lifestyles early in childhood.

Because almost all children receive their health care in primary care settings, developing effective and feasible strategies for preventing and treating childhood obesity in primary care settings offers an important opportunity for addressing this major public health problem. Giving the primary care provider a major role in preventing the onset of childhood obesity and in intervening promptly to correct excessive weight gain is critical. As noted, however, primary care pediatricians lack the training to care for obese patients. Few have time to assess, intervene, and monitor progress related to the child's dietary, behavioral, and physical activities, especially when the doctors are generally not reimbursed by third-party payers either to provide services themselves or to employ a multidisciplinary team within their practices to provide appropriate services.[51] The clinical system is well prepared to treat acute conditions but not chronic conditions like obesity.

Changing the Role of the Primary Health Care Provider: A Solution to the Prevention and Treatment of Childhood Obesity

The number of obese children and adolescents is large and growing. These young people are in need of intensive intervention, but clearly the burden is too large to be borne by specialty physicians. Thus the primary care provider's role must be changed.

As leading authorities on the health of children in their communities, pediatricians could play a unique role both in increasing community awareness of the problem of overweight and in identifying promising approaches that deserve additional testing.[52] Realizing that primary care centers are not now effectively preventing and treating obesity, the field needs to move forward. Although consensus on the best strategies for prevention and treatment is still evolving, the American Medical Association (AMA) has begun to take action. Working with the Council on Scientific Affairs (CSA) and other associations and experts, the AMA issued a report in 2004 on the epidemiology of obesity and the problems it causes.[53] The report included recommendations on labor force and training, on costs and reimbursement, and on racial disparities in treatment.

Labor Force and Training

Among its recommendations the AMA urges physicians, managed care organizations, and other third-party payers to recognize obesity as a complex disorder that involves appetite

regulation and energy metabolism and that carries with it risks of various diseases. The AMA is working with federal agencies, medical specialty societies, and public health organizations to educate physicians about how to prevent and manage obesity in children and adults, including basic principles and practices of physical activity and nutrition counseling. It advises that such training should be included in undergraduate and graduate medical education and offered through accredited continuing medical education programs.

The AMA directs physicians to assess their patients for overweight and obesity during routine medical examinations and to discuss with their at-risk patients the health consequences of further weight gain. If treatment is indicated, physicians should encourage and facilitate their patients' weight-maintenance or reduction efforts or refer them to a physician with special interest in managing obesity. Physicians should also become knowledgeable about community resources and referral services that can help them manage obese patients.

The AMA urges federal support for research to determine the causes and mechanisms of overweight and obesity; the long-term safety and efficacy of voluntary weight maintenance and weight-loss practices and therapies, including surgery; and the effectiveness of interventions to prevent obesity in children and adults and of weight-loss counseling by physicians. Finally it encourages a national effort to educate Americans about the health risks of being overweight and obese and to provide information about how to achieve and maintain a preferred healthy weight.

Cost and Reimbursement

To promote reimbursement for care, the AMA exhorts federal agencies to work with organized medicine and the health insurance industry to develop coding and payment mechanisms for the evaluation and management of obesity. Reimbursement for obesity treatment is one of the great anomalies of the U.S. health care system. Despite the health risks associated with obesity, patients get little support from health insurers. The low reimbursement rates preclude the long-term financial feasibility of weight-management programs without other support or a significant proportion of patients who can pay for care "out-of-pocket." One study of 191 children in a hospital weight-management program found a median reimbursement rate of 11 percent, with variations from 0 to 100 percent.[54] Many insurers will not cover weight-loss treatments unless the patient has an obesity-related condition such as diabetes or hyperlipidemia.

Although the reimbursement problem has been and continues to be a critical barrier to treating child and adolescent obesity, signs of change are beginning to appear. The American Obesity Association (AOA), an advocacy organization, has committed itself to expanding insurance coverage for obesity treatment. And state policymakers are slowly beginning to allow Medicaid treatment options for their low-income citizens. This year, two of four bills introduced were enacted into law. In Iowa, Governor Tom Vilsak signed into law a bill that requires the state's Medicaid program to develop a strategy for providing dietary counseling to child and adult Medicaid enrollees by July 1, 2006. Counseling and support will be offered to assist enrollees in developing a personal weight-loss program. And Colorado's governor, Bill Owens, signed a measure establishing an obesity treatment pilot program for Medicaid beneficiaries who are older than fifteen and have a BMI equal to or greater than 30. On the private side, five states introduced legislation requiring insurers to provide or offer coverage for surgical procedures used to treat obesity.

In keeping with the guidelines of the National Institutes of Health and other organizations, obesity should be recognized as a disease and should receive coverage for its treatment just as other diseases do. Third-party payers should reimburse practitioners for preventive counseling and management

---

In keeping with the guidelines of the National Institutes of Health and other organizations, obesity should be recognized as a disease and should receive coverage for its treatment just as other diseases do.

---

programs for children that are known to be cost-effective.

The Future of Pediatric Obesity

The key to successfully treating childhood obesity ultimately lies in developing and funding a targeted research agenda. At the top of that agenda should be basic research into the biology and physiology of regulating appetite during the various developmental stages of childhood. Research should also focus on the mechanisms that regulate body fat distribution during adolescence as well as gender and ethnicity differences in body composition and fat distribution. Other key research areas include the differing susceptibility to weight gain during childhood and adolescence; the underlying changes in physical activity at puberty; more clinical studies on the efficacy of specific prevention and treatment programs; and the effort to move from efficacy to broad effectiveness.

Until recently, childhood obesity has been considered a clinical problem for specialist pediatricians. Now, however, the problem must be approached in a more global manner. The public health community must consider the urgent need to institute preventive programs. Given the reluctance of policymakers to institute changes, particularly those that are unpopular or expensive, it is important to establish objective evidence of the beneficial impact of any preventive or treatment programs. To stop the epidemic of childhood obesity, acting on all levels—medical, social, political, and educational—is fundamental. A broad range of action would include conducting nutrition education campaigns, regulating the marketing of junk food to children, eliminating energy-dense foods and sodas from schools, and promoting physical activity.

In an outstanding 2003 editorial in the *Archives of Pediatric and Adolescent Medicine*, Leona Cuttler, June Whittaker, and Eric Kodish suggested forming a national pediatric obesity panel under the aegis of the National Institutes of Health, the Centers for Disease Control and Prevention, or the Institute of Medicine.[55] Including representatives of major stakeholders, the panel would shape policy, analyze the best practices through rigorous evaluation, disseminate information accrued, revise policy at regular intervals as new information is gained, and become a central trusted voice. Under such a panel's leadership, the United States could transform its approach to treating childhood obesity and ultimately stem the epidemic that threatens so many of the nation's children.

Notes

1. C. L. Ogden and K. M. Flegal, "Prevalence and Trends in Overweight among U.S. Children and Adolescents, 1999–2000," *Journal of the American Medical Association* 288 (2002): 1728–32; R. P. Troiano and K. M. Flegal, "Overweight Children and Adolescents: Description, Epidemiology and Demographics," *Pediatrics* 101, no. 3, pt. 2 (1998): 497–504.

2. William Dietz, "Health Consequences of Obesity in Youth: Childhood Predictors of Adult Disease," *Pediatrics* 101 (1998): 518–25; A. R. Sinaiko and others, "Relation of Weight and Rate of Increase in Weight during Childhood and Adolescence to Body Size, Blood Pressure, Fasting Insulin, and Lipids in Young Adults—the Minneapolis Children's Blood Pressure Study," *Circulation* 99 (1996): 1471–76; Ram Weiss and others, "Obesity and the Metabolic Syndrome in Children and Adolescents," *New England Journal of Medicine* 350 (2004): 2362–74.

3. S. E. Barlow and others, "Treatment of Child and Adolescent Obesity: Reports from Pediatricians, Pediatric Nurse Practitioners, and Registered Dietitians," *Pediatrics* 110 (2002): 229–35.

4. Ibid.; T. Bodenheimer, E. H. Wagner, and K. Grumbach, "Improving Primary Care for Patients with Chronic Illness," *Journal of the American Medical Association* 288 (2002): 1775–79; C. T. Orleans and others, "Health Promotion in Primary Care: A Survey of U.S. Family Practitioners," *Preventive Medicine* 14 (1985): 636–47; R. F. Kushner, "Barriers to Providing Nutrition Counseling by Physicians," *Preventive Medicine* 24 (1995): 546–52.

5. David Young-Hyman and others, "Care Giver Perception of Children's Obesity-Related Health Risk: A Study of African American Families," *Obesity Research* 8 (2000): 241–48.

6. Sarah Barlow and William Dietz, "Obesity Evaluation and Treatment: Expert Committee Evaluation," *Pediatrics* 102, no. 3 (1998): 1–11.

7. I. Lissau and T. I. A. Sorensen, "Parental Neglect during Childhood and Increased Risk of Obesity in Young Adulthood," *Lancet* 343 (1994): 324–27; W. Kinston and others, "Interaction in Families with Obese Children," *Journal of Psychosomatic Research* 32 (1998): 513–32; S. L. Johnson and L. L. Birch, "Parents' and Children's Adiposity and Eating Style," *Pediatrics* 94 (1994): 653–61.

8. P. W. Speiser and others, "Consensus Statement: Childhood Obesity," *Journal of Clinical Endocrinology and Metabolism* 90 (2005): 1871–87.

9. S. R. Marder and others, "Physical Health Monitoring of Patients with Schizophrenia," *American Journal of Psychiatry* 161 (2004): 1334–49.

10. D. Ludwig, K. E. Peterson, and S. Gortmaker, "Relation between Consumption of Sugar Sweetened Drinks and Childhood Obesity: A Prospective and Observational Analysis," *Lancet* 357 (2001): 505–08.

11. S. A. Bowman and others, "Effects of Fast-Food Consumption on Energy Intake and Diet Quality among Children in a National Household Survey," *Pediatrics* 113 (2004): 112–18; S. A. French, L. Harmack, and R. W. Jeffery, "Fast-Food Restaurant Use among Women in the Pound of Prevention Study: Dietary, Behavioral and Demographic Correlates," *International Journal of Obesity-Related Metabolic Disorders* 24 (2000): 1353–55.

Sonia Caprio

12. L. L. Moore and others, "Does Early Physical Activity Predict Body Fat Change throughout Childhood?" *Preventive Medicine* 37 (2003): 10–17.

13. Henry J. Kaiser Foundation, "The Role of Media in Childhood Obesity" (www.kff.org/entmedia024404pkg.cfm [June 2, 2004]).

14. J. B. Schwimmer, T. M. Burwinkle, and J. W. Varni, "Health-Related Quality of Life of Severely Obese Children and Adolescents," *Journal of the American Medical Association* 289 (2003): 1813–19.

15. N. H. Falkner and others, "Social, Educational and Psychosocial Correlates of Weight Status in Adolescents," *Obesity Research* 9 (2001): 32–42.

16. C. L. Odgen and others, "Centers for Disease Control and Prevention 2000 Growth Charts for the United States: Improvements to the 1977 National Center for Health Statistics Version," *Pediatrics* 109 (2002): 45–60.

17. W. H. Dietz and T. Robinson, "Use of BMI as a Measure of Overweight in Children and Adolescents," *Journal of Pediatrics* 132 (1998): 191–93.

18. American Academy of Pediatrics, Committee on Nutrition, "Prevention of Pediatric Overweight and Obesity," *Pediatrics* 112 (2003): 424–30.

19. Barlow and others, "Treatment of Child and Adolescent Obesity" (see note 3).

20. Karen B. Dorsey and others, "Diagnosis, Evaluation and Treatment of Childhood Obesity in Pediatric Practice," *Archives of Pediatric and Adolescent Medicine* 159 (2005): 632–38; Stephen Cook and others, "Screening and Counseling Associated with Obesity Diagnosis in a National Survey of Ambulatory Pediatric Visits," *Pediatrics* 116 (2005): 112–16.

21. Evelyn P. Whitlock and others, "Screening and Interventions for Childhood Overweight: A Summary of Evidence for the U.S. Preventive Services Task Force," *Pediatrics* 116 (2005): 125–44.

22. Nancy Krebs, "Screening for Overweight in Children and Adolescents: A Call for Action," *Pediatrics* 116 (2005): 238–39.

23. A. L. Rosenbloom, "Emerging Epidemic of Type 2 Diabetes in Youth," *Diabetes Care* 22, no. 2 (1999): 345–54.

24. American Diabetes Association, "Type 2 Diabetes in Children and Adolescents: Consensus Conference Report," *Diabetes Care* 23 (2000): 381–89.

25. Speiser and others, "Consensus Statement: Childhood Obesity" (see note 8).

26. J. Anjal, "What Works for Obesity? A Summary of the Research behind Obesity Interventions," *British Medical Journal* (April 30, 2004).

27. L. H. Epstein and others, "Ten-Year Follow-up of Behavioral, Family-Based Treatment for Obese Children," *Journal of the American Medical Association* 264 (1990): 2519–23; H. Bjorvell and S. Rossner, "A Ten-Year Follow-up of Weight Change in Severely Obese Subjects Treated in a Combined Behavioral Modification Program," *International Journal of Obesity* 16 (1992): 623–25.

28. L. H. Epstein and others, "A Five-Year Follow-up of Family-Based Behavioral Treatments for Childhood Obesity," *Journal of Consulting and Clinical Psychology* 58 (1990): 661–64; L. H. Epstein and others, "Family-Based Behavioral Weight Control in Obese Young Children," *Journal of the American Dietetic Association* 86 (1986): 481–84.

29. Epstein, "Family-Based Behavioral Weight Control" (see note 28); A. Valoski and L. H. Epstein, "Nutrient Intake of Obese Children in a Family-Based Behavioral Weight Control Program," *International Journal of Obesity* 14 (1990): 667–77.

30. Epstein and others, "A Five-Year Follow-up" (see note 28).

31. G. D. Foster and others, "A Randomized Trial of a Low-Carbohydrate Diet for Obesity," *New England Journal of Medicine* 348 (2003): 2082–90; S. B. Sondike, N. Copperman, and M. S. Jacobson, "Effects of a Low-Carbohydrate Diet on Weight Loss and Cardiovascular Risk Factor in Overweight Adolescents," *Journal of Pediatrics* 142 (2003): 253–58.

32. Foster and others, "A Randomized Trial" (see note 31).

33. D. Ludwig, K. E. Peterson, and S. Gortmaker, "Relation between Consumption of Sugar-Sweetened Drinks and Childhood Obesity: A Prospective and Observational Analysis," *Lancet* 357 (2001): 505–08.

34. C. B. Ebbeling and others, "A Reduced–Glycemic Load Diet in the Treatment of Adolescent Obesity," *Archives of Pediatric and Adolescent Medicine* 157 (2003): 773–79.

35. W. H. Dietz and S. L. Gortmaker, "Do We Fatten Our Children at the Television Set?" *Pediatrics* 75, no. 5 (1985): 807–12; R. C. Kleges, M. L. Shelton, and L. M. Kleges, "Effects of Television on Metabolic Rate: Potential Implications for Childhood Obesity," *Pediatrics* 91 (1993): 281–86; T. N. Robinson, "Reducing Children's Television Viewing to Prevent Obesity: A Randomized Controlled Trial," *Journal of the American Medical Association* 282, no. 16 (1999): 1561–67.

36. Jack Yanovsky, "Intensive Therapies for Pediatric Obesity," *Pediatric Clinics of North America* 48 (2001): 1041–53.

37. "Clinical Guidelines on the Identification, Evaluation, and Treatment of Overweight and Obesity in Adults—the Evidence Report," *Obesity Research* suppl. 2 (1998): 51S–209S; "Consensus Statement: Childhood Obesity," *Journal of Clinical Endocrinology and Metabolism* 90 (2005): 1871–87.

38. R. I. Berkowitz and others, "Behavior Therapy and Sibutramine for the Treatment of Adolescent Obesity," *Journal of the American Medical Association* 289 (2003): 1805–12.

39. A. Matos-Godoy and others, "Treatment of Obese Adolescents with Sibutramine: A Randomized, Double-Blind, Controlled Study," *Journal of Clinical Endocrinology and Metabolism* 90 (2005): 1460–65.

40. Berkowitz and others, "Behavior Therapy and Sibutramine" (see note 38).

41. Jean-Pierre Chanoine and others, "Effect of Orlistat on Weight and Body Composition in Obese Adolescents," *Journal of the American Medical Association* 293 (2005): 2873–83.

42. R. A. DeFronzo, "Pharmacologic Therapy for Type 2 Diabetes Mellitus," *Annals of Internal Medicine* 133 (2000): 73–74.

43. M. Freemark and D. Bursey, "The Effects of Metformin on Body Mass Index and Glucose Tolerance in Obese Adolescents with Fasting Hyperinsulinemia and a Family History of Type 2 Diabetes," *Pediatrics* 107 (2001): 1–7; J. P. Kay and others, "Beneficial Effects of Metformin in Normoglycemic Morbidly Obese Adolescents," *Pediatrics* 50, no. 12 (2001): 1457–61.

44. I. S. Farooqi and S. O'Rahilly, "Recent Advances in the Genetics of Severe Childhood Obesity," *Archives of Disease in Childhood* 83 (2000): 31–34; C. Vaisse and others, "Melanocortin 4 Receptor Mutations Are a Frequent and Heterogeneous Cause of Morbid Obesity," *Journal of Clinical Investigation* 106 (2000): 253–62; C. D. Sjostrom and others, "Swedish Obese Subjects (SOS). Recruitment for an Intervention Study and Selection Description of the Obese State," *International Journal of Obesity-Related Metabolic Disorders* 16 (1992): 465–79.

45. Sjostrom and others, "Swedish Obese Subjects" (see note 44).

46. J. S. Torgerson and C. D. Sjostrom, "The Swedish Obese Study: Rationale and Results," *International Journal of Obesity-Related Metabolic Disorders* 25, suppl. 1 (2001): S2–S4.

47. T. H. Inge and others, "A Multidisciplinary Approach to the Adolescent Bariatric Surgical Patient," *Journal of Pediatric Surgery* 39 (2004): 442–47; H. J. Sugerman and others, "Bariatric Surgery for Severely Obese Adolescents," *Journal of Gastrointestinal Surgery* 7 (2003): 102–07.

48. T. Quattrin and others, "Obese Children Who Are Referred to the Pediatric Endocrinologist: Characteristics and Outcome," *Pediatrics* 115, no. 2 (2005): 348–51.

49. Speiser and others, "Consensus Statement" (see note 8).

50. Ibid.

51. A. M. Tershacovec and others, "Insurance Reimbursement for the Treatment of Obesity in Children," *Journal of Pediatrics* 134 (1999): 573–78.

52. Steven Teutsch and Peter Briss, "Spanning the Boundary between Clinics and Communities to Address Overweight and Obesity in Children," *Pediatrics* 116 (2005): 240–41.

53. American Medical Association, "Report 8 of the Council on Scientific Affairs (A-04)," *Actions on Obesity,* June 2004 (www.ama-assn.org/ama/pub/category/13653.html [December 12, 2005]).

54. Tershacovec and others, "Insurance Reimbursement" (see note 51).

55. Leona Cuttler, June Whittaker, and Eric Kodish, "Pediatric Obesity Policy: The Danger of Skepticism," *Archives of Pediatric and Adolescent Medicine* 157 (2003): 722-24.